# INTENSIVE CARE

# Concepts and Practices

## of

# INTENSIVE CARE

## FOR NURSE SPECIALISTS

*EDITORS*

**LAWRENCE E. MELTZER, M.D.**
*Director, Section of Clinical Investigation*
*Director, Coronary Care Unit, Presbyterian-*
*University of Pennsylvania Medical Center, Philadelphia*

**FAYE G. ABDELLAH, R.N., Ed.D., LL.D.**
*Chief, Research Grants Branch, Division of Nursing,*
*National Institutes of Health, U.S. Department of Health,*
*Education and Welfare, Washington*

**J. RODERICK KITCHELL, M.D.**
*Director of Medical Services, Abington Memorial Hospital,*
*Abington; Assistant Clinical Professor of Medicine, University*
*of Pennsylvania School of Medicine, Philadelphia*

**THE CHARLES PRESS** *Publishers Inc.*

**236 SOUTH 20th STREET • PHILADELPHIA, PA. 19103**

SECOND PRINTING, 1970

Library of Congress catalog card number: 70–76470

THE CHARLES PRESS *Publishers, Inc.*
236 South 20th Street, Philadelphia, Pa. 19103

Printed in the United States of America

# Contents

# Contributors

FAYE G. ABDELLAH, R.N., Ed.D., LL.D.
Chief, Research Grants Branch, Division of Nursing, National Institutes of Health, U.S. Department of Health, Education and Welfare, Washington, D.C.

MARILYN ABRAHAM, R.N., M.S.
Supervisor, Medical Neurological Unit, The New York Hospital-Cornell Medical Center, New York, New York

WALTER L. BARKER, M.D.
Assistant Chief of Surgery, Chicago State Tuberculosis Sanitarium, Chicago, Illinois

IRENE L. BELAND, R.N., M.S.
Professor of Nursing, College of Nursing, Wayne State University, Detroit, Michigan

MARY T. BIELSKI, R.N., M.S.
Associate Professor, Medical Nursing, New York Hospital-Cornell University, School of Nursing, New York, New York

CHRISTOPHER R. BLAGG, M.D.
Assistant Professor of Medicine, School of Medicine, University of Washington, Seattle, Washington

TRUMAN G. BLOCKER, Jr., M.D.
President, The University of Texas Medical Branch at Galveston, Texas

**LUCY BRAND, R.N., M.S.**
Assistant Professor, College of Nursing, Wayne State University and Head Nurse, Intensive Care Unit, Detroit General Hospital, Detroit, Michigan

**DELILAH BULLACHER BREEN, R.N., B.S.**
Instructor, Operating Room Technique, Hotel Dieu School of Nursing, El Paso, Texas

**ISABEL E. DUTCHER, R.N., M.A.**
Associate Professor, Medical-Surgical Nursing, College of Nursing, Rutgers University, The State University of New Jersey, Newark, New Jersey

**KATHLEEN S. FELIX, R.N.**
Head Nurse, Dialysis Transplant Team, The New York Hospital-Cornell Medical Center, New York, New York

**BARBARA FELLOWS, R.N., M.N.**
Renal Nursing Supervisor, University of Washington Hospital, Seattle, Washington

**M. ARLENE MARTIN GARDNER, R.N., M.A.**
Associate Professor of Nursing, Frances Payne Bolton School of Nursing, Case Western Reserve University, Cleveland, Ohio

**HAROLD C. HARDENBURG, Jr., M.D.**
Director, Artificial Kidney Unit, Overlook Hospital, Summit, New Jersey

**JOHN T. KIMBALL, M.D.**
Assistant Professor of Medicine, The New York Hospital-Cornell Medical Center, New York, New York

**J. RODERICK KITCHELL, M.D.**
Director of Medical Services, Abington Memorial Hospital, Abington, Pennsylvania; Assistant Clinical Professor of Medicine, University of Pennsylvania, School of Medicine, Philadelphia, Pennsylvania

**MARIE KURIHARA, R.N., M.A.**
Nursing Care Specialist in Cardiopulmonary Diseases and Medical Intensive Care Unit, Veterans Administration Hospital, Long Beach, California.

JOHN E. LEE, M.D.

Clinical Assistant Professor, The New York Hospital-Cornell
Medical Center, New York, New York

RITA GASTON LUNG, R.N., B.S., M.S.

Assistant Professor, Medical-Surgical Nursing, University of
Texas School of Nursing, University of Texas, Galveston,
Texas

JEAN Mac VICAR, R.N., M.S.

Associate Professor, School of Nursing, University of Maryland, Baltimore, Maryland

BETSY MARSHALL, R.N., B.S.

Nurse Member of Dialysis Transplant Team, The New York
Hospital-Cornell Medical Center, New York, New York

WILLIAM V. McDERMOTT, Jr., M.D.

Professor of Surgery, Harvard Medical School; Director Fifth
Harvard Surgical Service, Boston City Hospital, Boston,
Massachusetts

LAWRENCE E. MELTZER, M.D.

Director, Section of Clinical Investigation and Director,
Coronary Care Unit, Presbyterian-University of Pennsylvania
Medical Center, Philadelphia, Pennsylvania

HARVEY J. MENDELSOHN, M.D.

Director, Division of Thoracic Surgery; Associate Professor
of Thoracic Surgery, Department of Surgery, Case Western
Reserve University, Cleveland, Ohio

DORIS MOLBO, R.N., M.A.

Associate Director, Nursing Research, John Hartford Foundation Hyperbaric Oxygen Research Unit, Lutheran General
Hospital, Park Ridge, Illinois

FRANK MOODY, M.D.

Associate Professor, Department of Surgery and Chairman,
Gastrointestinal Division, University of Alabama, Birming-
ham, Alabama.

FRANK E. NULSEN, M.D.

Professor of Neurosurgery, School of Medicine, Case Western
Reserve University, Cleveland, Ohio

WILMA J. PHIPPS, R.N., A.M.

Associate Professor of Nursing, College of Nursing, University of Illinois Medical Center, Chicago, Illinois

**ROSE PINNEO, R.N., M.S.**
Assistant Professor of Nursing; Clinical Specialist in Cardiovascular Nursing, University of Rochester, School of Medicine and Dentistry, Department of Nursing, Rochester, New York

**LAWRENCE POWER, M.D.**
Associate Professor of Medicine; Chief, Section of Endocrinology and Metabolism, Wayne State University, School of Medicine and Attending Physician, Detroit General Hospital, Detroit, Michigan

**WILLIAM A. REED, M.D.**
Assistant Professor, Department of Surgery, University of Kansas Medical Center, Kansas City, Kansas

**VIRGINIA HILL RICE, R.N., M.S.N.**
Research Assistant, College of Nursing, Wayne State University, Detroit, Michigan

**ALBERT RUBIN, M.D.**
Associate Professor Biochemistry and Surgery, Rogosin Laboratory, The New York Hospital-Cornell Medical Center, New York, New York

**BELDING H. SCRIBNER, M.D.**
Professor of Medicine, School of Medicine, University of Washington and Head, Division of Nephrology, University of Washington Hospital, Seattle, Washington

**ANNA SUPPLE, R.N., B.S.N.**
Administrative Supervisor, Boston City Hospital, Boston, Massachusetts

**ALAN P. THAL, M.D.**
Professor of Surgery, Department of Surgery, University of Kansas Medical Center, Kansas City, Kansas

**JACK van ELK, M.D.**
Head, Section of Cardiology and Principal Investigator, John Hartford Foundation Hyperbaric Oxygen Research Unit, Lutheran General Hospital, Park Ridge, Illinois

**JEAN A. YOKES, R.N., M.S.N.**
Cardiovascular Nurse Specialist, University of Kansas Medical Center, Department of Nursing Education, Kansas City, Kansas

# Introduction

FAYE G. ABDELLAH, R.N., Ed.D

**INTENSIVE CARE AND THE PHYSICIAN–NURSE SPECIALIST TEAM**

Fundamentally, intensive care is a plan designed for critically or seriously ill patients who are unable to communicate their needs, or who require deliberate, planned observation and highly skilled nursing attention. The care is usually provided in a separate self-sufficient facility within which all necessary equipment and supplies are immediately at hand. The most distinguishing aspect of intensive care is, and must always be, the expertness of medical and nursing management. There is good evidence that patient care of this optimal type is best achieved through the cooperative efforts of a *physician–nurse specialist team.*

**Criteria for intensive care.** As a general rule, admission to an intensive care unit should be based on the level of patient care required rather than according to specific clinical disorders.[1, 2] (*Elements of Progressive Patient Care*[3] provides a useful method of classifying patient care needs.) No attempt should be made to quantitate the degree of illness beyond this basic denominator: the patient should have a problem, either medical, post-surgical, or traumatic which is presently, or potentially, life-threatening and may benefit from continuous, concentrated and specialized care. Each of the subjects considered in this book (e.g., respiratory failure, shock, hepatic failure, circulatory emergencies, etc.) represent typical conditions which demand intensive care.

More specifically, intensive care is required rather than customary, or routine care in any of the following circumstances:

1. When frequent or continuous nursing assessment of the patient's clinical status may have a direct influence on the course and outcome of an illness or injury, e.g., the early detection of progressive neurological findings indicating a cerebral contusion in a patient with head trauma.

2. When *immediate* action in response to a particular finding can spell the difference between life and death, e.g., the recognition of an arrhythmia such as ventricular fibrillation by a nurse who then defibrillates the patient within seconds and saves a life.

3. When specific, expert treatment must be given at frequent intervals, e.g., the treatment of patients with extensive burns.

4. When the patient's area, nurses' station, and facilities on the usual hospital floor are not adequate or efficiently arranged for comprehensive care, or if special equipment is required in the treatment program. (In an intensive care unit, special equipment should be standard equipment found at the bedside.)

**The physician–nurse specialist team concept.** An intensive care unit demands the highest form of cooperative endeavor between physician and nurse: the physician–nurse specialist team.

Ideally, this team is comprised of three members (or groups of members) one of whom is a physician and the other two, nurses (see Fig. 1). Both nurses have been trained as specialists, but one (the *nurse specialist*) is at a beginning level and the other (the *clinical nurse specialist*) is at an advanced level of specialization.*

*Physician.* The physician member of the team should be a certified specialist in his field. This implies that there may be several small teams within an intensive care unit, each with a different physician, e.g., a thoracic surgeon–nurse specialist team, a cardiologist–nurse specialist team, etc. The nurse specialist is the constant member of all teams.

*Clinical nurse specialist.* This advanced-level specialist is a professional nurse who has completed graduate clinical training and has received a master's degree in a particular specialty, e.g., surgical nursing, cardiovascular nursing.

The clinical nurse specialist serves in a "peer" relationship with a physician member of the team (Fig. 1). She is trained in

---

* This particular classification of nurses with specialty training is perhaps unfortunate and confusing. The similarity of titles (i.e. nurse specialist and clinical nurse specialist) is due to the lack of a more descriptive designation for the beginning specialist. However, the two levels of specialization are clearly distinguished by educational requirements and training as explained later in this introductory chapter. The term "nurse specialist" is used collectively to describe any nurse with training in a specialty.

PHYSICIAN–NURSE SPECIALIST TEAMS

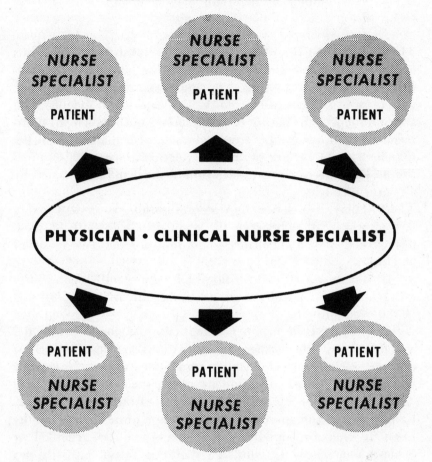

*Fig. 1*

depth to make highly responsible decisions about the nursing care of patients. Her recommendations will frequently influence the plan of medical care.

*Nurse specialist.* Nurses who are graduates of hospital diploma programs, or associate degree or baccalaureate programs, may qualify as nurse specialists on the basis of formal on-the-job training (designated as a clinical residency) in a specialized area of nursing.

The nurse specialist is involved in the direct care of the patient and communicates with the physician and clinical nurse specialist.

**The objectives of the physician–nurse specialist team.** The goals of the team are first, the preservation of life; second, the restoration of the patient to his maximal functional capacity; and third, a decrease in the overall morbidity. The dependent, independent, and interdependent nature of the relationship between the team members permits these purposes to be achieved. Some of the benefits which accrue because of the team relationship are:

1. The aims of care are clearly understood and appreciated by all of the members.

2. There is a deliberate decentralization of services and a lack of stratification between the team members. Both of these elements facilitate and enhance communication between physician and nurse.

3. There is a clear definition of function and responsibility for each member. This increases the probability that decisions will be followed through.

4. Because each member anticipates and complements the actions of the other, emergency situations are handled in an efficient, well-organized manner thus preventing unnecessary trauma to the patient and producing the most effective results.

5. Continuous education is inherent to the team approach. Both nurses and physicians are engaged in a project where guidelines are changing rapidly and where procedures, regarded as modern today, may be outdated within a few months. In an environment of this type, the members are challenged to keep abreast of advances in medical and surgical practices.

6. Each team member becomes cognizant of a responsibility to motivate his colleagues toward achieving excellence in patient care. Each becomes aware of the image conveyed to physician/nurse counterparts (staff nurses and house officers) as the "role model" of the team is emulated throughout the hospital.

**The responsibilities of the members of the team**

*Physician responsibilities.* In a broad sense, the physician's ultimate responsibility is to direct patient care. This involves prompt identification and diagnosis of the patient's problem, the selection of a method of treatment, and later, revision of the therapeutic plan in accordance with the clinical response. To fulfill these responsibilities, the physician depends heavily on nurse specialists to make pertinent observations and to consult with him continuously regarding the patient's clinical course and response to therapy. The physician also relies on the nurse specialist to anticipate, and have ready for use, the supplies and equipment needed in the care of the patient.

More specifically, the physician's primary responsibilities are as follows:

1. to direct the rapid, orderly, and effective mobilization of the physician–nurse specialist team, essential for prompt diagnosis and treatment. The team must make "deliberate haste" if maximal therapeutic benefits are to be realized.

2. to perform the medical evaluation and work-up to establish the correct diagnosis.

3. to make decisions with the nurse specialist regarding initial and subsequent treatment and care.

4. to plan for early emergency intervention to prevent increasing of irreversible damage (e. g., to relieve brain pressure by decompression, clot evacuation, etc.).

5. to attempt to stabilize the patient's condition (e. g., palliative measures).

6. to provide orders which are clear and concise. Any break in this form of communication can be disastrous. For example, if continous intravenous heparin is to be used for anticoagulation, the physician must describe the precise rate of administration and give specific instructions regarding serial blood clotting times so that the therapy is effective and bleeding complications prevented.

7. to make follow-up observations and adjustments in the overall management of the patient as indicated by changes in the clinical picture. Again, this is done cooperatively with the nurse specialist.

***Clinical nurse specialist responsibilities.*** As Pellegrino has pointed out, clinical nursing at a professional level is not something done to, or for, the patient but rather the perception of what needs to be done, and how, within the framework. The clinical nurse specialist's responsibilities can be categorized as follows:

1. to share with the physician the responsibility for patient care.

2. to identify systematically and accurately the nursing needs of patients.

3. to devise and implement appropriate nursing care plans for individual patients.

4. to organize subteams of nurse specialists and direct them in carrying out the nursing care plans.

5. to supervise nurse specialists on subteams.

6. to carry her own case load.

7. to make observational studies of patients' needs and evaluate nursing requirements.

8. to coordinate procedures, tests, and personnel for the patients for whom she is responsible.

9. to translate research findings into actual nursing practice.

10. to institute improvements in patient care.

11. to serve as a model of expert clinical nursing.

Viewing this role conceptually, the clinical nurse specialist is responsible for controlling and manipulating the patient's environment in a manner designed to promote his well being and comfort while carrying out the established objectives of care at the same time. To accomplish this ultimate goal, the clinical nurse specialist must provide for continous nursing assessment in order to detect pertinent changes in the clinical picture. To succeed in this purpose, the clinical nurse specialist collects data through careful, systematic observation; analyzes and interprets these data in the light of her training, experience and knowledge of physical and behavioral sciences, and, finally, translates the findings into expert nursing action to be taken by herself or delegated to nurse specialists on the team.

NURSING ASSESSMENT

It is apparent throughout this book that the various authors are in complete agreement that planned assessment of the patient's clinical state is the keystone to excellent care. The assessment begins as soon as the patient is admitted to the intensive care unit. These initial observations indicate the need for immediate nursing action and provide a basis for subsequent comparison. (Demands of the patient's condition naturally take immediate precedence over the assessment.) Observation must not be an isolated, independent nursing duty, but hopefully, should be carried out while the nurse continues to minister to the patient. This becomes part of a sustained interaction between the patient and nurse. Nevertheless, the clinical nurse specialist must employ a deliberate and conscious approach in securing the information needed, rather than discovering it accidentally.

From the data collected, the clinical nurse specialist formulates a plan of action designated as the Nursing Care Plan (NCP). In developing the NCP, the following factors are considered:

1. A profile of the patient: age, occupation, education, religion, marital status, ages of children, past behavior patterns, particular likes and dislikes, pertinent social and medical history.

2. The anatomy and physiology of the structures involved by the pathological process, injury, and/or surgery.

3. The basis and rationale of the treatment regimen being followed, diagnostic procedures, and the equipment used for diagnosis or treatment.

4. Possible complications of the pathological process, or injury, or surgical procedure.

5. Factors in the medical history which may influence the course of the present illness and/or surgical procedures, such as diabetes and pulmonary emphysema.

6. Attitudes of the patient and his family toward the particular illness, and/or surgical procedure.

7. Specific rehabilitation needs for this pathological process or injury, and/or surgical procedure.

8. Knowledge of research studies which either influence current concepts of care; clarify controversial aspects of care; or provide the basis for changing a current concept of care.

9. The legal responsibilities of the nurse practitioner.

*Nurse specialist responsibilities.* In scope and direction, the responsibilities of the beginning specialist are similar to those of the clinical nurse specialist; they differ, however, in degree and depth. Generally, nurse specialists are involved in the following duties:

1. assessment of the patient's clinical course

2. recognition of the patient's needs and initiation of steps toward meeting these needs

3. patient care, including the use of specialized equipment for monitoring or therapeutic purposes

4. making decisions and carrying out appropriate nursing actions

5. assisting in the development of a nursing care plan

6. initiating preventive measures to protect the patient from complications

To fulfill this role, the nurse specialist must be conversant with the pathophysiology of the patient's illness and must be able effectively to communicate her findings to the physician member of the team.

The proficiency requirements for a nurse specialist in an intensive care unit will depend to a large degree on the services the institution provides. For example, in hospitals where open heart surgery, renal dialysis, organ transplantation are performed, the nurse specialist will require additional training in these specialties. A detailed checklist of required proficiencies can be developed for an institution from the guide shown in Fig. 2.

In each chapter of this book, the specialist's role is described specifically.

**The present status of physician–nurse teams.** Although the physician–nurse specialist team approach is attractive in concept and undoubtedly effective in practice, many practical problems exist which make it difficult to fulfill the high aims of patient care this venture promises. Some of the major obstacles to implementing physician–nurse specialist teams at the present time are:

1. there are too few nurses qualified currently to serve as clinical nurse specialists or nurse specialists.

2. the number of programs designed to train specialists in nursing is still limited and in-depth source material is not readily available. (There are many books and articles containing "pieces" of subject matter; this makes it difficult for those involved in daily patient care to keep well informed.)

CHECKLIST OF PROFICIENCY REQUIREMENTS FOR THE NURSE SPECIALIST IN THE
INTENSIVE CARE UNIT

Check those areas in which you are proficient
_____Intensive Care Units concepts
_____General Nursing Care
_____Fundamentals of care in the specialty

Special technologies, e.g.,
_____Monitor usage
_____Ventilation/respiration
_____Cardiopulmonary resuscitation
_____Countershock
_____Pacing
_____Add others as indicated by the specialty

Other special procedures, e.g.,
_____I.V. infusions
_____Venipuncture
_____Rotating tourniquets
_____Hypothermia
_____ECG (reading and interpolation)
_____Add others as indicated by specialty

*Fig. 2*

3. there is a lack of specification of expectations of team members and poor definition of their respective roles. This vagueness often results in a lack of team leadership by the physician or clinical nurse specialist.
4. communication between physician and nurse regarding means for improving care for a specific patient population is not wholly effective.

Each of these barriers will certainly be crossed as more nurse specialists are trained, and as the medical and nursing professions coordinate and strengthen their efforts in improving patient care.

## The establishment and training of physician-nurse teams

1. It is essential that the Chief of the Medical Service, the Chief of the Surgical Service, the Director of Nursing, and the hospital administration all support the physician-nurse specialist concept; otherwise the plan is doomed.

2. Employing a clinical nurse specialist is an important step initially, particularly in those institutions which do not have schools of medicine or nursing.

3. The clinical nurse specialist in the specialty should meet with the nurse specialist and chief of that service (e.g., thoracic surgical service) to plan for the establishment of a small specific team.

4. The group should review any pertinent literature, e.g., *Intensive Coronary Care—A Manual for Nurses* (Meltzer et al), seeking plans which may be applicable to their institution.

5. Their charge should be to define the objectives of the team and the areas of knowledge and training required for medical and nursing personnel.

6. Teaching conferences should then be arranged.

7. The chief of the specific service then designates a physician as the leader of the small specialty team and work in a one-to-one relationship; similarly the clinical nurse specialist in a one-to-one relationship with the nurse specialist to coordinate plans.

8. Programs should be established for the training of additional nurse specialists.

**The patient care committee.** In an intensive care unit, where several small teams may function independently, it is important to have a permanent patient care committee. Some of the purposes of the group would be:

1. formulating objectives of care for a specific patient population.

2. on the basis of new knowledge, revising objectives and subsequently changing practices of care.

3. identifying areas for research in patient care.

4. identifying needs for staff development programs for medical and nursing personnel.

5. making lines of communication effective between personnel of other disciplines and the medical and nursing personnel on the intensive care unit.

6. reviewing medical-legal problems and determining policies accordingly.

Composition of a patient care committee is visualized thus:
*Core Group:*
    Chief, Clinical Nurse Specialist
    Chief, Surgical Service or his delegate
    Chief, Laboratories or his delegate
    Chief, Anesthesiology or his delegate
    Chief, Medicine or his delegate
*Subspecialty Members:*
    Chief of subspecialty
    An attending physician in the subspecialty
    Nurse specialist in the specialty

The core group should meet once every month or two months, depending upon the number of subspecialties represented in the institution, with the subspecialty members alternating. For example:

| *January* | *March* | *May* |
|---|---|---|
| Core group | Core group | Core group |
| Thoracic surgery team members | Neurosurgical team members | Cardiac surgery team members |

Other persons may be invited to attend as the need arises for consultation concerning specific problems, e.g., a pharmacologist, a physical therapist, or a microbiologist.

**The training of nurse specialists.** The physician–nurse specialist approach to patient care can only exist and be successful if those charged with meeting an institution's goal for excellence fully appreciate the philosophy of this concept, particularly the need for specialization in nursing. It is inherently implied in the team approach to patient care that the professional nurse must assume a *new* and different role; one which is clinically oriented and focuses on patient care. As Pellegrino has stated, ". . . we shall find little sympathy, and only empty refuge, if we divert our energies to a niggardly defense of our professional boundaries. What is needed is a considerate ordering of the best means of meeting the needs of society for those functions recognized as nursing."[4]

In attempting to implement physician-nurse specialist teams, the most obvious question which arises concerns the source of nurse specialists and their training. One logical method which may be adopted is that of Dr. William H. Stewart, the Surgeon General of the U.S. Public Health Service, who proposed that career ladders be devised to permit vertical mobility of all categories of health manpower.[5] This basic plan can be utilized in the training of nurse specialists as seen in Fig. 3.

According to this scheme, nurses (R.N.) would be classified, on the basis of education, as "professional" nurses (those graduat-

# Career Routes for Training of Nurse Specialists

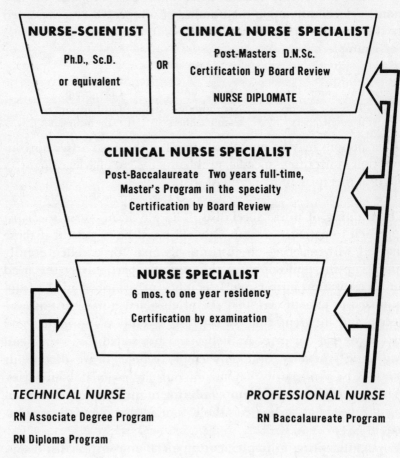

**NURSE-SCIENTIST**

Ph.D., Sc.D.

or equivalent

OR

**CLINICAL NURSE SPECIALIST**

Post-Masters D.N.Sc.

Certification by Board Review

NURSE DIPLOMATE

**CLINICAL NURSE SPECIALIST**

Post-Baccalaureate   Two years full-time,
Master's Program in the specialty

Certification by Board Review

**NURSE SPECIALIST**

6 mos. to one year residency

Certification by examination

**TECHNICAL NURSE**

RN Associate Degree Program

RN Diploma Program

**PROFESSIONAL NURSE**

RN Baccalaureate Program

*Fig. 3*

ing from baccalaureate programs), or "technical" nurses (those completing hospital diploma or associate degree programs).

From a starting level of competence as an R.N., both professional and technical nurses would be given the opportunity to move up the career ladder and become *nurse specialists* in a specialty. This step involves additional training in the form of a clinical residency.

**The clinical residency.** This training program (sometimes called a clinical internship rather than residency) can be six months to one year in duration and should provide concentrated, on-the-job instruction combining lectures, multimedia instructional systems, study by the individual, and clinical experience in the specialty; all under expert supervision. A one-year period as a staff nurse in an intensive care unit provides an invaluable background prior to starting a clinical residency in a specialty.

A clinical residency may be offered by a local institution or agency; whenever possible, there should be a close affiliation with a college or university to assure a high quality of education. It may be helpful (and perhaps necessary) for those institutions offering clinical residencies to have a full-time director of the residency program because considerable time and effort must be dedicated to plannning and evaluation. Since much of the instruction will involve preceptor-type training, it is essential that the institution have competent, functioning, physician-nurse specialist teams. Didactic training alone will prove insufficient for nurse specialist training.

Since most nurses (84%) are graduates of diploma programs, the clinical residency route to specialization will assume great importance. Nurses should be encouraged to climb this career ladder and hospitals must develop adequate programs for this purpose. (That local institutions can, and will, provide first-rate training is readily apparent from their successful experience with coronary care nursing.)

Upon completion of the residency training program, formal certification can be awarded the nurse specialist. This recognition should be based on both written and clinical examinations. (These examinations must be a firm requirement to assure that uniform standards of practice exist.)

**The graduate program.** In contrast to the nurse specialist, the clinical nurse specialist should be trained for this advanced level of specialization through a graduate program of education. In this career plan, the professional nurse with a baccalaureate degree would be required to enroll for two years of full-time study in an approved program leading to a master's degree in order to qualify as a clinical nurse specialist. This preparation is designed to provide the nurse with *breadth* training in medical and surgical nursing and *depth* training in a particular specialty.

At the completion of the master's program, the clinical nurse specialist would be eligible for certification by a Board in the specialty and then designated as a Diplomate.*

A few nurses contemplating a career in research and theory development in nursing may elect to continue their training to a doctoral level (see Fig. 3).

This proposed plan for the training of nurse specialists is in accord with the American Nurses' Association Position Paper, "The Educational Preparation for Nurse Practitioners and Assistants to Nurses,"[6] which states that the educational programs for professional nurses and their assistants should be upgraded and strengthened, and should take place within American educational institutions, with (1) beginning professional education occurring in colleges and universities; (2) beginning technical education in junior or community colleges; and (3) occupational training for nurses' aides and other health workers within general vocational programs of short-term duration.

Regardless of which route is chosen, it should be emphasized that continuing education programs need to be established to provide up-to-date information on recent developments in the specialty.

There are several barriers to the full utilization of specialists in nursing at the present time. Thus far only a few professional nurses, prepared at the baccalaureate level, have chosen to become clinical nurse specialists and there is an obvious shortage of these advanced specialists. In many hospital situations the nurse specialist will be the only nurse member of the team. (In such circumstances a head nurse may assume some of the responsibilities of

* Clinical Boards for certification of nurse specialists have been recommended by nursing leaders and will be developed as the demand for specialists increases.

the clinical nurse specialist.) Training programs for nurse specialists now exist in many centers but participation for staff nurses in these programs is still limited. This incomplete utilization relates partly to the fact that nurses from diploma programs often find themselves isolated from new knowledge (unless they are in clinical settings where ongoing research is conducted). Furthermore, most nurses tend to resist change as it creates a feeling of insecurity. This is unfortunate, because nurses at all levels have a contribution to make. It is within areas of specialization, particularly, that nurses can find their contributory roles.

**References:**

1. ABDELLAH, F. G. and STRACHAN, E. J.: Progressive Patient Care, *Amer. J. Nurs.,* 59:649, 1959.
2. U.S. Department of Health, Education, and Welfare: *Elements of Progressive Patient Care,* Public Health Service Publication No. 930-C-1, September, 1962.
3. Educational Preparation for Nurse Practitioners and Assistants to Nurses. A Position Paper, American Nurses' Association, 1965, p. 7.
4. PELLEGRINO, E. D.: The Changing Role of the Professional Nurse in the Hospital, *Hospitals,* 35:56, December 16, 1961.
5. PRESTON, RUTH, et al.: Patient Care Classification as a Basis for Estimating Graded Inpatient Hospital Facilities, *Medical Care Research,* K. L. White (ed.), New York, Pergamon Press, 1965, pp. 37–48.
6. STEWART, WILLIAM H.: Education for the Health Professions Speech presented at the White House Conference on Health, Washington, D.C., November 3, 1965, p. 5.

# Chapter I

# Respiratory Insufficiency and Failure

WILMA J. PHIPPS, R.N., A.M.
WALTER L. BARKER, M.D.

## THE PROBLEM

Respiratory insufficiency implies an inability of the lungs to exchange gases adequately to meet the demands of the body during effort. Respiratory failure denotes inadequate ventilation and exchange, even at rest. Usually, respiratory insufficiency can be compensated for by reduction in activity; however, if there are superimposed stresses, respiratory insufficiency may lead to respiratory failure and death.

This chapter is concerned with the management of progressive respiratory insufficiency and remediable (i.e., reversible) respiratory failure.

### Respiratory insufficiency

There are two types of respiratory insufficiency: acute and chronic. The former includes those disorders which rather abruptly compromise respiration, such as reflex bronchospasm with loss of airway integrity, acute left ventricular failure, and overwhelming pulmonary infections. Chronic respiratory insufficiency results from degenerative pulmonary parenchymal changes in the alveolar and capillary structures, and is usually progressive over a period of years. Diseases such as pulmonary fibrosis, emphysema, and other diffuse disorders that affect the lung structure lead not only to failure of gaseous exchange but, eventually, to increased pulmonary arterial pressure, the development of pulmonary heart disease (cor pulmonale), and ultimately to combined cardiorespiratory failure.

Because of the life-threatening nature of respiratory insufficiency, it is essential that the problem be recognized and treated as soon as possible. Whether respiratory insufficiency is first identified in an emergency room, after a surgical procedure, or elsewhere in the hospital, corrective measures must be instituted promptly, and ideally in a facility specifically equipped to handle the multiple problems anticipated, viz., a respiratory care unit or an intensive care unit.

**The pathophysiology of respiratory insufficiency.** To appreciate the problem of respiratory insufficiency and its treatment, it is necessary initially to consider certain principles of normal respiratory function as the basis of clinical and physiological abnormalities.

*Normal respiratory function.* Fundamentally, respiratory function is geared to the exchange of oxygen and carbon dioxide. Mechanical forces, engendered primarily by movement of the thoracic cage, bring air to the alveoli and carry the exchanged gases back for their expiration. This process constitutes the *ventilatory* phase of pulmonary function. In like fashion, these gases must be transported by the bloodstream to and from the lungs (alveoli) where they are exchanged. This movement of blood through the pulmonary capillaries is known as *pulmonary perfusion.*

The functional keystone of this exchange system is the alveolar-capillary unit. At these sites (there are millions of alveoli and billions of capillaries in the normal lung) inspired air is separated from capillary blood by a very thin semi-permeable barrier, the alveolar-capillary membrane. Diffusion of oxygen and carbon dioxide takes place across this membrane, with the direction of movement dependent on the relative partial pressure and solubility of the gases on each side of the membrane.

For normal diffusion to occur (along with adequate oxygenation of venous blood) the phases of ventilation and perfusion must function effectively. In addition, the alveolar-capillary membrane must be permeable to those gases. Finally, if blood returning to the arterial circulation is to be fully oxygenated, venous blood cannot be shunted around alveolar capillary units.

***The basis of respiratory insufficiency.*** *Hypoxia,* or inadequate concentration of oxygen, can result from the following causes:

1. Decreased movement of gases to and from the lungs (hypoventilation).
2. Abnormalities of the flow of blood in the pulmonary capillaries (perfusion).
3. Uneven distribution of blood flow in relationship to ventilation (ventilation-perfusion disorders).
4. Impairment in alveolar-capillary membrane permeability.
5. Arterial-venous shunting.

It is important to recognize that hypoxia may develop from any of these disturbances in pulmonary function. On the other hand, *hypercarbia,* abnormal carbon dioxide retention in the blood, can only result from hypoventilation and/or ventilation–perfusion disorders.

***Clinical disorders of respiratory function.*** There are four general clinical conditions that can be correlated with the disorders of pulmonary function just described:

### 1. RESTRICTIVE LUNG DISEASE

In restrictive diseases, the total lung capacity is reduced; in other words, there is a decrease in the number of alveoli available for the normal exchange of oxygen and carbon dioxide. Restriction may result from diseases that deform the bony thorax, e.g., kyphoscoliosis and rheumatoid spondylitis, or from conditions which limit thoracic mobility, e.g., abdominal distention due to tumor, ascites, or ileus, or splinting of the chest because of pain. Expansion of the lungs can also be restricted by fibrotic diseases that limit the distensibility of the lungs, e.g., collagen diseases, pleural fibrosis, and interstitial fibrosing pneumonitis.

### 2. OBSTRUCTIVE LUNG DISEASE

These diseases are characterized by a reduction in the normal flow of gases to and from the lung. The most common causes of obstructive lung disease include severe pulmonary emphysema, chronic bronchitis, and bronchospastic crises such as bronchial asthma.

3. DISEASES ASSOCIATED WITH MEMBRANE PERMEABILITY DIS-
ORDERS

There are two groups of diseases that affect the alveolar capillary membrane and interfere with the exchange of oxygen. The first includes diseases in which the total area of alveolar-capillary membrane is reduced, such as far-advanced tuberculosis, or pneumoconiosis. The second group involves a primary abnormality of the alveolar capillary membrane as seen in progressive granulomatous diseases and interstitial fibrosis of the Hamman-Rich type.

4. ARTERIO-VENOUS SHUNTING

As noted, if venous blood bypasses functioning alveoli, hypoxia will result from venous dilution of the arterial stream. Arterio-venous (A-V) shunting may be the result of a true communication between the pulmonary artery and vein or the right and left heart chambers. A-V shunting may also occur when groups of alveoli become non-functioning and blood perfusing the pulmonary capillaries passes through without gaseous exchange taking place (physiologic shunting).

*The control of respiration.* The rate and volume of respiration are controlled by both chemical and neurologic means, which are interrelated.

The transport of oxygen and carbon dioxide by the blood, to and from the tissues, involves a system of buffers and other biochemical means. Oxygen is carried in the hemoglobin molecule, as oxyhemoglobin, while carbon dioxide is transported either in physical solution or by buffered salts. These mechanisms play an important role in the control of respiration. Changes in oxygen and carbon dioxide tensions, as well as pH, stimulate chemoreceptors located in the arch of the aorta and at the bifurcation of the carotid arteries (carotid bodies). These peripheral stimuli are relayed to the respiratory centers of the brain (in the medulla) where reflex neurologic control of respiration is effected. In addition to this basic control, the periodicity of pulmonary ventilation is also influenced by stretch reflexes arising within the lung.

The peripheral chemoreceptor areas may be narcotized by a variety of substances, including excessive amounts of analgesics and sedatives, resulting in the loss of control of ventilation through this mechanism. Central (neurological) control of respiration can be inhibited by very high carbon dioxide tensions which are anesthetic to the medullary centers. In the presence of severe hypercarbia, the only stimulus for spontaneous respiration will be those peripheral chemoreceptors which respond to oxygen-lack and reflexly stimulate ventilation. The administration of high concentrations of oxygen to a patient with markedly elevated carbon dioxide levels has obvious danger: the sole remaining stimulus to respiration (i.e., low oxygen tension) is lost, and respiration will cease. This vicious cycle of events is referred to as *carbon dioxide narcosis* or oxygen poisoning.

### *Respiratory failure*

Respiratory failure usually develops as a sequela of respiratory insufficiency. If insufficiency is not recognized and adequately treated near its onset, ventilatory and perfusion functions may decrease rapidly and hypoxia and hypercarbia ensue. The clinical picture of such progression is quite distinct: the patient develops marked anxiety, mental confusion, and even tremors or frank convulsions. The respiratory rate increases (tachypnea) as does the heart rate (tachycardia). As the hypoxia worsens, cyanosis becomes evident. Hypotension may be present and, depending on the degree of peripheral vasoconstriction, the skin will often be cold and clammy. Ultimately, the patient's compensatory mechanisms fail. At this point, hypotension becomes profound and irreversible; mental confusion progresses to stupor and coma; tachypnea leads to irregularity of respiratory effort; and the heart rate slows markedly. Irreversible cardiorespiratory failure and death are almost inevitable.

There are two other causes of respiratory failure:

#### UPPER AIRWAY OBSTRUCTION

Obstruction of the airway is most likely to occur in a patient whose sensorium is depressed as a result of overdosages of analgesics or sedatives, head injury, or metabolic disturbances. The cardinal signs of laryngeal and tracheal obstruction are rattling and gurgling respirations, rib retraction, use of accessory muscles of respiration, stridor, cyanosis, and regurgitation of oral fluids through nose (occasionally).

RESPIRATORY PARALYSIS

Paralysis of the muscles of respiration may develop during the course of such neurological diseases as poliomyelitis, myasthenia gravis, and Guillain-Barré syndrome. This possibility should be suspected among patients with these disorders who show evidence of progressive skeletal muscle paralysis, rapid, shallow breathing, and a feeling of impending dissolution (angor animi).

## ASSESSMENT OF THE PROBLEM

**1. Clinical manifestations of respiratory insufficiency.** The most important findings related to acute respiratory insufficiency are hypoxia, hypercarbia, hypotension, and dyspnea. These abnormalities may occur singly or in combination.

*Hypoxia.* By definition, hypoxia refers to an inadequate supply of oxygen to the tissues. Although cyanosis is a common manifestation of hypoxia, its presence cannot be regarded as a reliable index of the true state of arterial oxygenation. Ordinarily, cyanosis does not become apparent until the arterial oxygen saturation is below 85%. Severe tissue hypoxia may exist despite oxygen saturations that are above cyanotic levels.

The *earliest signs of hypoxia* are tachycardia, hypertension, and hyperventilation. (The elevated blood pressure is explained by an increase in sympathetic nervous system activity induced by hypoxia which leads to selective tissue vasoconstriction and increased peripheral resistance.) In *advanced* stages of hypoxia, or among old, debilitated patients, where the sympathetic response fails, the heart rate decreases markedly and the blood pressure falls to hypotensive levels. These effects are a prelude to circulatory arrest, the usual cause of death with prolonged hypoxia.

*Hypercarbia.* Hypercarbia, or carbon dioxide retention, causes two antagonistic responses, a local depressant effect on tissue function and a stimulation of the autonomic nervous system.

As a result of the *local* effect of increased carbon dioxide, varying degrees of circulatory failure and hypotension may develop along with cerebral depression (ranging from mild sedation to deep coma). In contrast, the *stimulatory* effect mediated through the sympathetic nervous system results in an increase in cardiac output and pulse rate. The balance between the stimulatory and depressant effects of excess carbon dioxide determines the ultimate clinical picture.

Other signs and symptoms of hypercarbia include muscle twitching, visual defects, increased cutaneous blood flow with erythema and sweating, and cardiac arrhythmias.

As the partial pressure of carbon dioxide ($pCO_2$) increases to over 100 mm Hg, the patient becomes progressively drowsy and then lapses into severe coma with eventual respiratory arrest.

*Hypotension.* Both hypoxia and hypercarbia can produce hypotension. The hypotension may result from either a decreased cardiac output or a reduction in peripheral resistance or both.

Hypotension *not* associated with peripheral vasoconstriction is characterized by warm, dry skin of natural color and a pulse rate that is not grossly increased. In patients with increasing levels of retained carbon dioxide, where peripheral vasoconstriction is marked, hypotension is accompanied by cold, pale, sweaty skin, tachycardia, and a thready peripheral pulse. Oliguria or anuria is common in this situation.

*Dyspnea.* Difficult or labored breathing is one of the cardinal subjective criteria of respiratory insufficiency. This symptom indicates that the patient is unsuccessfully attempting to increase his pulmonary ventilation.

**2. Pulmonary function tests.** Qualitative and quantitative evaluation of pulmonary function has become a routine part of the evaluation of patients with pulmonary disease. This discussion will briefly consider the customary pulmonary function tests employed today to determine the adequacy of ventilation.

The basic instrument for this evaluation is the spirometer, which records respiratory volumes on a fast-moving drum. Using this device, the total gas content of the lung can be separated into four distinct *volumes* as follows: (1) *tidal volume*—that volume of gas inspired and expired with each normal breath; (2) *the inspiratory reserve volume*—the additional volume of gas which can be inspired over and above the tidal volume by maximal inspiration; (3) *expiratory reserve volume*—that volume of gas which can be expired by forced expiration after completion of a normal expiration; and, finally, (4) *the residual volume*—that gas remaining in the lungs at the end of a forced expiration.

In addition, the gas content in the lungs is also evaluated in terms of four *capacities.* These are: (1) *the total lung capacity* —the total volume of the lung at maximal inspiration (which contains all four lung volumes); (2) *the vital capacity*—the maximum amount of air which can be expired following maximal inspiration (which includes the inspiratory reserve volume, the tidal volume, and the expiratory reserve volume); (3) *the inspiratory capacity*—the amount of air which can be maximally inspired after completion of normal expiration (which includes tidal and inspiratory reserve volumes); and (4) *the functional residual capacity*—the gas remaining in the lungs at the end of a normal expiration (or the sum of the expiratory reserve and residual volumes).

The normal total lung capacity is about 6 liters. Of this the vital capacity comprises approximately 4.5 liters, and the residual volume between 1.0 and 1.5 liters. The tidal volume is normally about 0.5 liters. These volumes and capacities are illustrated by a normal spirogram (Fig. 1).

Two other ventilatory parameters are of clinical significance: (1) *a timed vital capacity* or forced expiratory volume (FEV). By measuring the volume of maximally-fast expiration at specified periods of time starting after a full inspiration (one, two, or three seconds), an index of ventilatory efficiency can be obtained. Normally, the one-second vital capacity is about 80 per cent of the forced expiratory volume, the two-second between 85 and 90 per cent, and the three-second, 95 per cent or higher. (2) *The maximum breathing capacity* (MBC), also referred to as maximal voluntary ventilation (MVV). This capacity represents the maximal amount the patient can exchange per minute by voluntary hyperventilation.

The values for forced expiratory volume (FEV) and maximal voluntary ventilation (MVV) obtained from the patient are compared with a prediction nomogram permitting an evaluation of the patient's ventilatory efficiency versus that anticipated according to sex, age, and height.

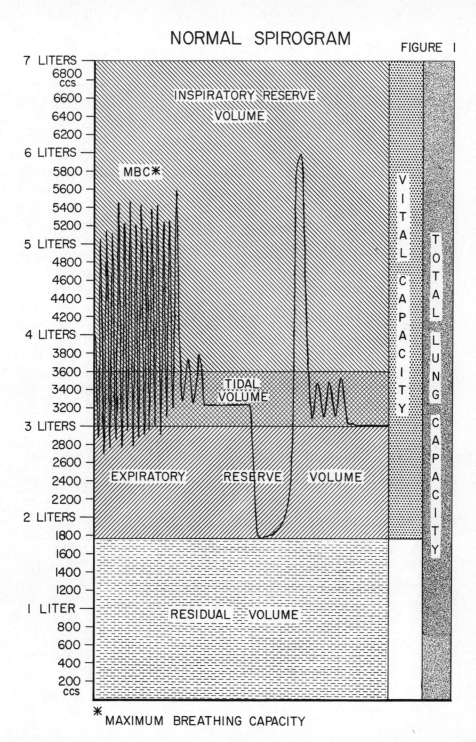

# NORMAL SPIROGRAM

FIGURE I

* MAXIMUM BREATHING CAPACITY

Table 1
PARTIAL PRESSURES OF BLOOD GASES (AS MM. HG)

|  | $pO_2$ | $pCO_2$ |
|---|---|---|
| Arterial | 95 | 40 |
| Venous | 40 | 46 |
| Tissues | <30 | >50 |

By comparing the residual volume of the lung (as determined by nitrogen or helium washout techniques) with the total lung capacity, a useful ratio can be obtained. The RV/TLC is normally under 25%. This implies that the bulk of the total lung capacity is represented by the vital capacity.

**3. Blood gas studies.** Blood gas measurements are important indices in the assessment of respiratory function.

As previously noted, the diffusion of oxygen and carbon dioxide across the alveolar-capillary membrane is dependent primarily on the tension (partial pressures) of these gases in the alveoli and blood. The partial pressure of oxygen ($pO_2$) and carbon dioxide ($pCO_2$) can be measured simply from *arterial* blood samples. The values obtained from venous blood are quite different (Table 1), and do not reflect the true state at the pulmonary capillary level. Venous samples should not be used for blood gas determinations. The normal values of arterial blood gases are found in Table 2.

Table 2
ARTERIAL BLOOD GASES—NORMAL VALUES

| | |
|---|---|
| $O_2$ content (breathing room air at sea level) | 17.5 to 20.5 vol. % |
| $O_2$ per cent saturation (breathing room air at sea level—resting or exercise) | 94% |
| $O_2$ per cent saturation (breathing 100% $O_2$) (plus 1.9 ml. $O_2$ dissolved in plasma/100 ml. blood) | 100% |
| $O_2$ capacity | 1.34 X Hb. (in gm./100 ml.) / 0.3 |
| $O_2$ tension (breathing room air) | 95 to 100 mm. Hg |
| $O_2$ tension (breathing 100% $O_2$) | 600 to 640 mm. Hg |
| $CO_2$ content, whole blood | 49 vol. % or 21.9 mM./L. |
| $CO_2$ content, plasma | 59.6 vol. % |
| $CO_2$ tension | 40 mm. Hg |
| pH | 7.4 |

## 4. Correlation of pulmonary function tests, blood gases, and clinical disorders.

### RESTRICTIVE LUNG DISEASES

A *total* reduction in lung volumes is found in patients with restrictive lung diseases; however, there is no disparity in the relative ratios of these values. The $pCO_2$ is usually normal.

### OBSTRUCTIVE LUNG DISEASES

In these ventilatory defects a disparity is found between lung volumes, as vital capacity, and the maximum breathing capacity. If the MBC is low in the presence of a normal VC, it can be assumed that an obstructive disorder exists (usually the result of pulmonary emphysema). In keeping with the above disparity, the timed vital capacity is distinctly abnormal. (The 1-second timed vital capacity may be as low as 35%–40% of normal.) In other words, patients with obstructive airway disease may be capable of taking in a normal volume of air, provided they have sufficient time to do so. The low MBC and the low timed vital capacity result because of the inability to move air in and out of the lungs rapidly. For this reason there is a high residual volume, so that the RV/TLC may be as high as 40%.

Patients with chronic obstructive disease may be perfectly comfortable as long as their effort requirements are not exceeded. (Spirograms demonstrating restrictive and obstructive defects are shown in Fig. 2.)

### ABNORMAL MEMBRANE PERMEABILITY

Diseases that affect membrane permeability may result in hypoxia at rest, but more often they are manifested by decreased arterial saturation with exercise. The lung volumes are usually reduced, but the MBC is maintained at a relatively normal level. The diagnosis is suspected from radiologic examination of the chest where fine, diffuse lesions are noted in the lung fields.

### ARTERIO-VENOUS SHUNTS

The existence of either direct or physiologic shunting in the lungs can be ascertained by the detection of a low $pO_2$ in the presence of normal pulmonary function tests.

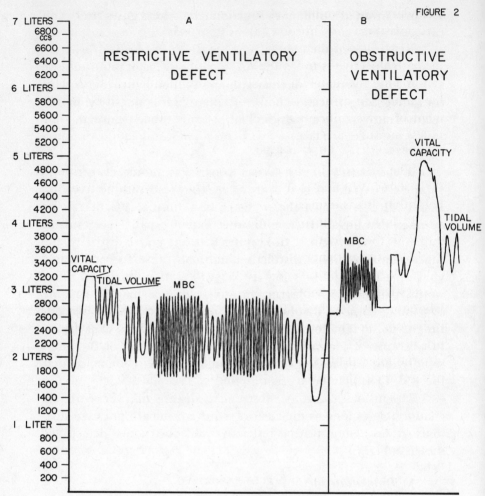

FIGURE 2

*Fig. 2*

## PRINCIPLES OF TREATMENT

Candidates likely to develop respiratory insufficiency and/or respiratory failure include those with the following medical conditions: trauma, either surgical or accidental; acute suppurative problems of systemic or pulmonary etiology; extensive burns; airway obstructions; neuromuscular diseases, including myasthenia gravis, Guillain-Barré syndrome, peripheral neuropathies, and poliomyelitis; profound anemia; central respiratory depression secondary to poisoning (barbiturate poisoning); or bronchial or cardiac asthma; *any* unconscious patient may also be a candidate.

Regardless of the etiology of respiratory insufficiency, the immediate objective is to maintain the patient's respiration until he can breathe adequately on his own, and simultaneously to support his circulation as necessary. Any patient with respiratory impairment of any significant degree will become unconscious in time unless measures are taken to clear his airway and support respirations.

The first step in the treatment of these patients is to assess their status. We find that answers to the following questions are helpful in this assessment:

1. Is the patient conscious or unconscious?
2. Is the patient's airway obstructed?
3. Is the patient apneic?
4. What is the cause of the respiratory insufficiency?

As emergency measures are being performed, confirmatory laboratory studies, including a chest x-ray, an electrocardiogram, urinalyses, blood counts, and determination of blood electrolytes, pH, and gases ($pCO_2$ and $pO_2$), should be done. Determination of serial arterial blood gases is particularly valuable in evaluating the status of the patient and assessing the effectiveness of the therapy.

**Treatment of the conscious patient who has respiratory insufficiency**

**A.** *Immediate measures*

1. Most patients can breathe best when sitting in a supported forward-leaning position.

2. Be sure the patient has a clear airway. Upper airway obstruction prevents oxygen from reaching the alveolar level.

3. Administer oxygen by mask or catheter. If oxygen is effectively reaching the cellular level, tachycardia can be expected to be controlled.

4. Semiconscious patients may require an oropharyngeal airway to prevent the tongue from falling back and obstructing the airway. Use of such an airway also facilitates removal of secretions from the pharynx.

5. Patients capable of responding should be encouraged to cough. This provides the best exodus for tracheal and bronchial secretions. The natural airway supplies adequate humidification and prevents the introduction of contaminants into the tracheobronchial tree (which is basically sterile). A significant degree of intratracheal pressure may be developed with a closed glottis in the act of coughing. It may reach 60 to 100 mm Hg on good expiratory effort. Effective methods for assisting the patient to cough are described in the chapter on "Chest Surgery."

## B. *Other measures*
### INTRATRACHEAL ASPIRATION

If the patient is unable to cough effectively, intratracheal aspiration is the next most useful method of cleansing the tracheobronchial tree. Basically, clean technique should be employed. The catheters and equipment should be housed in containers of 70% ethyl alcohol. The usual technique for intratracheal aspiration involves "blind" intubation of the trachea. The catheter is introduced into the nose and makes the curve through the inferior turbinate into the posterior pharynx. While the patient's tongue is held forward, he is instructed to take a deep breath or to give any kind of explosive cough. This tends to open the glottis and permits the catheter to be inserted between the vocal cords and into the trachea. Several attempts may be required in order to effect entrance. With practice, facility may be achieved in introducing a nasotracheal catheter in this manner. Distortion of the nasal passages and inability of the patient to control his gag reflex may make this technique difficult; however, by merely stimulating the posterior pharynx, a cough of significant intensity may be produced to allow the catheter to be passed.

Once the trachea is entered, the aspirating suction machine is attached, either to a Y tube or fenestrated catheter (so that no suction is applied while the patient is being intubated). The catheter is advanced gently to avoid bleeding or irritation. Prolonged aspiration is undesirable, because of the undue loss of alveolar gas it engenders. Five to ten ml of normal sterile saline may be introduced through the tube, and the liquid or liquefied secretions are then aspirated. Although a nurse specialist should be capable of performing true intratracheal suctioning of this type, hospital policies may interdict. In this circumstance, or if untrained in this procedure, the nurse can readily insert a catheter through the nose into the oropharynx to stimulate the cough reflex.

*Principles and precautions in the use of intratracheal aspiration*

1. The procedure should be performed with the use of as clean a technique as possible. Wash hands well, wear sterile gloves, or use a sterile hemostat to grasp catheter. Tracheobronchial suctioning requires two persons, one to pull the patient's tongue forward while the other introduces the catheter through the nose.

2. Raise the bed backrest so that the patient is sitting upright.

3. A No. 14 or No. 16 curved-tip rubber catheter is attached to the suction machine, preferably with a Y tube connector. The catheter should be inserted *without* suction and can be guided into either bronchus by turning the head away from the side from which it is desired to catheterize.

4. Suction is applied once the catheter is in place, by placing the thumb over the open end of the Y tube. Suction should be performed for only 10–15 seconds at a time. Once the catheter is in place, the trachea may be irrigated with 5–10 ml of saline and then aspirated.

5. The catheter may be left in place between periods of suctioning, and oxygen should be administered in these intervals.

6. As the catheter is withdrawn, suction should be applied, so that secretions will not be left in the oropharynx.

BEDSIDE BRONCHOSCOPY

Bronchoscopy is indicated when secretions are retained and obstructive atelectasis persists, despite coughing or suctioning. The use of intermittent positive pressure breathing in such patients will not usually dislodge the plug and, in fact, may impact secretions. Under these conditions, *bedside* bronchoscopy is the preferred treatment, particularly in postsurgical patients where movement to an operating room is impractical.

A tray with the following equipment should be available.

7 x 40 Bronchoscope with #40 light carrier in place

40 Suction Tip with rubber tubing attached and a multi-fit connector placed on the tray

Battery Box Cord to fit the bronchoscope attached to the battery box on the connecting end and the other end coiled beneath the scope itself

(Attach the cord to the scope at time of use.)

#16 Laryngoscope with a #16 light carrier in place

Extra Battery Box Cord in the lid of the box

Extra #40 Light Carrier

Extra Bulbs for scope

Endotracheal Tube #7 with cuff and Yon adaptor (or plain needle)

Medium adult airway

Laryngeal Mirror

Finger Tip Control Syringe with cannula attached

DeVilbiss Spray Set

Alcohol Lamp

Tongue Blade

Bottle Tetracaine 2% (Pontocaine)

30 cc Vial Injectable Saline

Plain Gauze 4 x 4's

Tube Lubricating Jelly

O.R. Caps

O.R. Gowns

Surgical Gloves

Masks

An adequate source of light and suction is required. Minimal anesthesia with one to two per cent Pontocaine may be used to spray the oropharynx (with a drop or two on the vocal cords) to avert laryngospasm. The patient is propped up in bed at about a 30° angle and the head allowed to drop back over the backrest. Ordinarily, these patients are weakened from pain, sedation, and previous attempts to clear the airway; as such the bronchoscope may be introduced with ease.

Upon entering the trachea, oxygen may be delivered through the sidearm of the bronchoscope. Secretions are aspirated, some of which may be sent to the bacteriology laboratory for culture after being trapped in a Luken's tube. Both main stem bronchi are then inspected and all secretions are aspirated, preferably with an open-end suction tip. If a plug is encountered, it is dislodged and removed.

Sterile saline may be introduced through the bronchoscope and aspirated to humidify and liquefy the secretions. In certain instances a dilute solution of Tergemist may be introduced to assist in the liquefaction of thick bronchial secretions. When the airway appears patent, the bronchoscope is removed, oxygen is administered, and intermittent positive pressure breathing and aerosols are continued.

INTESTINAL AND GASTRIC DECOMPRESSION

Abdominal distention with gastric dilatation or ileus causes an elevation of the diaphragm and a decrease in ventilation. In such instances, temporary decompression of the stomach and intestine will improve ventilation and prevent aspiration and vomiting. In the marginal respiratory patient, protracted nasogastric intubation is harmful, because of the production of excess pharyngeal secretions. (In the comatose patient who has lost his airway and requires more definitive measures to control secretions and ventilation, nasogastric intubation may be accomplished easily and with safety once the airway is definitely secured. This, however, may require tracheostomy.)

## Treatment of the unconscious patient

*Emergency measures* (see Table 3). The unconscious patient who loses his airway requires immediate attention. Secretions must be aspirated promptly from the oropharynx and ventilation started. Ventilation can be accomplished at first by mouth-to-mouth or mouth-to-nose techniques. An oropharyngeal airway is used to keep the tongue from falling back; it may have an extension on it (S-shaped tube) so that mouth-to-tube resuscitation can be given. Once secretions are aspirated from the oropharynx and an airway is established, an elastic bag (Ambu or anesthesia type) is used to carry out emergency ventilation. However, these are only temporary measures, and either endotracheal intubation or tracheostomy should be performed promptly.

1. ENDOTRACHEAL INTUBATION

Whenever in doubt about a patient's ability to maintain his airway, it is best to proceed with endotracheal intubation. These patients are marginal, and unless ideal facilities are readily available for performing immediate tracheostomy, difficulty may be encountered and an airway (which is critical to begin with) may be entirely lost during the tracheostomy procedure. A far safer method in experienced hands is to introduce an endotracheal tube and later to perform elective tracheostomy if more prolonged respiratory support is indicated.

Endotracheal intubation is indicated for the following reasons:

     a. to establish and maintain a free airway in patients who cannot be treated adequately with lesser means;

     b. to permit positive pressure ventilation which cannot be done effectively by mask;

     c. to prevent aspiration by sealing off the trachea from the digestive tract; and

     d. to permit effective removal of retained tracheobronchial secretions.

*Technique and precautions of endotracheal intubation.*

Most hospitals have personnel who can perform emergency endotracheal intubation. Ordinarily, a tube 8–9 mm in diameter is adequate to provide ventilation and egress of secretions. An oral airway (Guedell) should be used to prevent occlusion of the tube by the patient's bite; it is secured with tape. The cuff on the endotracheal tube is inflated sufficiently to occlude the main tract and prevent air leak and aspiration around the tube. Adequately humidified oxygen may be introduced through the tube once the secretions have been aspirated, and a variety of respirators may be attached to ventilate the patient.

Continued inflation of an endotracheal cuff cannot be allowed indefinitely, because of the possibility of tracheal wall necrosis. We have adopted the policy that 24–36 hours of continuous cuffed intubation is maximal. After this time, if the patient does not have spontaneous return of respiration, or if additional support is required, tracheostomy is performed. The endotracheal tube is not removed until this is accomplished.

If a cuff is inflated longer than 24 hours and additional time is desired to decide on tracheostomy, the cuff should be deflated for at least 15 minutes every two hours and the tube slightly rotated to avoid any pressure points.

The most common complications of endotracheal intubation are vocal cord damage and edema of the larynx and trachea. While edema is often transient and of no consequence, severe degrees of edema with associated stridor and increased respiratory effort may develop hours or even days after removal of the endotracheal tube, necessitating tracheostomy. Milder forms of obstruction may be treated conservatively. High humidity and large doses of corticosteroids have been helpful in some patients. Tracheal slough and stenosis are rare complications resulting from pressure necrosis of the tracheal wall. A further danger of intubation is the possibility of placing the tube in one lung, with subsequent obstruction and atelectasis of the other lung. On occasion, the tube may be inserted too close to the carina (the ridge between the orifices of the two main bronchi), causing dry secretions which obstruct *both* bronchi. This situation is immediately life-threatening.

With proper placement of the tube, gentle aspiration, and adequate humidification, these complications may be avoided almost universally.

It is important that periodic suctioning be performed to keep the airway patent. The method is the same as described with tracheostomy care.

## 2. TRACHEOSTOMY

### Indications for tracheostomy

Tracheostomy should be done electively with the full benefits of an established airway whenever possible. For this reason endotracheal intubation is the primary and initial treatment in emergency situations.

The indications for tracheostomy overlap those for endotracheal intubation, namely to maintain a free airway whenever the need is expected to persist for more than 36 hours, and to permit the use of positive pressure ventilators.

A tracheostomy is also needed whenever an endotracheal tube cannot be tolerated by a conscious patient, or if the passage of an endotracheal tube is impossible or undesirable (e.g., with pharyngeal or laryngeal obstruction due to tumor, infection or vocal cord paralysis).

In patients with chronic respiratory insufficiency, permanent tracheostomy may be indicated. The procedure, however, should not be done for the sole purpose of reducing the anatomical dead space, since this saving is trivial compared to the enormous alveolar dead space found in chronic lung disease.

In burn patients, where the oropharyngeal passages and even the trachea itself is damaged, endotracheal intubation may be quite hazardous, and tracheostomy is the treatment of choice.

### Types of tracheostomy

A variety of tracheostomy cannulae is available. The Jackson (or Hollinger) silver tube is the most common. With the advent of respirators, however, numerous adaptations and modifications have been added to the basic cannula. The Morch tracheostomy tube is essentially the same as a Jackson silver tube, except that it has a screw-on swivel adaptor on the inner cannula which serves as a connector to the respirator and allows suctioning without disconnecting the respirator. All of these tubes may have an endotracheal cuff attached to provide a closed system. A large cannula is preferred, and in most adults, one with an internal diameter of 6–8 mm is suitable. When a cuff is used, it should fit the tracheostomy tube snugly. We use a 3/8" endotracheal cuff on a No. 7 Jackson tracheostomy tube.

A malleable plastic tracheostomy tube with a bonded cuff which inflates evenly has been developed. It is similar in design and construction to the classical tracheostomy tube, but has the added advantage of having a built-in cuff. More recently, a double-cuff system has been employed on this tube, allowing the cuffs to be inflated alternately, so that two pressure points are involved rather than one.

*Tracheal fenestration*

Rockey has devised a technique of tracheal fenestration which provides for a permanent tracheostomy *without* the insertion of a tube. In this procedure, muscle and skin flaps are used to create a permanent opening into the trachea.

A plastic cannula with a detachable one-way flap valve is available for aspiration purposes only. The flange on the plastic tracheostomy tube is sutured to the anterior wall of the trachea and is introduced in much the same manner as a routine tracheostomy. It has the advantage of simple aspiration without introduction of a hollow tube into the lumen of the trachea, and, in addition, with the detachable one-way flap valve, the patient can ventilate adequately and still cough and use the normal pathway for removal of secretions.

*Technique of tracheostomy*

One or two per cent procaine provides adequate local anesthesia. A high tracheostomy is preferable in order to maintain the tip of the cannula well above the carina. The incision may be midline and vertical or a curved collar type. Cosmetically, a curved collar incision is preferable; however, the limited exposure that is gained from it, especially in emergencies, may reduce the speed with which the tracheostomy can be performed. In the more urgent cases, and in particular in patients with thick, heavy necks, a midline vertical incision provides for extension of the incision upward or downward as may be required. In general, an emergency tracheostomy is best performed with the use of this vertical incision.

It is important that hemostasis be obtained before opening the tracheal wall, to avoid aspiration of blood. If the pyramidal lobe of the thyroid overrides the area for tracheostomy, it should be dissected off and/or transected with adequate hemostasis prior to opening into the tracheal lumen. It is preferable to expose and enter the pretracheal fascia, which is relatively avascular, and identify the third tracheal ring. A portion of this tracheal ring is excised to provide an adequate opening. It is important to firmly grasp the small portion of cartilage to be removed in order to prevent slippage of this fragment into the tracheal lumen. Prior to incision of the trachea, a tracheal hook is used to grasp the trachea and elevate it so that its position will not vary with respiration or swallowing. A Jackson dilator spreads the tracheal opening so that a cannula, No. 7 or No. 8, with or without the attached cuff, may be readily introduced and immediate aspiration begun. If a bacteriologic specimen is desired, a Luken's tube is spliced into the system to trap secretions.

The incision is loosely closed around the tracheostomy tube, and usually a single silk suture is used to approximate the skin so the tracheostomy tube rests evenly without abutment against the posterior tracheal wall. The tube is firmly secured with ties around the neck. By appropriately folding an uncut 4 x 4 gauze pad, a pantaloon type of dressing may be inserted around the flange of the tube to make a neat and safe padding.

### Dangers and complications of tracheostomy

Upon opening the trachea, the natural humidifying mechanisms of the oral nasopharynx are lost. As a result, drying and crusting may occur unless adequate humidification is provided. In addition, the patient loses the effectiveness of his own cough mechanism and requires tracheal aspiration to remove secretions. Gentle suctioning will prevent damage to the ciliated epithelium and trauma to the trachea. Excellent care is essential once a tracheostomy has been performed; lesser care may lead to catastrophe.

### Removal of tracheostomy cannula

The following criteria serve as a guide as to the proper time for removal of the tracheostomy cannula:

1. The patient must have demonstrated complete independence of the respirator support over a 24-hour period and be able to deep-breathe and cough effectively. Expressed in physiological terms, this means that the patient has a vital capacity of approximately three times the predicted normal tidal volume.

2. The patient must possess adequate cough, gag, and swallow reflexes.

3. The patient must be able to bring up his secretions well

enough so that deep tracheal aspiration has been unnecessary for at least 24 hours.

4. The tracheostomy tube may be corked so that the patient has essentially a normal airway around the tracheostomy tube with normal glottic function. If he tolerates such intermittent occlusion (which is gradually increased in time), the tracheal cannula can be removed and a dry sponge placed over the stoma. Ordinarily, the tracheal stoma heals without secondary closure.

In most patients we feel it desirable to remove the tracheostomy tube as early as is consistent with their safety, in order to avoid complications of protracted tracheal intubation. We have

*Table 3*

THE EMERGENCY TREATMENT OF
THE UNCONSCIOUS PATIENT

*Means of Ventilation*

| Device | Driving Force | Airway | Gas Delivered |
|---|---|---|---|
| Mouth-to-mouth | Resuscitator's expiratory efforts | Lift chin or resuscitube | Expired Air 13% $O_2$ 3.5% $CO_2$ |
| Bag (Ambu, etc.) | Resuscitator's hand | Lift chin or use oropharyngeal airway or endo-tracheal tube | Air 21% $O_2$ 79% N |
| Anesthesia bag plus oxygen (Better than Ambu—but less portable) | Resuscitator's hand | Same as above | 100% $O_2$ |
| *After Airway Is Cleared* | | | |
| Gas operated respirators (Bird, Bennett) | Oxygen under pressure | Any airway: mouth, endo-tracheal tube, tracheostomy | Oxygen 40–100% |
| Electric-operated respirator— piston-driven (Morch, Emerson, Air Shields, etc.) | Piston-driven by electric motor | Tracheostomy cuffed or uncuffed endotrachael tube (Uncuffed patient may talk with air going by) | Air (21%) or additional oxygen |

Devised by Dr. Ronald Rosenberg, Department of Anesthesia, University of Illinois.

found that early removal, perhaps four to five days after introduction of the tracheostomy tube, can be very well tolerated by patients who are not in chronic respiratory insufficiency.


### 3. OXYGEN THERAPY

Minor decreases in arterial oxygen tension may be undesirable or dangerous in a patient with limited cardiac reserve. Oxygen therapy is used to insure adequate oxygenation, especially of the heart and brain, and to eliminate the compensatory responses to hypoxia. Postanesthetic, unconscious, anemic, hypovolemic, and acidotic patients require oxygen support irrespective of the level of hypoxia.

The optimal concentration of oxygen is that which permits full use of the oxygen-carrying capacity of the arterial blood. In the sick or debilitated patient, increased physiological shunting is frequently present to such a variable degree that it is impossible to predict the arterial oxygenation that can be achieved by any given inspired concentration of oxygen. In general, a margin of safety is desirable and, as a rule, the optimal inspired concentration of oxygen is that which results in an arterial oxygen tension of approximately 100–150 mm Hg with normal hemoglobin levels. Only in acute situations is a higher arterial oxygen tension desirable. In some cases of chronic obstructive pulmonary disease it may be necessary to regulate the inspired oxygen concentration very carefully to avoid respiratory depression. In such patients arterial oxygen tension of approximately 80 mm Hg is optimal.

In the presence of very severe pulmonary disease with large physiological shunts, it may be impossible at times to reach an arterial oxygen tension higher than 50–60 mm Hg, even when 100 per cent oxygen is inspired. Since it is dangerous to overload the vascular system in these patients, transfusion is seldom indicated. It becomes obvious that oxygen therapy by itself is never definitive treatment, and underlying physiologic derangements must be corrected.

### Complications of oxygen therapy

1. *Respiratory depression.* Respiratory depression may develop when hypoxia is the principal stimulus to spontaneous res-

piration. This is likely to happen in patients under general anesthesia, and heavily narcotized, or who have been retaining carbon dioxide for long periods of time. Patients with profound respiratory depression and associated hypoventilation need some form of assistive or controlled ventilation to rid them of carbon dioxide and, at the same time, supply them with adequate oxygen. These patients are often given oxygen at flow rates of one to two liters per minute with respirators. Patients who are given high concentrations of oxygen, in an attempt to bring about satisfactory correction of underlying cyanosis, may become increasingly drowsy when receiving such therapy. In addition, they may complain of headache or visual disturbances, or become apneic. These symptoms indicate carbon dioxide retention with progressive respiratory acidosis.

2. *Circulatory depression*. Circulatory depression may follow oxygen administration. If the preceding period of hypoxia has led to pronounced sympathetic activation, the patient may undergo a circulatory rebound upon correction of his hypoxia, and collapse will ensue. If airway obstruction or respiratory failure is treated promptly with endotracheal intubation, adequate ventilation, and oxygenation, severe circulatory failure may be avoided.

3. *Atelectasis*. Atelectasis has been shown to occur more rapidly if pure oxygen rather than room air is present in the closed air space (i.e., the obstructed segment). This belief is not fully accepted; however, it can be said that the prolonged use of 100 per cent oxygen, for one reason or other, may be deleterious.

4. *Substernal pain*. Substernal pain occurring with high oxygen tensions may be attributed to tracheobronchitis resulting from inadequate humidification of oxygen.

In general, oxygen toxicity is a vague term. It may be concluded that prolonged administration of oxygen under pressure has serious potential side effects. In some patients the danger of oxygen toxicity is less threatening than the danger of tissue hypoxia; under those circumstances 100 per cent oxygen should be given.

*Techniques of oxygen administration*

A variety of methods is available to administer oxygen. A nasal catheter is the most common and least expensive. The only precaution to observe with its use is to insure that the tip of the catheter is kept just below the soft palate above the level of the uvula, to avoid undue drying and gastric distention. A 6–8 liter per minute flow provides oxygen concentrations of approximately 30–40 per cent.

A disposable plastic face mask is readily acceptable to most patients; it is simple and comfortable. The flows must be equal to, or larger than, the patient's minute ventilation. With a reasonably tight fit, oxygen concentrations will be in the range of 60–80 per cent at a flow of 8–10 liters per minute.

A plastic face hood provides an open system and does not deliver as high a concentration of oxygen as other devices. Because of the effectiveness of high humidification achieved with the face hood, it is useful for short periods of time to treat laryngeal edema and thick tracheobronchial secretions.

Masks with non-rebreathing and reservoir bags should fit tightly and are indicated when administering 100 per cent oxygen. They may be used in conjunction with positive pressure and are useful in the treatment of pulmonary edema, asthma, and emphysema.

With the availability of newer devices, air-conditioned suites, and respiratory units, oxygen tents have become unnecessary.

#### 4. MECHANICAL RESPIRATOR THERAPY

A large number of mechanical respirators are commercially available including the Bird, Bennett, Emerson, Morch, Air Shields, and Engstrom respirators. Classified as either pressure-cycled or volume-controlled ventilators, they may be used intermittently or continuously for assistance or control of respiration. It is evident that any good respirator must have a mechanical setup which is easy to maintain, clean, and sterilize together with an adequate humidifying system.

Undoubtedly, each of the commercially available respirators will have its proponents. The Bennett respirator combines inexpensiveness and simplicity of function. The Morch respirator may be used with an uncuffed tube and still provide adequate alveolar ventilation; because it is mechanically cycled, the patient often breathes out of phase with the machine. The Engstrom respirator with its multiplicity of functional control for pressure, flow, volume, and rate is perhaps the most complex of the respirators.

In general, we have found that the Bird respirators of the Mark VII, VIII, X, and XVII types are the most useful and versatile of instruments. With these respirators, one may adjust flow rate and cycling sensitivities optimally to the individual patient; although the controls are somewhat complicated, they can be used in respiratory units with trained personnel. Their humidifying systems are excellent.

### Pressure-cycled or pressure-limited ventilators

This type of respirator will inflate the patient's lungs until a preset pressure has been reached, at which time the inspiratory phase stops and expiration begins. With the use of a pressure-limited ventilator, the tidal volume produced by the preset pressure will be a function of the resistance of the patient's lungs and of the inspiratory flow rate. Since pulmonary compliance and airway resistance may change considerably in a given patient from day to day, or even from hour to hour, the expired minute and tidal volumes must be monitored frequently to insure that pressure settings are adequate.

The Bennett and Bird machines are pressure-controlled ventilators. There are several models of each available. Most models can be used either for treatment (e.g., deep-breathing exercises, delivery of aerosols, etc.) or for continuous ventilation of the apneic patient. A small Bennett machine without controls for automatic cycling is available solely for treatments. The usual force for both the Bennett and Bird is oxygen under pressure; however, both are available in an electric model which utilizes compressed air instead of oxygen. Of the pressure-limited ventilators, we prefer the Bird respirator.

Both the Bennett and Bird respirators have a sensitivity control knob which should be able to trigger the machine with the least amount of effort. With the Bird respirator the normal patient triggers the machine without difficulty at a setting of 10–15 (with 5 representing maximum sensitivity). Beyond a setting of 20, the patient cannot trigger the machine at all. This level is used in patients who require increased resistance to slow their respiratory rate.

With the Bennett respirator the sensitivity valve is turned counterclockwise to increase sensitivity, and clockwise to decrease sensitivity. If turned all the way off, patients with normal respirations can usually trigger it satisfactorily. A one-quarter to one-half turn counterclockwise makes it sensitive enough for most patients in respiratory distress.

The pressure gauge should register 1–2 cm of negative pressure at the beginning of each inspiration. If the negative pressure registered is greater than this, the patient is required to make too vigorous an inspiratory effort. This can be relieved by increasing the sensitivity of the machine.

*Intermittent positive pressure breathing with pressure-cycled machines.* When treatments are being administered, the patient himself cycles the machine. The pressure gauge on the machine is set to deliver a predetermined amount of positive pressure on inhalation. This is usually in the range of 10–20 cm $H_2O$ pressure. When this pressure is reached, the machine shuts off and exhalation is accomplished by the elastic recoil of the lungs.

The amount of positive pressure administered should be determined by the needs of the individual patient. Lower pressures will be required in patients with a non-restricted airway and good pulmonary compliance; higher pressures will be necessary when there is increased resistance to air flow (as in asthma and emphysema), and when there is decreased compliance of the lung and chest wall.

Most patients will not require pressure greater than 25 cm $H_2O$, and the average pressure used (by us) for treatment is 15–17 cm $H_2O$.

Patients in respiratory distress who have not lost their ability to breathe are very likely to resist positive pressure devices. The procedure should be fully explained to them before treatment is begun, and the pressure should be started at low levels (5–10 cm $H_2O$) and gradually increased. The ideal pressure for a patient is that which will expand his lungs well but will not cause hyperventilation.

During treatment the pressure should be increased gradually, then reduced for a short period of time, and then increased again and finally brought down to a normal ventilatory level for the prescribed treatment period. The purpose of the change in pressure is more adequately to ventilate dependent portions of the lungs and prevent atelectasis. The frequency and length of the treatment periods depend on the needs of the patient. In some patients 10–15 minutes of treatment every 6 hours is sufficient, while others require treatment at least every 4 hours. Occasionally, patients with conditions such as status asthmaticus may require treatment every 1–2 hours for a period of time.

*Continuous ventilation with pressure-controlled machines.*

*Pressure setting.* Normally a slightly higher pressure is necessary than that used for treatments. This increase in pressure is required to lift the apneic chest. We find that 15–25 cm $H_2O$ pressure is usually sufficient although higher pressures are sometimes necessary, especially in patients with poor pulmonary compliance.

*Rate.* The rate for automatic cycling is usually at 12–16 respirations per minute. The patient should be closely monitored with spirometry and blood gas studies and the rate adjusted accordingly.

We feel that patients on continuous ventilation should have the pressure increased by 10–20 cm $H_2O$ pressure for a few breaths ("sigh effect") at least every hour. This assures more adequate ventilation of dependent portions of the lungs and helps prevent segmental atelectasis.

*Humidification.* As discussed previously, adequate humidification is mandatory. With the use of the ultrasonic nebulizer, secretions are thinned more rapidly and more frequent suctioning is necessary. In addition, condensation of moisture on the inside of the respirator tubing (especially when it is non-corrugated) is a problem and can cause occlusion of the tubing. Although many of the respirators have trap bottles to collect moisture, adjusting the angle of the tubing may prevent this. Therefore, we disconnect the tubing periodically during the exhalation phase, empty it, and rapidly reconnect it.

*Volume-controlled ventilators.*

The Morch, Emerson, Air Shields, and Engstrom are volume-controlled ventilators. These automatic respirators are used only for patients in acute respiratory distress and are not used for intermittent positive pressure-breathing treatments. They differ from pressure-controlled ventilators in that they deliver a predetermined volume of air with each inspiration which can vary from zero to 2½–3 liters. The volume used is determined by an estimated normal tidal volume for the patient. The volume must be great enough to overcome airway resistance and decreased pulmonary compliance, and to compensate for leaks in the system, especially when the respirator is used with an uncuffed tracheostomy tube. Use of a volume-cycled respirator permits maintenance of relatively constant minute and tidal ventilation regardless of changes in pulmonary compliances and airway resistance. The accuracy of tidal volume administration depends, of course, on the size of the air leak between the respirator and the trachea. A volume-limited respirator should have incorporated in it a safety valve that will bleed the system when a preset pressure has been reached if a closed (cuffed) system is employed. The respiration rate is the same as that used in pressure-controlled ventilation, or 12–16 respirations per minute.

*Differences in the various volume-controlled respirators.* The *Morch* respirator is an electrically-controlled, piston-driven machine which can be operated manually in the event of a power failure. It operates on room air, or oxygen can be added. When we use the Morch respirator, we do not cuff the tracheostomy tube, since the volume of air delivered is sufficient to overcome the leaks in the system. The pressure necessary to deliver the predetermined volume of gas builds up to the limit of pulmonary compliance. When this is reached, the remaining volume will shunt through the mouth or around the tracheostomy tube.

Older models of these machines require the addition of a Venturi nebulizer to supply adequate humidity; however, newer models have a heated aerosol system with a built-in water trap, eliminating condensation in the tubing.

The *Emerson* volume-controlled respirator is also an electrically-driven piston machine which can operate on room air or with oxygen added; it may be used either with a cuffed or uncuffed tracheostomy tube. One of the advantages of the Emerson ventilator is a variable inspiration-expiration time control. This instrument also has an automatic "sigh" mechanism which increases the tidal volume being delivered approximately every seven minutes. Another advantage of the Emerson is the bleed-off valve which prevents the pressure (necessary to deliver the predetermined volume) from going above 45 cm $H_2O$. This added safety factor is especially important if a cuffed tracheostomy tube is being used. In addition, if leaks in tubing occur, an automatic warning alarm rings.

The Emerson has a high humidity system with heat of the blow-over type. A collection bottle prevents the build-up of condensation in the tubing as long as the angle of the tubing going to the patient is not greater than 45°.

The *Air Shields* volume-controlled ventilator is an electrically operated bellows respirator with a variable inspiration-expiration time control. Like the other volume-controlled respirators, it operates on room air or with added oxygen. It has a heated aerosol system which utilizes the spinning technique to achieve gas humidification, and an automatic alarm system (which detects prolonged inspiration or expiration, increases in pressure above predetermined levels, and power failures), and may be used with either a cuffed or uncuffed tracheostomy tube.

*Benefits of positive pressure breathing.* Not only may alveolar ventilation be improved, but control of ventilation in the apneic patient is possible with the use of positive pressure instrumentation. In addition, aerosolization and humidification can be brought down to lower bronchial levels or even to the alveoli. With these machines, a variety of gases other than oxygen may be used, depending on the therapeutic problem. Carbon dioxide may be obtained in 5, 7, and 10 per cent mixtures with oxygen. While in the past the use of carbon dioxide as a respiratory stimulant has sometimes been suggested, more recent concepts negate its use in respiratory failure. It is still sometimes used in the treatment of hiccoughs. Helium is commonly used, in an 80 per cent mixture combined with oxygen, on the theory that replacement of the nitrogen content of the air with a light inert gas will provide a gas mixture that may be transported through the airway with less ventilatory effort. Unfortunately, this thesis is only partially true.

No patient should be maintained on continuous respirator control unless superior technical and medical supervision is available. Obstruction to the airway and mechanical failure of the respirator are disastrous complications. A respirator is no substitute for assiduous mechanical cleansing of the tracheobronchial tree. It is indeed unwise to attempt to clear out the lower recesses of the lung by using positive pressure respirators alone. It is our feeling that the drying effect of the positive pressure in the face of *obstructive secretions* (mucus plug) will further impact and inspissate the patient's secretions, leading to progressive segmental or subsegmental atelectasis. The prime prerequisite for successful use of respirators is an adequately cleansed and patent airway. Another complication of respirators, particularly when used for protracted periods of time, is the rupture of capillaries and hyalinization of the alveolar-capillary membrane producing progressive alveolar-capillary block. This will be discussed more fully below.

We feel that respirators, although life-saving, like tracheostomy, should be used for finite periods of time and the patient returned to his normal mechanisms for ventilation and humidification as soon as possible. Patients with carbon-dioxide retention who are suddenly placed on respirators in order to improve ventilation may rapidly reverse carbon dioxide tensions. Gordon and others have shown that rapid reversal of carbon dioxide may lead to sudden ventricular fibrillation and death. Patients should gradually be brought to optimal levels of volume pressure flows.

In an intensive care unit all medical and nursing personnel should be acquainted with the use of these machines. In many hospitals the Department of Inhalation Therapy or the Department of Anesthesia has direct control of this equipment. Despite this hierarchy of administration, the exigencies of emergency on a 24-hour basis demand that all medical and nursing personnel have the same ability to use these respirators as do the members of the Departments of Anesthesia and Inhalation Therapy.

MANAGEMENT OF PATIENTS UNDERGOING PROLONGED
ARTIFICIAL VENTILATION

Systemic circulatory effects of protracted artificial ventilation
are well documented. Cournand and others have shown that mean
airway pressure must be as low as possible in order to avoid interference with circulation. *A low mean airway pressure can be maintained when the duration of positive airway pressure on inspiration is less than, or equal to, the expiration phase when no positive
pressure is applied.* It is obvious that an increased mean airway
pressure may impede venous return to the right heart.

Ordinarily, about 15 respirations per minute is the optimal
rate. If this frequency in combination with a desired tidal volume
is inadequate, the rate is adjusted upward. If more than 20–25
breaths per minute are required to maintain adequate carbon
dioxide removal, then the tidal volume must be increased. It is
important to produce periodic hyperinflation to simulate the
normal sigh mechanism.

### Complications of prolonged artificial ventilation

*Diffuse atelectasis.* Diffuse atelectasis occurs normally during
a constant volume ventilation with normal, or smaller than normal, tidal volumes; this becomes particularly apparent in patients
who are maintained on protracted controlled ventilation. It is
obvious that the prevention of diffuse air-space collapse requires
a correct ventilatory pattern. Patients who are not attuned or
adapted to controlled ventilation and cannot cycle with the machine may require sedation, psychologic reassurance, and even 100
per cent oxygen to block their respiratory drive. (In the latter
situation the patient should be observed closely for carbon dioxide
accumulation attendant upon high oxygen tensions.) All other
therapeutic adjuvants, including adequate aspiration, humidification of the inspired gases, chest physiotherapy, and hourly to two-
hourly turning of patients are mandatory. If the atelectasis cannot
be remedied, therapeutic bronchoscopy should be done.

*Gastrointestinal complications.* Gastric dilatation and ileus
are common sequelae among comatose patients maintained on
respirators. Such distention leads to elevation of the left hemidia-
phragm, with subsequent reduction in ventilation, and may cause

hypotension and hypokalemia in extreme cases. Vomiting with aspiration can be disastrous, in this circumstance, and gastric decompression should be used to prevent this catastrophe. When the airway is protected with a tracheostomy, a nasogastric tube may be kept in place with safety; without a tracheostomy, periodic removal of the nasogastric tube is desirable. The problem can be minimized by the use of a cuffed tube and by decreasing the inspiratory pressure.

*Alveolar capillary block*. Because of failure of adequate cycling, or the nature of the underlying pulmonary disease, patients may require controlled respiration for indefinite periods of time (upward of several months). In one instance of which we are aware, a patient developed an increasingly severe alveolar-capillary block, probably due to hyalinization of the alveolar-capillary membrane, and required progressive increases in the rate and volume of ventilation. Despite all ventilatory maneuvers, the patient could not adequately exchange all his gases and eventually succumbed, both to the underlying disease and, no doubt, to the therapy used to treat it initially.

*Hyperventilation*. Hyperventilation and respiratory alkalosis occasionally occur in patients receiving continuous respiratory assistance. This condition is suggested by chest pain, syncope, tingling and numbness of fingers and toes, vertigo, carpopedal spasm, and even tetany. To avoid this hyperventilation syndrome, the respiratory rate of the machine should be periodically decreased by 6–8 respirations per minute.

*Excessive adrenergic response to bronchodilating drugs*. When palpitation or nervousness occurs during or immediately following an intermittent positive pressure breathing treatment with bronchodilating agents such as Isuprel, excessive absorption of the drug is suggested. When these agents are administered by intermittent positive pressure breathing, they should be diluted and not administered more often than every three hours because of their vasoconstrictor effects.

*Bronchospasm or paroxysmal cough*. If bronchospasm develops during treatment with intermittent positive pressure breathing, it may indicate hypersensitivity to the aerosol medication being used. In these instances, treatment should be stopped immediately and the regimen revised.

*Weaning from respirator support*

As a rule, weaning from the respirator should start as soon as possible, not only because the muscles of breathing may be restored to normal tone more quickly, but also because of the psychological benefit to the patient as he recognizes his improvement. On the other hand, premature attempts at weaning are inadvisable. The precise time for weaning requires considerable judgment and experience.

Our experience has shown that the average patient is unable to be off the respirator for any appreciable time if his vital capacity is less than twice his normal tidal volume. When weaning is initially attempted, the patient should be off the respirator for three to four minutes every half hour, and if this is tolerated, these periods can be increased. Adequately humidified oxygen should be provided when the patient is off the respirator. This progressive removal from respirator control may require mild sedation to allay the patient's anxiety. Few patients become independent of respirator support until their vital capacity has increased to 30–35 per cent of predicted normal values. It is quite obvious that chest physiotherapy, postural drainage, antibiotics, and oxygen support should be maintained during this weaning process. Even when weaning appears complete, patients (particularly those who are old and debilitated) should remain under close observation for several days. Generally speaking, the longer the period of respirator support, the slower the weaning process.

DRUG THERAPY

Drugs often constitute a part of the total treatment program for respiratory insufficiency. The following classes of drugs are those most frequently employed:

*Antibiotics*

These agents should be used judiciously in conjunction with culture and sensitivity control. In emergency states, however, antibiotic therapy can be given prophylactically to protect against superinfection without the benefit of culture and sensitivity studies. When antibiotics are indicated, they should be administered with adequate dosage for finite periods of time; cultures and sensitivities should be repeated at frequent intervals. Prolonged or indiscriminate use of antibiotics may produce bacteriologic resistance, complicating fungal infections, and system reaction, such as enteritis.

### Bronchodilators

Aminophylline, administered either intravenously, orally, or rectally, is often given in conjunction with such expectorants as potassium iodide, ammonium chloride, as well as a host of commercial preparations to assist in liquefying secretions. We do not advocate the continued use of expectorants because of the bronchorrhea they may induce. Water is still a most effective liquefying agent.

### Ventilatory stimulants

Coramine and caffeine sodium benzoate have been used in the past to stimulate respiration, but in most instances, these drugs had only limited value at best. Newer agents, such as vanillic diethylamide (Emivan), have also been tried for this purpose; however, their true efficacy remains uncertain.

### Adrenocortical steroids

Steroid therapy has proved valuable in the treatment of certain inflammatory or bronchospastic pulmonary diseases. In these patients who have alveolar-capillary membrane thickening, the inflammatory process may be arrested or even reversed with this regimen. The adverse systemic consequences of adrenocortical steroid therapy are well documented, and patients must be observed carefully while receiving these drugs. Adequate antibiotic and chemotherapeutic drugs should be administered to patients with respiratory infections who are also receiving steroids.

### Summary of management

A schema of the management of patients with acute and chronic respiratory insufficiency is found in Fig. 3.

*Fig. 3*

SCHEMA OF MANAGEMENT OF ACUTE AND CHRONIC RESPIRATORY FAILURE

| | DIAGNOSIS | | TREATMENT | | | |
|---|---|---|---|---|---|---|
| Status of Patient | Clinical Findings | Laboratory Findings | Airway Control | Oxygen | Drugs | Miscellaneous |
| *Conscious*<br>1. Unobstructed Airway | Tachypnea (occ. hypoventilation)<br>Tachycardia or Bradycardia<br>Dyspnea<br>Cyanosis<br>Hyper or Hypotension<br>Mental confusion<br>Somnolence<br>Neurological manifestations<br>Warm, dry, or cold, clammy skin<br>Wheezing | $pCO_2 \uparrow > 40$ mm Hg<br>$pO_2 \downarrow < 90$ mm Hg<br>pH $\downarrow < 7.36$<br>Hct $\uparrow\downarrow$ 40<br>Base deficit | Respiratory support<br>Aspirate secretions prn<br>IPPB (pressure cycled) | Low flow, humidified about 40% or less | Liquefying agents:<br>Alevaire<br>Mucomyst<br>Respiratory stimulants<br>Digitalis, diuretics prn (for CHF)<br>Antibiotics<br>Bronchodilators<br>Vasopressors prn<br>Volume replacement | |
| 2. Obstructed Airway | Same as #1, plus:<br>Noisy respirations<br>Intercostal retraction | Variable findings | Secure airway<br>Tracheal aspiration<br>Bronchoscopy<br>Endotracheal intubation<br>Tracheostomy<br>Respiratory support prn | Same | Same as above, plus:<br>Sedation, once airway secured | |
| *Unconscious*<br>3. Partially Obstructed Airway | Same as #1, plus:<br>Irregular Respirations:<br>Cheyne-Stokes<br>Biots<br>Hyporeflexia or Areflexia<br>Pupillary Reaction<br>Odors | Same as #1<br>Generally Acidotic<br>Rule out:<br>Hyperventilation alkalosis | Maintain and secure airway<br>Tracheal aspiration<br>IPPB<br>Respiratory support<br>Endotracheal intubation<br>Tracheostomy if prolonged support is necessary | Same | Same as #1 | Feeding tube<br>I.V. fluids<br>Turn patient<br>Gastric decompression<br>Foley catheter (monitor urine output)<br>Cardiac monitoring |
| 4. Completely Obstructed Airway | Same as #1, plus:<br>Stertorous respirations<br>Intercostal retraction<br>Severe cyanosis<br>Apnea ± | Same as #1 | Immediate:<br>Endotracheal intubation<br>Tracheostomy<br>Continued ventilation necessary | Humidified <40% (especially if $pCO_2$ is very elevated) | Same as #1 | Same as above |

## THE NURSING ROLE

### The patient with a tracheostomy

The nursing care of the tracheostomy patient is of prime importance. These patients are totally dependent on the personnel in attendance, not only for assiduous care, but also for emotional reassurance.

*Principles and precautions in the care of the tracheostomy*

1. Sterile technique should be used, and either sterile gloves or forceps employed, when suctioning the tracheostomy.

2. The catheter should be of such size as not to occlude the stoma. Ordinarily, a No. 14 or No. 16 French catheter is adequate.

3. Between each suctioning, the catheter should be kept in disinfectant solution in a covered container. Studies in our medical center indicate that 70% ethyl alcohol is the best disinfecting agent for this purpose. Despite the cost, using a catheter only once is ideal.

4. Most patients also require suctioning of mouth and pharynx. It is important that a separate catheter be used for this purpose. It, too, should be in a covered container in 70% ethyl alcohol. The containers should be clearly labeled "oral" and "tracheostomy," and care should be taken to assure that the catheters are not switched inadvertently during the suctioning procedure.

5. *Catheters should be rinsed with normal saline or sterile distilled water after removing from the disinfectant and before suctioning.* Separate bottles of rinsing solution should be used for the oral and tracheostomy catheters.

6. Ideally, the suction catheters, the disinfectant solution and container, and the normal saline or distilled water used for rinsing the catheters should be changed every four hours. If this procedure is not followed, the risk of contamination is high. We have become increasingly concerned about this "breeding ground" for gram-negative bacteria and therefore are very careful in avoiding possible means for contamination to occur. If a bottle of sterile solution is opened and the contents not fully used initially, the remainder should be discarded promptly.

e of not requiring oxygen (an important asset in those patients
vhom oxygen therapy is undesirable).

Another efficient method for providing humidity is by means
nebulizers that utilize the Venturi principle. The nebulizer is
nected, by large-bore tubing, to a tracheostomy mask which
around the tracheostomy tube. This technique provides mois-
e at the rate of 0.5–1.0 cc per minute.

As stated, the addition of heat to the nebulization process in-
ases the effectiveness of the system. By delivering the aerosol to
trachea at body temperature, or slightly above, the saturation
be increased to maximal levels; accordingly, the tracheal wall
s not have to contribute additional moisture as it might if the
osol temperature was less than 98° F.

The installation of sterile saline solution into the trache-
omy tube at frequent intervals may assist in moisture produc-
n. We commonly instill 10–15 cc of saline into the tracheostomy
e just prior to suctioning, with care being taken to aspirate this
mediately, especially in patients without a cough reflex. Exces-
e washing of the lung with normal saline will cause a loss of
face action and result in decreased compliance, increased inter-
tial edema, and other microscopic alveolar changes.

13. The inner cannula should be removed at least every two
urs for cleaning. It should be reinserted as soon as cleaned.
eaning is effected with a test tube brush and detergent solutions,
er which the cannula is rinsed in sterile water. If the inner can-
la becomes difficult to reinsert, the physician should be notified
once.

14. The outer cannula should be changed only by the physi-
n. An additional tracheostomy tube should be kept at the pa-
nt's bedside for emergency use. We change tracheostomy tubes
ery 7–10 days unless indicated more frequently.

15. There is no prescribed timetable for suctioning the tra-
eostomy tube. The frequency of suctioning depends entirely on
e amount of secretion present. Some patients may require suc-
ning every 15 minutes; most are suctioned at one to two-hour
tervals. Suctioning will be most effective following change in
sition or after treatment with mucolytic agents.

To avoid hypoxia, the patient should not be suctioned more

7. The method of suctioning has alre
this chapter.

8. The suction catheter should be inse
the bronchus to stimulate coughing. This di
range of 10–15 cm. In our experience, th
cautious and limit her suctioning to the en
is inadequate, and patients suctioned in this
pools of secretion just beyond the tip of t
come thickened and inspissated and obstr
tube.

9. The catheter should be rotated 360
with suction on.

10. The catheter should be guided in
turning the patient's head opposite to the

11. Patients should be turned from side
hour; this is particularly important in the
prevent pooling of secretions in dependent p

12. Adequate humidification is mandat
midification is to maintain a normal physic
for the respiratory mucosa and to restore ade
retained dry secretions. Obviously, the be
patient's intact airway mechanisms. Once a
formed, this natural mechanism is lost an
must be used.

The most effective way of increasing the
spired gas involves the use of water particle
conjunction with heat. Ordinarily, the parti
vapor in expired air is about 47 mm Hg. In o
level, the optimum droplet size should be 0.5
small enough to minimize trapping of the pa
through the upper airway, yet large enough
in the finer bronchi and alveoli. With this
tling rate is slow, and only minimal wetting o
is directed against a smooth surface.

We feel that the ultrasonic nebulizer aff
tive humidification. This nebulizer produces
micra and can deliver up to 3–6 cc of moist
addition to providing a greater degree of ne
other method, the ultrasonic nebulizer has th

7. The method of suctioning has already been described in this chapter.

8. The suction catheter should be inserted deep enough into the bronchus to stimulate coughing. This distance is usually in the range of 10–15 cm. In our experience, the nurse may be overcautious and limit her suctioning to the end of the cannula. This is inadequate, and patients suctioned in this manner may develop pools of secretion just beyond the tip of the cannula which become thickened and inspissated and obstruct the tracheostomy tube.

9. The catheter should be rotated 360° as it is withdrawn, with suction on.

10. The catheter should be guided into each bronchus by turning the patient's head opposite to the side to be intubated.

11. Patients should be turned from side to side at least every hour; this is particularly important in the comatose patient to prevent pooling of secretions in dependent portions of lung.

12. Adequate humidification is mandatory. The aim of humidification is to maintain a normal physiological environment for the respiratory mucosa and to restore adequate liquefaction of retained dry secretions. Obviously, the best humidifier is the patient's intact airway mechanisms. Once a tracheostomy is performed, this natural mechanism is lost and artificial methods must be used.

The most effective way of increasing the water content of inspired gas involves the use of water particles of minimal size in conjunction with heat. Ordinarily, the partial pressure of water vapor in expired air is about 47 mm Hg. In order to maintain this level, the optimum droplet size should be 0.5–1.5 micra, which is small enough to minimize trapping of the particles during transit through the upper airway, yet large enough to insure deposition in the finer bronchi and alveoli. With this particle size the settling rate is slow, and only minimal wetting occurs when the mist is directed against a smooth surface.

We feel that the ultrasonic nebulizer affords the most effective humidification. This nebulizer produces particles of 0.8–1.0 micra and can deliver up to 3–6 cc of moisture per minute. In addition to providing a greater degree of nebulization than any other method, the ultrasonic nebulizer has the additional advantage of not requiring oxygen (an important asset in those patients in whom oxygen therapy is undesirable).

Another efficient method for providing humidity is by means of nebulizers that utilize the Venturi principle. The nebulizer is connected, by large-bore tubing, to a tracheostomy mask which fits around the tracheostomy tube. This technique provides moisture at the rate of 0.5–1.0 cc per minute.

As stated, the addition of heat to the nebulization process increases the effectiveness of the system. By delivering the aerosol to the trachea at body temperature, or slightly above, the saturation can be increased to maximal levels; accordingly, the tracheal wall does not have to contribute additional moisture as it might if the aerosol temperature was less than 98° F.

The installation of sterile saline solution into the tracheostomy tube at frequent intervals may assist in moisture production. We commonly instill 10–15 cc of saline into the tracheostomy tube just prior to suctioning, with care being taken to aspirate this immediately, especially in patients without a cough reflex. Excessive washing of the lung with normal saline will cause a loss of surface action and result in decreased compliance, increased interstitial edema, and other microscopic alveolar changes.

13. The inner cannula should be removed at least every two hours for cleaning. It should be reinserted as soon as cleaned. Cleaning is effected with a test tube brush and detergent solutions, after which the cannula is rinsed in sterile water. If the inner cannula becomes difficult to reinsert, the physician should be notified at once.

14. The outer cannula should be changed only by the physician. An additional tracheostomy tube should be kept at the patient's bedside for emergency use. We change tracheostomy tubes every 7–10 days unless indicated more frequently.

15. There is no prescribed timetable for suctioning the tracheostomy tube. The frequency of suctioning depends entirely on the amount of secretion present. Some patients may require suctioning every 15 minutes; most are suctioned at one to two-hour intervals. Suctioning will be most effective following change in position or after treatment with mucolytic agents.

To avoid hypoxia, the patient should not be suctioned more

than 10–15 seconds without a breath. If repeated suctioning is necessary, the patient should receive oxygen, preferably 100 per cent, for a few minutes between aspirations.

CUFFED TRACHEOSTOMY TUBES

Because the patient in respiratory failure may require controlled ventilatory assistance at some point during his treatment, a cuffed tracheostomy tube is usually used. If the patient is able to ventilate adequately, the cuff need not be inflated. Should assisted ventilation become necessary, the cuff may then be inflated. It is also inflated during treatment with medicated aerosols delivered by pressure-cycle respirators.

*Precautions related to cuffed tracheostomy tubes*

1. The inflated cuff may cause pressure necrosis of the tracheal wall. Therefore, the cuff should be deflated for 15 minutes at two-hour intervals. Patients on continuous respirator support should be watched very closely during this time.
2. The pharynx should be aspirated before the cuff is deflated.
3. When reinflating cuff, use just enough air to prevent an air leak around the cannula or through the mouth. Under ordinary circumstances, 5–7 cc of air is sufficient.

*Tube feedings in patients with tracheostomy*

Patients requiring tracheostomies often need tube feedings. A few precautions bear mentioning.

1. Tube feedings are best administered cold or at room temperature. This appears to cause less abdominal distention.
2. Feedings should be given slowly via gravity. Forced or rapid feeding can produce emesis and aspiration. As a precaution against aspiration, the cuff on the tracheostomy tube should be inflated before the tube feedings are given.
3. If difficulties are encountered, the nasogastric tube should be removed and a feeding gastrostomy or jejunonostomy created.

**Nursing care of patients on pressure-controlled respirators**

1. Ensure that an airtight system exists. When a face mask is used, it must fit securely; in unconscious patients an oropharyngeal airway may be necessary. With a cuffed tracheostomy an adaptor is attached, making it possible to suction the trachea without disconnecting the respirator.

2. Respirators make characteristic sounds on inspiration and expiration, which personnel soon learn to recognize. Attention to the pattern of these sounds should alert the nurse that problems may have developed. This is especially important in patients on automatic cycling. An obstructed airway should be suspected any time the respirations become "noisy." In addition, the ventilator will increase its rate as airway resistance increases. If there is complete obstruction, the inhalation valve will "chatter." When there is a leak in the airway, the machine will "hiss" or the pressure gauge dial will fail to reach the preset level.

3. The length of the inspiratory phase of respiration should not exceed the expiratory phase. During the administration of positive pressure, the intrathoracic pressure is increased so that the right atrial filling is reduced which, in turn, causes a decreased stroke volume and cardiac output. For this reason, the expiratory phase needs to be of sufficient duration to allow adequate atrial and ventricular filling before the start of the next inspiration. To this end, we attempt to maintain a ratio of 1–1 and ½ seconds of inhalation to 3 seconds of exhalation.

In patients with underlying problems that decrease cardiac output (shock, hemorrhage, acute pulmonary edema, congestive heart failure), the pressure administered should be in the range of 10–15 cm $H_2O$; higher pressures tend to compromise cardiac output and increase hypoxia.

4. Pressure-controlled ventilators can deliver 100 per cent oxygen; however, the dilution valve on the machine allows for the mixture of room air with the oxygen to a concentration of 40 per cent. As stated previously, 100 per cent $O_2$ may be extremely hazardous in some patients and should never be administered without a specific order from the physician, including a specified period of time. In patients with chronic respiratory disease, such as asthma

and emphysema, oxygen should be maximally diluted (40 per cent). It is well to remember that 40 per cent oxygen represents twice the concentration of room air and is usually sufficient except in situations of severe hypoxia.

5. Since these ventilators operate on oxygen under pressure, an auxiliary gas supply should be available to maintain the patient on continuous ventilation in case the wall oxygen supply fails.

## Nursing care of patients on volume-controlled respirators

1. These machines are used in conjunction with a tracheostomy, either cuffed or uncuffed, or an endotracheal tube. There is no way to breathe patients adequately by face mask.

2. The intensive care unit must have an auxiliary electrical power supply should the main power source fail. With a power failure the patient should be disconnected from the respirator and ventilated by either mouth-to-mouth or mouth-to-tube technique, or by Ambu-bag or hand bellows, until the respirator is connected to the auxiliary power source. Personnel should be taught to push the bag or bellows slowly and to count out a normal respiratory rate. In an emergency some individuals push the bag so rapidly that the patient is receiving little effective ventilation. Once the patient is reconnected to the respirator, 100 per cent oxygen should be given for a period of time to overcome the hypoxia which may have developed during the power failure.

### Observations Which Confirm That Patients on Respirators Are Being Adequately Ventilated

1. Improvement in skin color or absence of cyanosis.

2. Rhythmic expansion of the chest with expiratory phase longer than inspiratory phase.

3. Normal pulse; a change in pulse rate may indicate decreased cardiac output due to the increase in intrathoracic pressure.

4. Stationary blood pressure; a drop of the blood pressure may reflect decreased cardiac output.

5. Absence of any abnormal neurologic signs.

6. Audible rhythmicity of respiration.

7. Normal function of respirator.

8. Absence of hyperventilation or hypoventilation.

***Observations Which Indicate That the Patient Is Not Being Adequately Ventilated***

1. *Impaired ventilatory excursion.* The following causes should be considered:
    a. kinking of connecting tubes;
    b. occlusion of tubing with water, blood, or mucus;
    c. low volume flow, and/or pressure settings;
    d. obstructed tracheostomy;
    e. bronchospasm;
    f. pulmonary edema.
2. *Prolonged expiratory phase with delay in inspiratory cycle.* The usual causes of this problem are:
    a. connecting leaks;
    b. excessive pressure setting;
    c. low rates.
3. *Absent inspiratory cycle.*
    This may result from:
    a. failure to connect respirator to electrical outlet or to oxygen supply;
    b. sensitivity control set too low;
    c. leak between the patient and the machine;
    d. incorrect respiratory rate.
4. *Absent expiratory cycle.*
    a. "sticky" or malfunctioning exhalation valve;
    b. air leak in system.
5. *Hyperventilation resulting from:*
    a. high respiratory rate;
    b. high pressure control;
    c. high volume control;
    d. high flow rate.
6. *Hypoventilation resulting from:*
    a. low respiratory rate;
    b. low pressure control;
    c. low volume control;
    d. low flow rate.

## Sterilization of respirators

The increasing incidence of gram-negative pulmonary infections has led to a closer evaluation of the techniques involved in the cleansing of respirators equipped with mainstream reservoirs. Unlike staphylococcus, these organisms thrive in areas of high humidity, so that attention must be paid to stagnant condensates which can be aerosolized into the patient. Reinarz and others have demonstrated that respirators *without* reservoir nebulizers do not contain more bacteria than the number found in ambient air.

We employ the following methods currently for sterilization:

### RESPIRATORS USED INTERMITTENTLY FOR TREATMENTS

Ideally, each patient should have an exhalation valve assembly (breathing head) and mouthpiece of his own stored in a plastic bag at his bedside. The exhalation valve should be cleaned with a detergent and hot water after each use and stored in a plastic bag. Every fourth day the exhalation valve should be exchanged for a sterilized one and the contaminated valve should be cold-sterilized.

### RESPIRATORS USED FOR CONTINUOUS VENTILATION

The exhalation valve and tubing should be changed every three days. When respirators are not in use, they should be covered with a plastic bag or sterile sheet. Cultures of exhalation valves, before and after cold sterilization, should be taken frequently.

### PROCEDURE FOR COLD STERILIZATION

a. Rinse parts under cold running water to remove foreign matter.

b. Soak in O-Syl solution, 2–3 per cent, for 10–15 minutes; (plastics will become soft if soaked longer).

c. Rinse in mouthwash solution to remove the odor of disinfectant.

d. Rinse in water.

e. Scrub in hot soapy water.

f. Rinse in hot water.

g. Air-dry on clean surface or rack.

h. Store parts in plastic bags in a closed container.

If a separate exhalation valve assembly is not available for each patient, the valve should be cold-sterilized before the ventilator is used by another patient.

## Prevention of Pulmonary Infection

Prevention of pulmonary infection in patients with protracted controlled ventilation requires:

1. meticulous removal of secretions;
2. prevention and prompt treatment of atelectasis;
3. aseptic and atraumatic tracheostomy care;
4. frequent sterilizations of intermittent positive pressure breathing equipment humidifiers, tubes, valves, and tracheostomy implements;
5. prevention of cross-infection with isolation precautions;
6. maintenance of maximum host-resistance to infection by insuring an adequate state of hydration and nutrition with adequate blood volume, tissue perfusion, and oxygenation;
7. employment of specific antibiotic therapy based on bacteriologic culture and sensitivity control.

Resistant strains of *Staphylococcus aureus, Bacillus proteus, Pseudomonas aeruginosa,* and *Klebsiella* are the predominating pathogens encountered. On occasion, aerosol antibiotics may be employed. Aerosolized Polymyxin B Sulfate, which is systemically toxic, may be used in doses of 50 mgm every 6 hours for the treatment of *Pseudomonas* respiratory infections.

*Isolation techniques.* Certain patients may require isolation, and the intensive care unit should have one or two rooms for this purpose.

REQUIREMENTS FOR AN ISOLATION ROOM

a. The isolation room should be located out of the usual flow of traffic. The door to the room should be kept closed.

b. The patient should be visible to the nurse from outside the room.

c. The room should be self-contained with its own oxygen and suction supply utility room or bathroom, handwashing facilities, and communication system.

d. A separate ventilation system with adequate air

changes per minute is highly desirable. The air from this room should not be mixed with the air supply to the remainder of the unit.

ISOLATION PRACTICES

Gown, mask, and hand-washing techniques must not be violated. We feel the discard-gown technique is a necessity. A supply of sterile masks and clean gowns should be kept on a table immediately outside the isolation room.

Since the patient in respiratory failure who develops a superimposed infection is often gravely ill, it is often necessary to assign one nurse per shift to the isolation room. When the patient is less ill, but still requires isolation, he can be left alone for short periods, as long as the nurse is close enough to observe him.

Only those supplies needed in the immediate care of the patient should be taken into the isolation room. Additional supplies and equipment may be brought by other personnel as the need arises.

Because of the extreme vulnerability of patients in respiratory failure to infection, care must be taken to keep anyone with an upper respiratory infection away from the unit.

## Psychologic Support of the Patient with Respiratory Insufficiency

As with any other critical illness, emotional support of both the patient in respiratory distress and his family must be one of the prime considerations of the nursing and medical staff. The dyspneic patient is frightened; he often expresses a feeling of doom and desires constant attention. One of the main advantages of an intensive care unit is the constancy of attention and the reassurance to the patient of the presence of trained personnel. A simple explanation of the type of respiratory assistance being provided and its specific purpose should be given to the patient's family. This is particularly helpful to the anxious and resistive patient, who may rely heavily on family support.

The majority of patients in respiratory distress are conscious and alert during most of their illness. They are apprehensive and may be depressed and frustrated by their inability to communicate. Generally, encouragement of the patient and adequate explanations before beginning various procedures help to allay apprehension. The lack of sleep associated with constant care may be exhausting to the patient. Assuring him that he is being watched at all times and giving him adequate sedation are helpful in this regard. Mood-changing drugs, such as Tofranil, have been employed more recently. Morphine, despite its potential depressant effect on respiration, relieves apprehension and fear of the numerous mechanical devices employed in the management of these patients.

## Bibliography

BATES, DAVID V. and CHRISTIE, RONALD V.: *Respiratory Function in Disease.* W. B. Saunders Co., Philadelphia, 1964.

BENDIXEN, H. H., EGBERT, L. D., HEDLEY-WHYTE, J., LAVER, M. B., and PONTOPPIDAN, H.: *Respiratory Care.* C. V. Mosby Company, St. Louis, 1965.

HERCUS, VICTOR: Planning A Respiratory Unit. *British Medical Journal,* December 15, 1964, pp. 604–606.

*Medical Clinics of North America:* Diseases of the Respiratory Tract. V. 48, No. 4, July, 1964.

McARDLE, K. H.: The Patient and the Bennett. *Nurs. Clin. N. Am.* 1:143–152, March 1966.

McCLELLAND, R. M. A.: Mechanical Means of Artificial Respiration. *Nursing Times,* 59:541–543, May 3, 1963.

National Research Council, *Cardiopulmonary Resuscitation Conference Proceedings.* National Academy of Science, Washington, D.C., 1966.

PACE, WILLIAM R.: *Pulmonary Physiology in Clinical Practice.* F. A. Davis Company, Philadelphia, 1965.

REINARZ, JAMES ALLEN, et al.: The Potential Role of Inhalation Therapy Equipment in Nosocomial Pulmonary Infection." *Journal of Clinical Investigation,* 44:5:831–839, 1965.

RUBIN, C.: Nursing the Patient Who Cannot Breathe. *Nursing Times,* 59:1088–1089, August 30, 1963.

SADOVE, MAX S. and CROSS, JAMES H.: *Recovery Room.* Chapter VII, Hiram T. Langston, M.D. W. B. Saunders Co., Philadelphia, 1956.

SANDIFORD, H. B. C.: The Management of the Airway of the Unconscious Patient. *Nursing Mirror,* 114:xi–xiii, April 20, 1962.

SEETIM, L., "The Patient with a Tracheotomy." *Nursing Times,* 61: 206, February 5, 1965.

SMITH, K. H.: Tracheostomy in Head Injuries. *Nursing Times,* 59: 1512–1513, November 29, 1963.

TOTMAN, LAWRENCE E. and LEHMAN, ROGER H.: Tracheostomy Care. *Amer. J. Nursing,* 64:96–99, March 1964.

# Chapter II

# Acute Myocardial Infarction

LAWRENCE E. MELTZER, M.D.
ROSE PINNEO, R.N., M.S.
J. RODERICK KITCHELL, M.D.

Because of its extraordinary incidence and awesome mortality, the problem of acute myocardial infarction will be considered apart from the cardiovascular emergencies to be discussed in the next chapter.

Until the advent of intensive coronary care (1962), the anticipated mortality of patients admitted to hospitals with acute myocardial infarction was 30%–35%. However, as a result of this new system of specialized care, the expected mortality in hospitals with coronary care facilities is now about 20% (a relative reduction in mortality of 35%). This remarkable success makes it quite clear that acute myocardial infarction can be treated best by a trained team in a coronary care unit setting. Currently, however, there are only 500–600 such units in operation among the 7,000 hospitals in this country; therefore, a high percentage of patients with myocardial infarction are still being managed in general intensive care areas or (less desirably) in customary hospital facilities.

The purpose of this chapter is to present some proven principles of the system of intensive coronary care as they apply to general intensive care facilities.

## THE PROBLEM

The sole blood supply to the myocardium is through the coronary arteries. When these arteries or their branches are obstructed, the myocardium is deprived of adequate blood and oxygen; this results in anoxia, followed by *local* death of portions of the heart musculature. This tissue destruction is termed "acute myocardial infarction."

In most instances myocardial infarction is the result of a progressive narrowing of the coronary arteries, caused by atherosclerotic plaques which develop over a period of years. Actual occlusion of the artery usually occurs suddenly as a result of either a thrombus forming on the rough surface of a plaque or bleeding beneath the plaque, which causes it to become dislodged (subintimal hemorrhage).

When coronary circulation is interrupted in this way, the series of events which follows places life and death in balance. The immediate effect of the deprivation of blood and oxygen to the myocardium is by no means predictable. However, it is clear that an occlusion of the coronary artery is not death producing in its own right; rather, death results from *complications* of the occlusion. It is the presence or absence of these complications that determines the ultimate course of acute myocardial infarction.

There are four major complications which may result in death:

**1. Arrhythmias.** Disturbances in the rate, rhythm, and conduction of the heart's electrical impulses (collectively called arrhythmias) represent the most common complication of acute myocardial infarction. About 80% of patients with infarction develop some type of arrhythmia within the first few days of the attack. The two major dangers of arrhythmias are their ability to produce sudden death and the reduction in pumping efficiency which they may engender. Only certain arrhythmias pose these threats, while others can be tolerated without obviously serious consequences.

Before the era of intensive coronary care, nearly one-half of the deaths from acute myocardial infarction were the direct result of arrhythmias. Recognizing that many of these arrhythmic deaths could be prevented, if patients were kept under continuous electrocardiographic surveillance in a specialized unit where trained personnel and resuscitative equipment were centered, the system of coronary care was developed. In an effective intensive coronary care unit sudden unanticipated death from arrhythmia should seldom occur.

**2. Left Ventricular Failure.** Following myocardial infarction, the strength of contraction of the left ventricle is often decreased so that the heart fails as an effective pump. This failure may be manifested as congestive heart failure, in which the left ventricle is unable to expel the full volume of blood returned to it from the venous system. This incomplete ventricular emptying results in a backflow of pressure in the pulmonary circuit, producing the clinical picture of left ventricular failure. (See page 121.) When there are obvious clinical findings indicating that left ventricular failure exists, the anticipated mortality is approximately 40%.

When left ventricular function is severely reduced to a point where ineffective perfusion occurs in the brain, heart, and kidneys, cardiogenic shock is said to exist. If this perfusion deficit is uncorrected within a critical period, shock is *irreversible* and death occurs. At least 80% of patients with cardiogenic shock die with present methods of treatment. (The system of intensive coronary care, while predictably effective in preventing arrhythmic deaths, has proved disappointing in reducing mortality from cardiogenic shock).

**3. Thromboembolism.** Less than 5% of deaths from acute myocardial infarctions are the result of thromboembolic complications. Clots arising on the injured surface of the left ventricle (mural thrombi) may escape from this chamber and obstruct arteries in the brain or peripheral vessels. Other thrombi may originate in the deep veins of the legs and produce pulmonary embolization (see page 138).

**4. Rupture of the left ventricle.** This is the least common complication of acute myocardial infarction and accounts for 2%–3% of the total mortality. As a result of necrosis of the myocardium, the ventricular wall weakens and then ruptures, allowing blood to fill the surrounding pericardial sac. This external pressure created against the heart (cardiac tamponade) prevents the return of blood to the ventricle and death follows within minutes.

The fundamental approach to the problem of acute myocardial infarction is to combat these death-producing complications. Ideally, this would be accomplished by *preventing* catastrophic situations from developing. If prevention fails, or is not possible, the alternative hope is to recognize these complications at their onset and to initiate therapy as soon as possible in an attempt to reverse their lethal effects. The methods for prevention, early recognition, and therapy of complications are presented in the following pages.

## ASSESSMENT OF THE PROBLEM

### The diagnosis of acute myocardial infarction

A decision must be made as to whether the patient has actually sustained an acute myocardial infarction or whether the symptoms that prompted his admission were from some other cause. There are several other diseases which produce symptoms suggesting acute infarction (e.g., acute cholecystitis, pulmonary embolism, etc.). Confirmation of the diagnosis of acute myocardial infarction cannot always be made at the time of admission: nevertheless, patients must be treated as if an infarction has occurred, even though this diagnosis may ultimately prove to be incorrect.

The diagnosis of acute myocardial infarction is established from three types of evidence:

*The history of the attack.* The principal symptom suggesting acute myocardial infarction is chest pain which is ordinarily quite distinctive. It usually occurs abruptly and is of a severe, crushing character. The patient may describe the pain as a heavy weight, a tightness. or a "knot" in his chest. Most often the pain is concentrated beneath the sternum, but frequently it radiates across the chest to the arms or to the neck. The pain is continuous and is not relieved by changing the body position, breath holding, or remedies such as antacids (taken by the patient in the mistaken belief that the pain is that of indigestion). Most patients develop great fear and apprehension because of the persistence of the pain and its oppressive quality.

Shortly after the onset of the pain, profuse perspiration may occur along with the onset of nausea and vomiting. Dyspnea frequently accompanies this picture.

Not all patients with acute myocardial infarction present such typical histories, and there are many variants. On some occasions the major pain may be in the arms, jaw, throat, or back, rather than in the chest. Sweating, nausea, vomiting, fear, or dyspnea

may *not* be present. In other patients the pain may be masked
(e.g., by anesthesia during the course of surgery).

Certain patients develop serious complications immediately
after the occlusion. Those with ventricular fibrillation or ventricular standstill die within minutes, while others with sudden
left ventricular failure may succumb before they can be brought
to the hospital.

Perhaps the most difficult aspect of the historical component
for diagnosis is the problem of distinguishing the pain of myocardial infarction from that due to *transient* forms of myocardial
ischemia. Many patients with coronary atherosclerosis develop
chest pain when the demands of the heart muscle for oxygen are
increased by physical exertion, excitement, etc. In many instances
myocardial ischemia is of short duration, and adequate blood
supply is restored to the myocardium before tissue destruction
can occur. Transient ischemia of this type is described as *angina
pectoris*. It is understandable that a narrow zone may exist between severe angina and actual myocardial infarction, and thus
the diagnosis may be uncertain in the initial period.

The history by itself is not diagnostic of acute infarction;
however, it is the distinctiveness of the history which promotes a
suspicion that myocardial infarction may have occurred.

*Electrocardiography.* A definitive diagnosis of acute myocardial
infarction can be made only on the basis of characteristic electrocardiographic changes which reflect myocardial injury and local
death of tissue. Regardless of the history, it is an unacceptable
practice to conclude that myocardial infarction has occurred unless specific electrocardiographic criteria are demonstrated. These
electrocardiographic changes may not be evident at the time of admission, or for several days thereafter. For this reason, repeated
(serial) electrocardiograms are usually required for accurate diagnosis.

*Enzyme studies.* When myocardial cells are destroyed, enzymes, normally found in the heart muscle, escape into the blood
stream, where they can be detected by laboratory tests. Thus, in
the presence of acute myocardial infarction, significant rises in
these enzymes should be found in blood samples. There are several enzymes that can be measured in this regard. Probably the
most commonly used are serum glutamic oxaloacetic transaminase

(SGOT), lactic dehydrogenase (LDH), and creatine phosphokinase (CPK). Each of these enzymes reaches peak levels in the blood at different times after the infarction and then returns to normal thereafter (Table 1).

*Table 1*

SERUM ENZYME VALUES
ACUTE MYOCARDIAL INFARCTION

| Enzyme | Peak Elevation following Myocardial Infarction | Return to Normal |
|---|---|---|
| CPK (Creatine Phosphokinase) | 6–24 hours | 2–3 days |
| SGOT (Serum Glutamic-Oxaloacetic Transaminase) | 1–2 days | 4–6 days |
| LDH (Lactic Dehydrogenase) | 2–3 days | 7–10 days |
| HBD (Hydroxybutyric Dehydrogenase) | 3–4 days | 1–3 weeks |

Enzyme studies are used only to *confirm* the diagnosis of acute infarction; they should never be considered diagnostic in the absence of electrocardiographic and historical evidence. These determinations are of most importance when the electrocardiographic changes are not wholly diagnostic or are equivocal. In these instances distinctive enzyme patterns may clarify the diagnostic dilemma.

## Evaluation of clinical status

The clinical status of the patient is assessed in two ways: first, by continuous cardiac monitoring and second, by direct observation of the patient.

*Cardiac monitoring.* Because of the extreme importance of arrhythmias, it is essential that all patients with acute myocardial infarction be kept under continuous electrocardiographic surveillance during the first several days after admission. By observing the electrocardiographic pattern on a cardiac monitor, arrhythmias can be detected at their onset and treatment instituted immediately.

There are dozens of monitors commercially available for this purpose. While they differ in design and operation, their fundamental components and basic functions are essentially the same.

The fundamental monitoring system has the following components:

a. *Skin electrodes* attached to the chest wall, which pick up the electrical impulses originating in the heart. Because these signals are too small to be visualized on an oscilloscope, they are directed through an amplifier, which markedly increases their dimensions.

b. *An oscilloscope,* which permits direct visual observation of these electrical signals.

c. *A rate meter,* which counts the number of heart beats per minute and displays this rate.

d. *An alarm system,* which is integrated with the rate meter to alert the observer to changes in the heart rate which exceed or fall below preset levels.

**Direct observation of the patient.** Cardiac monitoring merely gives information about one complication of myocardial infarction, namely arrhythmias. The remaining complications are recognized by repeated clinical observation of the patient (sometimes in conjunction with certain physiologic measurements). The importance of this particular phase of assessment is sometimes underestimated and too much emphasis given to mechanical monitoring methods. At the present time careful examination of the patient in a planned repeated manner represents the wisest approach to the detection of most complications other than arrhythmias.

*Physical examination.* The following findings are indicative of complications:

1. Severe, continuous chest pain.
2. Profuse sweating.
3. Cold, clammy skin.
4. Hypotension.
5. Dyspnea and tachypnea.

6. Slow heart rates (less than 60/min.)
7. Rapid heart rates (above 100/min.).
8. Distended neck veins (when patient is positioned at a 45° angle).
9. Gallop rhythm.
10. Cardiac enlargement.
11. Rales.
12. The appearance of cardiac murmurs.
13. Pericardial friction rub.
14. Peripheral edema.
15. Decreased or absent peripheral pulses.

## Assessment of specific complications

1. *Arrhythmias.* While the electrical system of the heart and its disorders cannot be considered in detail in this discussion, it is important to review briefly this subject. (Because the detection and treatment of arrhythmias are fundamental in the management of myocardial infarction, it is essential that the reader have a clear understanding of these disturbances. Several sources of such information are listed at the end of this chapter.)

Each normal heart beat is the result of an electrical impulse that originates in a specialized area of tissue in the right atrium described as the sinoatrial (SA) node. Under normal conditions the SA node discharges an electrical impulse 60 to 100 times each minute in a regular, rhythmic fashion. In this way, the SA node controls the heart rate and is called the "pacemaker." Other areas of the heart can also serve as the pacemaker, but they assume this role only under abnormal circumstances.

The path of the original impulse is shown in Fig. 1.*

a. The impulse begins in the SA node (1).

b. It spreads through the atrial muscles (2), which then contract.

c. It crosses the atrioventricular (AV) node (3) and passes down the Bundle of His (4).

d. Descending through the left and right bundle

---

* This diagram and explanation are reproduced from *Intensive Coronary Care —A Manual for Nurses.* Meltzer, L. E., Pinneo, R., and Kitchell, J. R. The Charles Press, Philadelphia, Pa.

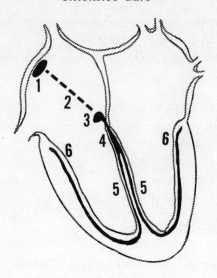

*Fig. 1*

branches (5), the impulse finally reaches the terminal Pur-
kinje fibers in the ventricular wall (6).

e. Ventricular contraction then occurs in response to
this stimulus.

As stated, disturbances in either the rate, rhythm, or conduction of these electrical impulses are called arrhythmias.

A. ARRHYTHMIAS WHICH PRODUCE SUDDEN DEATH

1. *Ventricular fibrillation.*

In ventricular fibrillation an abnormal focus within the ventricle serves as the pacemaker. This focus of extraordinary electrical force fires at an incredibly rapid rate and repeatedly stimulates the ventricles so that the recovery period after contraction
completely disappears. As a result, the individual muscle fibers
that comprise the ventricular wall merely twitch continuously,
but do not contract. Because the twitching is totally ineffective in
propelling blood from the ventricle, the circulation stops abruptly
and death follows within minutes.

The electrocardiographic pattern of ventricular fibrillation
(see Fig 2) is distinctive and can hardly be mistaken for any other
arrhythmia. In that the electrical activity within the ventricle is

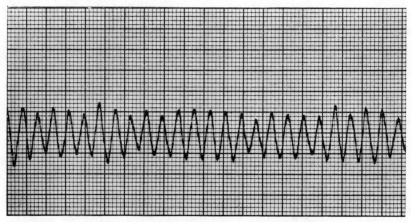

Fig. 2. Ventricular Fibrillation

totally chaotic, the normal P, Q, R, S, and T waves cannot be identified and each complex differs from the next. The waves occur in completely irregular fashion.

Within seconds of the onset of ventricular fibrillation, the patient loses consciousness and death can be anticipated, usually within two minutes.

Death from ventricular fibrillation can be prevented if an electric shock is delivered to the heart through the chest wall (precordial shock), within the two-minute period. After this critically short time, irreversible brain damage usually occurs.

When ventricular fibrillation develops spontaneously, it is termed *primary ventricular fibrillation.* In contrast, ventricular fibrillation that occurs as part of the terminal picture of left ventricular failure or shock is classified as *secondary* ventricular fibrillation. Precordial shock is almost always successful in the treatment of primary ventricular fibrillation, but is seldom of value in the secondary form, where the underlying disorder (shock or congestive failure) persists.

### 2. *Ventricular standstill*

When the electrical activity within the heart becomes inadequate to stimulate the muscles, the ventricles cease to contract, or contract ineffectively. This state is designated as *ventricular standstill*, Fig. 3. The result of this catastrophe is the same as with

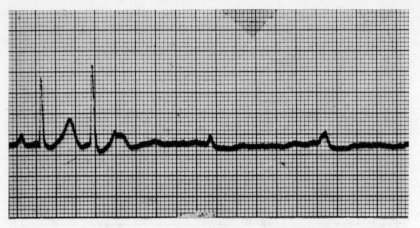

Fig. 3.  Ventricular Standstill

ventricular fibrillation, namely cessation of the circulation, and death.

Ventricular standstill can occur as a primary event or as secondary to advanced circulatory failure. The secondary form is far more common. Primary ventricular standstill can be treated successfully by means of cardiac pacing.

B. ARRHYTHMIAS THAT REDUCE CIRCULATORY EFFICIENCY

When the heart rate is significantly greater than 100 beats per minute or less than 60 per minute, the pumping efficiency of the heart is adversely affected. Rapid-rate arrhythmias with this potential include: ventricular tachycardia, Fig. 4; paroxysmal atrial tachycardia, Fig. 5; atrial flutter, Fig 6; atrial fibrillation, Fig. 7.

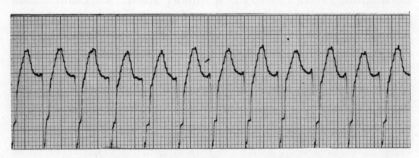

Fig. 4.  Ventricular Tachycardia

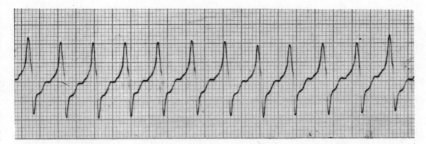

Fig. 5. Paroxysmal Atrial Tachycardia

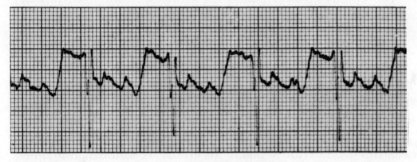

Fig. 6. Atrial Flutter

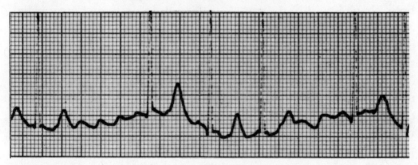

Fig. 7. Atrial Fibrillation

When these arrhythmias exist, ventricular filling time (the period between contractions) is obviously shortened. As a result, the amount of blood ejected by the ventricle with each contraction (the stroke volume) is decreased. A persistent decrease in the stroke volume and cardiac output (stroke volume times number of beats per minute) may lead to left ventricular failure and shock.

Slow-rate arrhythmias have similar hemodynamic consequences, but the mechanism differs. With acute myocardial infarction, where myocardial weakness exists, the stroke volume may often fail to increase, despite the prolonged filling period. If the stroke volume becomes relatively fixed for this reason, a slow rate may cause a decrease in cardiac output, with the same end result as noted with rapid-rate arrhythmias, namely left ventricular failure. Slow-rate arrhythmias capable of producing such effects are: marked sinus bradycardia (rate less than 50/min); advanced heart block; slow nodal rhythms.

Each of these rhythm disturbances can be readily detected by continuous cardiac monitoring. Sudden death from primary arrhythmias should seldom, if ever, occur with effective intensive care.

**2. *Congestive heart failure and cardiogenic shock.*** At least 60% of all patients with acute myocardial infarction show some evidence of left ventricular failure within the first few days after the attack; the degree of this failure varies considerably.

The precise etiology of left ventricular failure after acute myocardial infarction remains uncertain. It would appear, however, that either structural damage to the myocardium or metabolic changes within the muscle cells leads to decreased myocardial contractility. The loss of contractile strength results in incomplete emptying of the left ventricle, which, in turn, produces a back pressure in the pulmonary venous system.

When the left ventricle fails in this way, a complex of symptoms and physical findings develop. The most common (and classic) symptom of left ventricular failure is dyspnea. This may range from a mere awareness of breathing to the desperate respiration of acute pulmonary edema. Less obvious, but significant, symptoms which may suggest left ventricular failure are cough, restlessness, insomnia, and anorexia.

The physical signs of left ventricular failure include:
   a. the presence of rales in the lung fields;
   b. distended neck veins (with the patient positioned at a 45° angle);
   c. a third or fourth heart sound creating a gallop rhythm.

In some instances left ventricular failure may exist in the absence of these overt signs and symptoms. This subclinical form of failure (representing the earliest stages of the failing heart) can be recognized by x-ray examination of the chest or with simple hemodynamic measurements.

When the heart fails after myocardial infarction, the failure involves the left heart (the site of infarction) and the right heart may not be affected. For this reason peripheral edema and liver tenderness (typical findings of right-sided failure) may not be seen originally. If left ventricular failure persists, the right heart may fail subsequently and these latter signs will then be apparent.

CARDIOGENIC SHOCK

The etiology of cardiogenic shock is still uncertain, but the primary problem would appear to be advanced left ventricular failure. In this sense congestive heart failure and cardiogenic shock may represent only varying degrees of severity of left ventricular failure. Congestive failure and cardiogenic shock are jointly described as *"power failure."*

When the cardiac output is severely reduced, the amount of blood and oxygen reaching the vital organs is diminished to a point where adequate tissue perfusion no longer exists. (The problem of shock is considered separately in Chapter IV, "Shock."

Inadequate tissue perfusion results in a combination of clinical findings which collectively are categorized as cardiogenic shock. The major manifestations of cardiogenic shock are:

a. *A significant decrease in arterial blood pressure*

The systolic blood pressure usually falls below 90 mm Hg. It is important to realize that hypotension, *by itself,* is not synonymous with cardiogenic shock. Many patients with acute myocardial infarction have systolic blood pressures of 70–90 mm Hg and are not in shock, because these pressures are often sufficient to preserve adequate perfusion. Unless hypotension is accompanied by other clinical findings (described below), the diagnosis of cardiogenic shock should not be made. The problem of assessing the significance of hypotension is compounded by the fact that blood pressure determined by the usual cuff-stethoscope method may be spuriously low. When measured by direct arterial puncture techniques, the pressure may be considerably higher.

In the early stages of shock the systolic pressure usually falls before the diastolic pressure, and as a result, the pulse pressure (i.e., the difference between systolic and diastolic pressure) becomes narrow. As shock progresses, the diastolic pressure falls as well.

b. *Oliguria*

As a result of decreased cardiac output, there is reduced per-fusion of the kidneys. This is reflected by an oliguria or anuria. Normally, the kidneys should excrete at least 1 cc/min (or 60 cc/hr). In the presence of cardiogenic shock there is a marked diminution of the urinary output (usually less than 20 cc/hr) or the flow stops completely. Accurate urine measurements are there-fore vital in assessing the clinical course of shock.

c. *Mental changes*

Patients with shock develop apathy, confusion, restlessness, and agitation, all secondary to ineffective perfusion of the brain. When the cerebral ischemia persists, coma usually develops.

d. *Skin*

As a reflex response to hypotension, the peripheral blood ves-sels constrict in an attempt to preserve the circulation for the vital organs. For this reason the skin is usually cold and pale. This re-action, in association with increased sympathetic nervous system activity (an early sign of shock), produces the pale, cold, clammy sweat typical of cardiogenic shock.

e. *Congestive heart failure*

When the cardiac output falls, the blood supply to the myo-cardium is further embarrassed and signs of left ventricular failure (distended neck veins, rales, dyspnea) are usually noted. In car-diogenic shock the central venous pressure, which indirectly re-flects such left ventricular failure, is usually markedly elevated. (In other forms of shock, the central venous pressure may be normal or low; see Chapter IV "Shock").

**3. *Ventricular rupture.*** This complication occurs in most in-stances as a sudden, unexpected event which produces death within minutes. The reason that the ventricular wall ruptures in certain patients is not entirely clear. It has been suggested that physical exertion during the period of early healing, sustained hypertension, and anticoagulant therapy may be causative factors. However, the evidence for any of these explanations is question-able. Most ventricular ruptures occur with extensive infarction where the degree of necrosis is marked.

Rupture of the ventricular wall can seldom be recognized clinically. In most instances death occurs abruptly and appears clinically to be the result of an arrhythmia. In addition to rupture of the free ventricular wall, rupture may also involve the interventricular wall. In this event a diagnosis can be made by the sudden appearance of a loud murmur in conjunction with the onset of congestive heart failure. Surgical correction of this latter defect may be attempted if time permits.

Ventricular rupture can occur at any time after the infarction, but is most frequent between the fifth and tenth days.

4. *Thromboembolism.* Patients with acute myocardial infarction have a high risk of developing thromboemboli, but these seldom produce death. A full discussion of thromboembolic complications is found in the following chapter and is omitted here.

## PRINCIPLES OF TREATMENT

### General principles of intensive care

Because of the high incidence of complications and the unpredictability of the clinical course during the early period of hospitalization, it is vital that patients with acute myocardial infarction be treated in an intensive care facility. Experience in several centers has shown that the anticipated mortality of patients treated in coronary care units is at least one-third less than that found with customary hospital care. This reduction in mortality is dependent primarily on the training and competence of the intensive care team, particularly the nurse members who are in constant attendance; equipment and physical surroundings are of much less significance. Unless nurses are specifically capable of assessing the patient's course and recognizing the first evidences (or warnings) of complications, little reduction in mortality will be achieved.

*Selection of patients.* Since complications may develop in *any* patient with myocardial infarction, it is wise to admit *all* patients with this *suspected* diagnosis to intensive care facilities. It is poor judgment to assume that high-risk or low-risk candidates for complications can be distinguished at the time of admission.

*Duration of intensive care.* Approximately 75% of all deaths from acute myocardial infarction occur during the first five days after the attack. The mortality after this initial critical period is substantially lower, as is the incidence of complications. On this basis, patients should be treated in an intensive care facility for at least five days, after which they can be transferred to usual hospital care.

## Immediate care

As soon as the patient reaches the unit, a planned treatment program should be put into effect. The exact plan of therapy will depend on the clinical picture presented. Those patients admitted with overt left ventricular failure, cardiogenic shock, or serious arrhythmias must obviously be treated for these life-threatening complications immediately, while those reaching the unit in less critical condition can be treated with a more standardized approach, as follows:

*Cardiac monitoring.* Since the risk of serious arrhythmias is highest in the immediate hours after the attack, it is essential that cardiac monitoring be initiated as soon as the patient is admitted. In this way catastrophic arrhythmias can be recognized at their onset and terminated immediately. Cardiac monitoring is the first step in the treatment program, regardless of the patient's condition on admission.

*Clinical assessment.* Careful physical examination should be performed promptly to ascertain the presence of complications, particularly that of left ventricular failure. These findings serve as a baseline for future reference. If left ventricular failure or cardiogenic shock is present, treatment is immediately directed toward these problems, as described in subsequent pages.

*Symptomatic treatment.*
RELIEF OF PAIN

It is undesirable to allow chest pain to persist, and analgesics or narcotics should be employed to control this distressing symptom. Meperidine (Demerol) in dosages of 75 to 100 mgm administered either intramuscularly or intravenously (depending on the severity of pain) is probably the agent of choice for this purpose. Morphine, long a standard therapy in this situation, has seemingly fallen into disfavor because of its effect in slowing the heart rate to dangerously bradycardic levels. All opiates can cause nausea, vomiting, urinary retention, hypotension, and respiratory depression; overdosages must be avoided.

OXYGEN

Although oxygen is commonly given to all patients with acute infarctions, this practice need not be routine, and should be reserved for those who exhibit dyspnea or physical findings of left ventricular failure or cardiogenic shock. When oxygen is required, it is best administered with a face mask, which provides a satisfactory oxygen concentration. Oxygen tents should not be used.

***Establishment of an intravenous conduit.*** It is clear that an intravenous route should be established and maintained in all patients with acute myocardial infarction. Perhaps the most popular technique for this purpose involves the insertion of a small polyethylene catheter into a large peripheral vein. The system is kept patent with a slow infusion of 5% D/W. This indwelling catheter permits rapid administration of drugs in life-threatening situations. (Establishing an intravenous infusion *after* a catastrophic event has occurred is often a futile experience, and the time lost in this procedure may be disastrous).

## The treatment of complications

***The warning arrhythmias.*** The most obvious benefit of intensive care is the *prevention* of arrhythmic deaths. Rather than directing the treatment program toward resuscitation of lethal arrhythmias, the objective should be to *prevent* the development of these catastrophes. Both ventricular fibrillation and ventricular standstill are preceded by specific *warning* arrhythmias. By recognizing and treating these lesser disturbances, unexpected death-producing arrhythmias can be prevented in almost every instance.

A. WARNINGS OF VENTRICULAR FIBRILLATION

1. *Premature ventricular contractions*

These ectopic beats are the forerunners of ventricular fibrillation, and every effort must be made to control them. Since at

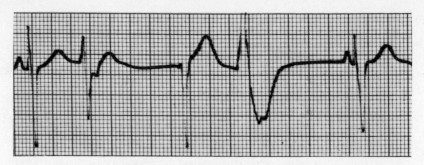

**Fig. 8. Multifocal PVC's**

least 75% of all patients with acute myocardial infarction show premature ventricular contractions (PVCs), it is apparent that this arrhythmia is not dangerous in every instance. It is only when PVCs occur in the following patterns that they have special danger and require vigorous therapy: PVCs occurring more than 6 times per minute; multifocal PVCs, Fig. 8; PVCs that strike near the T wave of the preceding cycle; bigeminy (where every other beat is a PVC), Fig. 9.

Premature ventricular beats of these types are best treated with lidocaine or procainamide in the following manner:

Lidocaine is injected intravenously, as rapidly as possible, in a dosage equivalent to 1 milligram of lidocaine per kilogram of body weight. The customary dosage is therefore 50 to 100 mgm delivered as a "push dose." In most instances this single injection will terminate the ectopic beats; if not, a second injection of a similar dosage can be given. Once the ectopic beats are controlled by this injection, additional lidocaine is given in the form of a

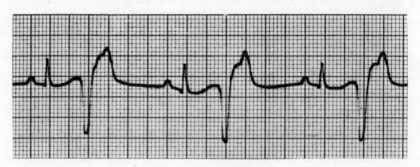

**Fig. 9. Bigeminy**

continuous intravenous infusion with a drip rate calculated to deliver 1–3 mgm per minute.

Procainamide can also be used for this purpose; however, it is considered a less desirable drug because of its ability to induce hypotension. If procainamide is used, the push dose contains 300 to 500 mgm of the agent.

Both of these drugs are highly effective in controlling PVCs, but failures do occur, necessitating other measures. Perhaps the most important of these alternative methods involves the use of potassium. Myocardial irritability is distinctly increased when cellular potassium becomes inadequate. This irritability, reflected by PVCs, can be controlled by the replacement of the potassium deficit. The cation is administered in dosages of 40 mEq in a 500 cc solution of dextrose in water. Potassium should never be given as direct, undiluted injection.

### 2. *Ventricular tachycardia*

The presence of four or more *consecutive* premature ventricular contractions, or ventricular tachycardia, is the most serious warning of the development of ventricular fibrillation.

Ventricular tachycardia may stop spontaneously, after seconds or minutes, or else may become an established rhythm. Even if the arrhythmia is of short duration and ceases without therapy, treatment is nevertheless indicated. A continuous infusion of lidocaine should be started promptly to prevent recurrences of this serious disorder. If the arrhythmia is not self-limited and continues, lidocaine should be given immediately as a "push dose" according to the regimen described above. Failure to convert ventricular tachycardia to normal sinus rhythm by the push dose is indication for electrical termination of the arrhythmia by means of precordial shock. Although some patients are unaware of the presence of ventricular tachycardia and the clinical picture may not appear desperately serious, precordial shock should nevertheless be given immediately if the arrhythmia persists, because of the high potential for development of ventricular fibrillation.

#### PRECORDIAL SHOCK

The use of a powerful electrical shock of very brief duration, delivered through the chest wall, has proved to be an excellent method for terminating certain rapid-rate arrhythmias. The technique, popularly called cardioversion, is particularly useful in the treatment of ventricular tachycardia, atrial flutter, atrial fibrillation, and paroxysmal atrial tachycardia. Its most important use is as a life-saving measure in terminating ventricular fibrillation.

When used to treat arrhythmias other than ventricular fibrillation, this choice of therapy is selected in preference to drugs because of its immediate effect. Thus for a patient with a rapid-rate arrhythmia, in whom adverse hemodynamic effects are apparent, elective cardioversion can correct the underlying arrhythmia instantly, saving precious time before drugs could be effective.

The principle of precordial shock is clearcut: the electric shock depolarizes the entire heart for a fraction of a second. This halts the ectopic pacemaker (which created the arrhythmia), after which the SA node can regain control, thus establishing normal rhythm.

When cardioversion is used electively to terminate arrhythmias (in contrast to its emergency use in treating ventricular fibrillation), it is important that the electrical impulse be synchronized with the "R" wave of the cardiac cycle in order to prevent the possible creation of ventricular fibrillation (a possibility if the impulse strikes during the vulnerable period which corresponds to the "T" wave). This synchronization is accomplished automatically when the synchronizer switch of the machine is in the "ON" position. Regardless of when the discharge button is pushed, the machine will wait for the next "R" wave before discharging the energy.

When precordial shock is used to terminate ventricular fibrillation, it is mandatory that the synchronizer be turned to the "OFF" position; otherwise the machine will not discharge, as there are no "R" waves with ventricular fibrillation. With elective cardioversion it is customary to anesthetize the patient for a very brief time because of the discomfort of the shock.

B. WARNINGS OF VENTRICULAR STANDSTILL

1. *Advanced heart block*

Disturbances of conduction manifest as second-degree or third-degree heart block (Fig. 10) are the forerunners of ventricular standstill in nearly every instance. Unless these forms of heart

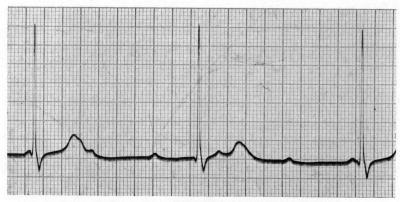

Fig. 10. Complete Heart Block

block (collectively called "advanced" heart block) are recognized and treated promptly, ventricular standstill can occur at any time. In complete heart block, impulses from the SA, or A-V node, are totally interrupted and the ventricle must rely on its own electrical rhythmicity. The rate in this circumstance is only 30–40 beats per minute. This poses two serious problems. First, the ventricular pacemaker is not dependable and, should it fail, ventricular standstill develops instantly. Secondly, the inherent ventricular rate, of 30–40 per minute, is fixed and cannot be increased to meet the body's demands. This severe bradycardia is usually associated with a significant reduction of cardiac output which leads to left ventricular failure. For both of these reasons, it is essential that advanced heart block not be tolerated. While drug therapy, particularly isoproterenol, may be attempted as a means of increasing the heart rate (or decreasing the degree of block), the results are, most often, unpredictable and there is no assurance that ventricular standstill will not occur despite such treatment.

At present the best method for treating advanced heart block and preventing ventricular standstill involves the use of electrical pacing of the heart; the technique is described in subsequent paragraphs.

### 2. *Marked bradycardias*

When the heart rate is less than 50, even in the absence of complete heart block, the threat of ventricular standstill is distinctly increased.

In those bradycardias that are not due to heart block, treatment is initially directed toward increasing the heart rate with drug therapy. The use of atropine is usually the first method attempted in combating these bradycardias. The drug is administered by rapid, direct intravenous injection in a dosage of 1 mgm. By inhibiting vagal influences on the heart, atropine causes an acceleration of the heart rate. The response to atropine usually occurs within seconds and may last for several hours. The drug must be used cautiously in patients with prostatic disease or glaucoma. If atropine fails in this task, or is contraindicated, isoproterenol can be used. The response to this latter agent is usually excellent. If drug therapy is unsuccessful, cardiac pacing can be employed.

TRANSVENOUS PACING

Transvenous pacing is accomplished by placing an electrode (situated at the tip of a catheter) into the right ventricular cavity by way of a large vein (see Fig. 11). The usual sites for catheter electrode insertion are an arm vein, a jugular vein, or a subclavian vein. Usually, the insertion is made following percutaneous needle puncture of the vein; occasionally, when the vein cannot be entered percutaneously, a surgical cutdown is used. The catheter electrode must be positioned against the endocardial wall of the right ventricle. This placement can be effected by either fluoroscopic guidance or by electrocardiographic means. In the latter situation the electrode position is determined by the electrocardiogram obtained from within the heart, using the catheter as an exploring electrode.

Once the catheter has been properly positioned, the free end is connected to a battery-powered device, a pacemaker which delivers electrical impulses of a desired rate and intensity through the catheter to the heart wall. By setting the pacemaker rate beyond the existing heart rate, the pacemaker controls (captures) the electrical activity of the heart and thus determines the heart rate. As with any electrical circuit, current must flow between two poles. With cardiac pacing the two poles can be situated about 1–2 cm apart at the tip of the catheter (a bipolar catheter), or the catheter can have a single pole or electrode (unipolar) at its tip and the circuit is completed by placing the second electrode in the skin.

Transvenous catheters are inserted as soon as second-degree or third-degree heart block is identified. The pacemaker may be left in place for long periods without difficulty. The great advantage derived from the insertion of a transvenous catheter is that pacing can be initiated prophylactically before ventricular standstill occurs. Because heart block associated with myocardial infarction is usually transient, pacing is continued until normal conduction returns; at that time the catheter can be removed. In 5 to 10 per cent of patients, heart block persists, necessitating the placement of a permanent implanted pacemaker.

### *Treatment of Ventricular Fibrillation*

RECOGNITION

The initial step in the treatment of ventricular fibrillation is the immediate identification of the arrhythmia. When ventricular fibrillation develops, the alarm mechanism of the cardiac monitor is triggered and both audio and visual signals are activated. (Either the high-rate or the low-rate alarm may sound.)

The electrocardiographic pattern of this lethal arrhythmia is distinctive (Fig. 2). However, even if the observer is unable to specifically identify this pattern, no time should be spent in further observation of the monitor. Instead, the nurse or physician should proceed immediately to the bedside and examine the patient. Ventricular fibrillation produces unconsciousness within seconds; if the patient is conscious, it can be concluded that ventricular fibrillation is not present.

If the patient is unconscious and the heart beat and peripheral pulses are not detectable, the planned program for treatment of ventricular fibrillation should begin instantly.

TERMINATION OF THE ARRHYTHMIA

Once ventricular fibrillation is identified, precordial shock should be performed *by the first person to reach the bedside.* The sooner the shock is delivered, the greater the chance for recovery.

In an intensive care unit every nurse and physician should be capable of defibrillating the heart in this dire emergency. It is vitally important that the entire team understand that defibrillation should be accomplished *before any other procedure* is undertaken. Specifically, *no time* should be lost by starting oxygen therapy, establishing an airway, or giving closed-chest cardiac massage when ventricular fibrillation occurs in an intensive care unit where personnel and equipment are in readiness to terminate the arrhythmia. Personnel accustomed to resuscitation techniques practiced in ordinary hospital rooms or wards, often find it difficult to disregard the need of closed-chest cardiac massage and oxygen therapy when ventricular fibrillation develops. These procedures, while often life saving in other surroundings, are time-wasting in the setting of an intensive care facility.

Defibrillation can be performed with either alternating-current or direct-current equipment. Regardless of the defibrillator used, *the maximal electrical energy that can be delivered by the machine* should be employed. There is absolutely no benefit in using lesser energies in this particular circumstance. The synchronizer must be in "OFF" position.

### CORRECTION OF LACTIC ACIDOSIS

When the circulation ceases as a result of ventricular fibrillation, acidosis can inevitably be expected, even though prompt restoration of an effective heartbeat may have been achieved by defibrillation. This acidosis, classified as lactic acidosis, occurs as the result of inadequate oxygen supply to cells throughout the body. When the circulation fails, normal aerobic cellular metabolism ceases and, attempting to survive, the cells utilize an alternative metabolic pathway not demanding oxygen (anaerobic metabolism). One of the products of this latter metabolism is lactic acid. Unlike carbon dioxide and water (the products of aerobic metabolism), which can be removed from the body by the lungs and kidneys, lactic acid cannot be disposed of in these ways and accumulates very rapidly. This produces a profound acidosis which can be controlled only by the use of alkalis, particularly sodium bicarbonate. Sodium bicarbonate should be administered immediately to every patient who has sustained ventricular fibrillation. Because of the severe degree of acidosis, it is wise to give about 80 mEq of sodium bicarbonate by direct intravenous injection. As the effect of bicarbonate lasts for only 6 to 10 minutes, it is necessary to administer additional dosages of 40 mEq at least every 10 minutes until adequate circulation is restored and the acidosis controlled.

The degree of acidosis and the amount of bicarbonate required are best determined by repeated measurement of blood pH and carbon dioxide. For this purpose we have found the Astrup equipment, which utilizes capillary blood (by finger puncture techniques), to be an ideal method. The test can be performed within minutes, and repeated determinations can be obtained simply.

Most patients with ventricular fibrillation require several hundred mEq of sodium bicarbonate to combat the acidosis. For this reason some manufacturers have prepared a 5% solution of sodium bicarbonate which contains approximately 300 mEq of bicarbonate in a 500 cc volume. The use of these flasks permits continuous intravenous infusion of bicarbonate and obviates the need for injecting the contents of multiple vials (which normally contain only 40 mEq).

PREVENTION OF RECURRENCE OF VENTRICULAR FIBRILLATION

Patients who have sustained one episode of ventricular fibrillation are high risks for subsequent attacks, and it is essential that this threat be controlled immediately. Recurrent ventricular fibrillation can be attributed to two major causes:

1. The myocardial irritability that initially led to fibrillation still exists. Accordingly, it is important that vigorous antiarrhythmic therapy be instituted to combat such ventricular irritability. The aim of treatment is to stop, or at least to minimize, premature ventricular contractions. This is best accomplished by the use of a continuous infusion of lidocaine or procainamide. If premature beats occur despite this preventive therapy, additional amounts of the agents can be injected as "push" doses. If the irritability continues despite this approach, other agents, including dilantin, digitalis, propranolol, or quinidine, can be tried; however, experience would suggest that if lidocaine or procainamide are unsuccessful for their intended purpose, other drugs will be similarly disappointing in their effectiveness. In this event some clinicians prefer to control premature beats by means of pacing

techniques in which the ectopic beats are eliminated by pacing the heart at a rate fast enough to prevent them.

2. A second cause of recurrent ventricular fibrillation is uncontrolled lactic acidosis. It is quite clear that myocardial irritability is greatly exaggerated and intensified in the presence of acidosis. When ventricular fibrillation recurs time after time following successful attempts at defibrillation, the problem is most likely the result of lactic acidosis and can be controlled by additional amounts of sodium bicarbonate.

### The Treatment of Ventricular Standstill

#### RECOGNITION

As noted in the discussion of warning arrhythmias, ventricular standstill seldom, if ever, occurs without previous electrocardiographic warning in the form of advanced heart block or extreme bradycardia. In this sense ventricular standstill is not truly an unexpected occurrence; only its onset is sudden.

When ventricular standstill occurs, the low-rate alarm of the monitor system is activated. While the electrocardiographic pattern of ventricular standstill is by no means as distinctive as ventricular fibrillation, it can nevertheless be recognized by a trained nurse-observer. The disappearance of the ventricular complex (QRS) in the presence of continuing atrial activity (P waves) is usually clear cut (see Fig. 3).

As with ventricular fibrillation, the observer should proceed immediately to the bedside once the alarm sounds, if there is any suspicion that the monitor pattern is that of ventricular standstill. Attempting to identify the pattern with certainty at this point is a tragic waste of time.

If ventricular standstill exists, the patient will be unconscious and pulseless, and no heart sounds will be audible.

#### TERMINATION OF THE ARRHYTHMIA

If the electrocardiographic warnings of *advanced heart block* were heeded and a transvenous pacemaker was inserted on a prophylactic basis, the obvious next step in treatment would be to turn on the pacemaker to initiate pacing impulses.

If a transvenous pacemaker has *not* been placed previously, the nurse or physician reaching the bedside first should punch the chest directly over the heart with a forceful blow. If this simple step is performed within seconds after standstill, the heartbeat may often resume. If this is ineffective the nurse or physician should begin external cardiac massage and mouth-to-mouth breathing (this valuable technique of cardiopulmonary resuscitation should be well known, not only to all medical personnel, but also to all paramedical personnel in an intensive care facility).

While cardiopulmonary resuscitation is being performed, *cardiac pacing* should be attempted. Three techniques may be employed:

### 1. *External cardiac pacing*

A pacing electrode is attached to the chest wall (near the apex of the heart) and the pacing impulse is delivered from either a separate external pacemaker device or from the pacemaker incorporated within the monitoring system. The energy level should be at its maximum and the rate set at about 70–80 impulses per minute. External pacing of this type can be successful if the electrical stimulation begins in from 15 to 30 seconds after the standstill; beyond this critical period, reactivation of the heartbeat is much less likely to occur.

### 2. *Transthoracic pacing*

The heart can also be stimulated by electrical impulses delivered through a thin wire inserted into the wall of the myocardium. This technique can be performed within seconds and requires minimal equipment. A long needle (spinal) is passed through the chest wall into the myocardium after which a fine wire, with a barb at the end, is inserted through the needle into the myocardial wall; the needle is then withdrawn. The wire is attached to a pacemaker for immediate pacing.

### 3. *Transvenous pacing*

Although transvenous pacing is by far the most predictably successful method of pacing the heart, the usefulness of this technique is limited in a catastrophic circumstance of ventricular standstill. Even in the hands of the most experienced physician, the insertion of a transvenous electrode is a time-consuming event and as such cannot be utilized as a primary treatment.

During the preparation and onset of cardiac pacing, cardio-pulmonary resuscitative technique should continue and should not be interrupted until an effective heartbeat is restored. This represents the only hope of survival, and all subsequent steps have little meaning unless brain function is preserved.

Prior to pacing attempts, or sometimes during pacing, epine-phrine (1 cc of 1:1000 solution) may be injected directly into the heart.

### CORRECTION OF LACTIC ACIDOSIS

For the reasons described with ventricular fibrillation, lactic acidosis should be anticipated in every instance of ventricular standstill. Because the period between the onset of standstill and its termination is usually much greater than in ventricular fibrilla-tion, the degree of acidosis is usually more profound, and sodium bicarbonate should be administered while cardiopulmonary resus-citation or pacing is in process. The total dosage of sodium bi-carbonate required to control the acidosis should be ascertained by repeated measurements of pH and carbon dioxide.

### PREVENTION OF RECURRENCE

Every patient who survives ventricular standstill should have a transvenous pacemaker inserted as soon as resuscitation is suc-cessful. The conduction disturbance that originally caused the standstill will still be present, and pacing must be continued (usually for several days or more) until the heart block subsides.

### The treatment of cardiogenic shock

As noted, the treatment of cardiogenic shock remains ineffec-tive and at least 80% of patients who develop shock after myo-cardial infarction die, with present therapeutic methods. Many believe that this incredible mortality will not be improved until usable mechanical means become available for assisting the failing ventricle.

At the present time the major hope for survival with cardiogenic shock centers about a program involving early recognition and a planned treatment regimen. The general principles of the assessment and treatment of all forms of shock are considered in a separate chapter. This discussion is limited to aspects of the treatment solely of cardiogenic shock. It is important to realize that the treatment of shock varies with its etiology and that a single approach cannot be used for all types of shock (e.g., hypovolemic, septic, cardiogenic, etc.).

### 1. EARLY RECOGNITION OF CARDIOGENIC SHOCK

Approximately 15% of all patients with myocardial infarction develop shock. In many instances, this state develops very shortly after the attack, and the patient is in moribund condition at the time of admission. In other patients, shock develops more insidiously and can be recognized in its early stages by planned, repeated observation of the clinical state. In addition to careful physical examination, simple measurement of the circulation time, urinary output, changes in central venous pressure, and pulse rate, and measuring of the pulse pressure may lead to early recognition of decreased cardiac output.

### 2. ENHANCEMENT OF CARDIAC OUTPUT

Although the precise mechanism of cardiogenic shock is still unknown, there is general agreement that the basic lesion is impaired left ventricular function, as manifested by decreased cardiac output and decreased stroke volume. The major aim of treatment is to improve left ventricular performance. This can be accomplished, in many instances, by the use of digitalis preparations and isoproterenol.

Digitalization must be achieved rapidly. In patients who have not had recent digitalis therapy, the use of Ouabain is recommended. The drug is administered intravenously in a dosage of 0.3 to 0.5 mgm.

Isoproterenol, the most effective inotropic agent known, is a valuable drug in the treatment of cardiogenic shock, and many clinicians believe that it should constitute the fundamental attack in combating this form of shock. The usual method of administration involves a slow, controlled intravenous drip of a solution containing 1 mgm of isoproterenol in 500 cc of 5% glucose in water. The rate of the infusion is titrated by the clinical response. The dosage is often limited by the development of ventricular irritability in the form of premature ventricular contractions or ventricular tachycardia.

### 3. MAINTENANCE OF ARTERIAL BLOOD PRESSURE

The use of vasopressor therapy has long been a standard part of the treatment program for cardiogenic shock. Some believe that the decrease in mortality, however small, that has occurred in the past decade can be attributed to the use of these pressor agents. In the past few years, nevertheless, considerable dissent has arisen about the need or value of vasopressors in this situation. Those who question the benefit of these pressor drugs suggest that vasoconstriction is already maximal in cardiogenic shock (as part of the body's natural response to decreased cardiac output), and that the administration of these agents (whose primary action is vasoconstriction) is to no avail, or even worse, may be dangerous. Those who advocate vasopressor therapy feel strongly that despite these objections, pressor agents are essential and are capable of increasing the blood pressure. They believe that unless arterial blood pressure is maintained, perfusion of the heart and brain is critically reduced and future therapy becomes meaningless when irreversible tissue changes occur. This dilemma is currently unresolved.

The most commonly used vasopressors are norepinephrine (Levophed), mephentermine (Wyamine), and metaraminol (Aramine); Wyamine and Aramine can be given either intramuscularly or intravenously. Levophed, perhaps the most popular of these agents, can be used only intravenously and is administered in the following way: one ampule containing 4 cc of norepinephrine solution is added to a flask of 500 cc of glucose in water. The infusion is initiated at a rate of 20 drops per minute and is increased to 30 drops per minute if no rise in blood pressure is noted. If this is ineffective, a second ampule is added to the solution and rate of infusion reduced to 20 drops a minute. A third and fourth ampule can be added in the same manner if the blood pressure has not increased. When the solution finally contains 4 ampules and is given at a rate of 30 drops per minute, and no response occurs, no benefit can be anticipated thereafter and the infusion should be discontinued. Extravasation of Levophed into the subcutaneous tissues can produce severe local reactions, including sloughing of the involved area.

### 4. PRESERVATION OF ADEQUATE OXYGENATION

The ultimate effect of decreased cardiac output is a marked reduction in tissue perfusion. This hypoxia leads to an irreversible phase of shock. While the basic approach to improving tissue perfusion is by enhancing cardiac output, the use of oxygen is undoubtedly beneficial in this circumstance. It is essential that a high oxygen concentration be furnished the patient if any benefit is to accrue. For this reason oxygen administered by nasal catheters or cannulae is of little value. While the use of tight-fitting face masks represents a more satisfactory method of administration of oxygen, this technique is often less than optimal in this situation. The use of pressure or volume-controlled ventilators is advisable (see Chapter I, "Respiratory Insufficiency and Failure").

### ADDITIONAL METHODS IN THE TREATMENT OF CARDIOGENIC SHOCK

While the concepts described above represent the basic therapy for cardiogenic shock, several other methods have been suggested. Many of these latter techniques have been attempted with other forms of shock and are not specific for shock accompanying myocardial infarction. The following comments represent current opinion of the benefit of these therapies in terms of cardiogenic shock:

### 1. *Steroids*

There is no secure evidence that corticosteroid therapy influences cardiogenic shock, but the practice of using these drugs has achieved some popularity.

### 2. *Hypothermia*

It has been hoped that by reducing the body temperature to 94° F. or less, the metabolic demands of vital tissues could be reduced, thus allowing the body to tolerate the reduction in perfusion. The benefit of hypothermia in this situation is still uncertain.

### 3. *Dextran*

Low molecular weight dextran has been proposed as an adjunctive therapy in the treatment of cardiogenic shock on the basis that it can improve the microcirculation by preventing "sludging" of blood. Because dextran is a volume expander, this complex sugar must be used with caution in the presence of myocardial infarction where congestive failure may be precipitated or aggravated. There is no specific evidence that dextran has a beneficial effect in this situation.

### 4. *Hyperbaric oxygen*

The concept of treating patients with cardiogenic shock by means of oxygen under pressure (Chapter XIV, "Hyperbaric Oxygenation") is theoretically attractive. Presumably, adequate tissue oxygenation could be preserved in this way; however, experience with this technique to date has been quite limited, and no conclusion can be made about the actual merit of this approach.

### 5. *Assisted circulation*

In principle, mechanical assistance of the circulation offers the most reasonable attack on the problem of cardiogenic shock. Several methods of such assistance have been attempted, including counterpulsation, extracorporeal pumping devices, and left ventricular assist systems. All of these techniques can be considered only experimental at this time, and no clearly effective method has evolved thus far.

METHODS OF ASSESSING THERAPY FOR CARDIOGENIC SHOCK

Selection of the specific methods of treatment in cardiogenic shock depends primarily on the clinical response, as well as certain physiological parameters. The most helpful determinations for guiding and assessing therapy include the following:

1. *Central venous pressure*

In most instances of cardiogenic shock, the CVP is markedly elevated, usually to levels of more than 20 cm $H_2O$. Occasionally, however, the CVP may be low. In this latter circumstance, the use of vasopressors or volume replacement may be helpful. The technique for measuring central venous pressure is described on page 293.

2. *Cardiac output determination*

Because cardiogenic shock results in decreased cardiac output, it is particularly valuable to know the degree of reduction (or subsequent improvement) of the cardiac output. Unfortunately, this determination is not completely reproducible in the shock state and the method must still be reserved for research purposes at this time. Rarely, the cardiac output may be near normal in cardiogenic shock, implying that treatment should be directed toward peripheral causes.

3. *Circulation time*

The measurement of the appearance time following the intravenous injection of dye or other substances (e.g., decholin) is a simple and effective method for estimating circulatory performance. Successful therapy is usually manifested by a progressive reduction in the circulation time.

4. *Urinary function*

An increase in urinary volume in response to therapy is most often a favorable sign. Continuous catheter drainage is essential for evaluation. The volume should be measured every 15 to 30 minutes during the course of treatment.

## The treatment of left ventricular failure

As already noted, at least 60% of patients with myocardial infarction develop physical signs of left ventricular failure during the course of hospitalization. This decompensation may present with an apparent suddenness, in the form of acute pulmonary edema, or more gradually.

The basic aims of therapy are:

### 1. TO REDUCE VENOUS RETURN TO THE LEFT VENTRICLE

This is accomplished with morphine, rotating tourniquets, venesection, and particularly, the use of the rapidly acting diuretic agents, ethacrynic acid and furosemide.

### 2. TO IMPROVE TISSUE OXYGENATION

Decreased cardiac output results in inadequate perfusion when left ventricular failure is severe. Oxygen is administered with a tight-fitting nasal mask to help combat this destructive process. On some occasions it is beneficial to deliver oxygen by means of positive pressure, using the Bird or Bennett machines.

### 3. TO IMPROVE MYOCARDIAL CONTRACTILITY

Digitalis preparations represent the cornerstone of this approach. The prompt-acting glycosides Ouabain and Cedilanid are the agents of choice.

The details of the treatment program for left ventricular failure are discussed in the next chapter, "Circulatory Emergencies."

## THE NURSING ROLE

### General principles

It should be apparent from the preceding discussion that the nursing role in the treatment of acute myocardial infarction can hardly be considered separately from the physician's role. Because of the rapid change of events that may occur at any time during the acute phase of the illness, the nurse is repeatedly confronted with situations which demand immediate decisions and action. In many instances these responsibilities must be assumed by the nurse.

The nursing role involves three interrelated functions:

1) Direct observation of the patient.
2) Continuous cardiac monitoring.
3) Routine nursing care and emotional support.

The first two of these duties have been described throughout the chapter as they relate to specific parts of the total treatment program. It is appropriate to consider the emotional aspects at this point.

An acute myocardial infarction creates an enormous response in most patients. This is readily understandable in view of the inherently life-threatening aspect of the illness. Even those patients who are unaware of the frightening mortality associated with the attack are nevertheless fearful and anxious because of the symbolic importance of the heart—the "vital" organ of life. For these reasons, as well as thoughts of invalidism and economic ruin, major psychologic reactions are prominent in almost every patient and constitute a serious disability in many. The nurse's skill in recognizing and helping to solve these problems represents an important part of the total program of therapy. The methods for accomplishing these aims are complex and certainly involve much more than mere reassurance. One central theme is to help the patient face his present limitation. The nurse-physician team can offer this help by treating the patient as a respected adult rather than as a child who must do as he is told.

## Specific complications

*Arrhythmias.* At least 80% of all patients with myocardial infarction have some type of arrhythmic disturbance during the acute part of the illness. It is essential that the nurse be able to recognize and distinguish the individual arrhythmias, as presented by the monitoring equipment, and to know their relative seriousness. In particular, the nurse has the responsibility of detecting those arrhythmias that serve as warnings of impending lethal arrhythmias. Above all, the nurse must be prepared to institute immediate treatment against those arrhythmias that threaten life when they occur.

WARNING ARRHYTHMIAS

*Premature ventricular contractions*

1. If the nurse detects any of the serious types of PVC's or notes a change in the frequency of these ectopic beats, the physician should be notified promptly.

2. A syringe, containing 100 mg of lidocaine, should be prepared and brought to the bedside for use by the physician.

3. A defibrillator should be near the patient and made ready for use in the event that ventricular fibrillation occurs before preventive therapy can be given.

4. After the undesirable PVC's have been controlled with lidocaine or procainamide, careful observation of the monitor is mandatory in order to detect recurrence of these ectopic beats.

*Ventricular tachycardia*

1. The occurrence of ventricular tachycardia should always be viewed as an emergency situation and the physician must be called at once.

2. Lidocaine should be prepared in the manner just described for PVC's, and the defibrillator should be turned on for immediate use in case lidocaine is unsuccessful.

3. In some instances ventricular tachycardia may be death-producing in its own right (without degenerating to ventricular fibrillation). If the patient becomes unconscious during the course of ventricular tachycardia, the nurse should use precordial shock in precisely the same manner as if ventricular fibrillation existed.

*Advanced heart block*

1. The nurse's ability to detect the first evidence of advancing heart block, or the sudden development of complete heart block, is of supreme importance in view of the high mortality anticipated once ventricular standstill occurs.

2. The physician members of the intensive care team should be alerted immediately.

3. Equipment and other materials needed for cardiac pacing should be assembled for the physician's use.

4. One mg of isoproterenol (Isuprel) should be diluted in 500 cc of 5% D/W for intravenous use prior to, and during, the insertion of the pacing catheter.

*Marked bradycardia*

1. A gradual or sudden decrease in the heart rate to 50 or less per minute is a potentially serious circumstance. However, the threat of a sudden catastrophe is considerably less than with advanced heart block. The nurse should keep the physician apprised of any reduction in the heart rate below 60/minute.

2. Atropine (1 mg) and pacing equipment should be readied.

*Prophylactic Transvenous Pacing*

1. The nursing role in prophylactic cardiac pacing begins before the procedure is contemplated or accomplished. It involves the detection of the electrocardiographic warnings of ventricular standstill by continuous cardiac monitoring. Because the nurse is in constant attendance, she has the greatest opportunity (and responsibility) to recognize the onset of advanced heart block or marked bradycardia. On the basis of this observation, the physician member of the intensive care team can be alerted to these danger signals before a lethal arrhythmia develops.

2. Once a decision is made to insert a pacemaker catheter, the nurse should promptly assemble the necessary materials. It is good practice to have the catheter, needles, syringes, and sterile drapes packaged in advance and ready for immediate use. The procedure should be explained to the patient by the nurse and physician.

3. The skin site selected for catheter insertion (arm, jugular, or subclavian areas) should be prepared in customary fashion with sterile techniques.

4. After the skin is infiltrated with a local anesthetic, a large needle (usually 14 gauge, with a cannula, stylus, and plastic sheath) is placed in the vein. The selected catheter is then introduced through this conduit, and advanced to the right ventricle (Fig. 11) by means of either fluoroscopic or electrocardiographic guidance. The nurse should assist in these phases of the procedure.

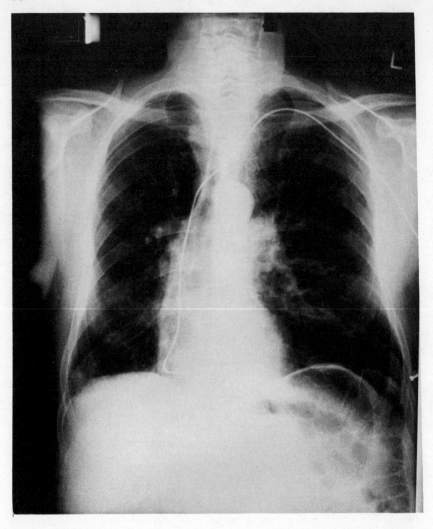

*Fig. 11*

5. The rate and intensity of the pacing impulse is set by the physician. The nurse must repeatedly observe the monitor thereafter to ascertain that the pacemaker continues to function properly. Because the tip of the catheter can be easily displaced by the patient's movements in bed, it is particularly important that the nurse explain to the patient the need for limited motion while the catheter is in place. Catheters inserted by way of arm veins

are especially subject to displacement and occasionally the arm must be immobilized to prevent this problem.

THE LETHAL ARRHYTHMIAS

*Ventricular Standstill*

Compared to ventricular fibrillation, the results of resuscitation after ventricular standstill are extremely poor. If life is to be saved when ventricular standstill occurs, the nurse-physician team must function at its most effective level.

In the event that ventricular standstill develops *before* a transvenous pacemaker has been inserted, the following steps should be taken by the nurse:

1. When the low-rate alarm sounds and the ECG pattern suggests ventricular standstill, the nurse should proceed instantly to the bedside to determine whether the patient is unconscious.

2. The chest should be punched directly over the heart with a forceful blow. As noted, this impact may re-establish the ventricular beat.

3. A call should be sounded for the physician and other personnel.

4. External cardiac massage and mouth-to-mouth breathing should be started by the nurse and continued until other assistance is available.

5. When the physician arrives, external, transthoracic, or transvenous pacing will be attempted.

6. Other nursing personnel should institute oxygen therapy and assemble and prepare the pacing equipment and drugs that will be used in the resuscitative attempt, as well as in the subsequent management program.

If an external pacemaker electrode is in place (a common practice in many institutions) when the catastrophe occurs, the pacemaker should be activated before any other step is taken. The sooner these impulses are initiated the greater the chance of reactivating the heartbeat. If the external pacemaker electrode is not already positioned on the chest wall when ventricular standstill begins, the nurse may still be able to attach it and start external pacing, provided all the necessary equipment is directly at hand. The nurse should not, however, spend time assembling this equipment at the expense of external cardiac massage and mouth-to-mouth breathing.

On some occasions ventricular standstill may begin in a patient who has a transvenous pacemaker catheter already positioned in the right ventricle. The development of ventricular standstill in this special circumstance indicates one of the following problems:

a. The pacemaker itself is not functioning, either as the result of a mechanical disorder or because the device is turned off. This latter situation may sometimes be deliberate. For example, a pacemaker catheter may be inserted prophylactically when the patient has a lesser degree of heart block and the equipment is not activated, but is kept in a "standby" position, to be used if the block progresses or if standstill develops. In this event instant activation of the pacemaker is often life-saving.

b. The terminals of the catheter electrode have become disconnected from the pacing device. The nurse should examine these two connections.

c. The electrode tip has become displaced from the endocardial wall of the ventricle, so that the stimulus does not reach the myocardium. Usually, this requires some repositioning of the catheter by the physician; however, if ventricular standstill occurs as a result of this displacement, the nurse should turn the patient on his side, in the hope that this will re-establish contact. If this is unsuccessful, external cardiac massage should be started and continued until the physician can re-establish the electrical circuit.

*Ventricular Fibrillation*

In most instances survival after ventricular fibrillation is directly dependent on the nurse's speed in reacting to the crisis and her competence in carrying out life-saving measures.

The nurse must never forget that the usual period between the onset of ventricular fibrillation and death is less than two minutes. Because of the desperate shortness of this period, the nurse must often defibrillate the patient before others arrive to assist. The ability of a nurse to recognize ventricular fibrillation and terminate this arrhythmia with precordial shock within the very short period of two minutes (or less) is clearly related to an understanding of the problem and previous training in handling this catastrophe.

The steps to be followed when ventricular fibrillation is identified on the monitor are as follows:

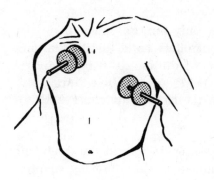

1. Observe the patient immediately to ascertain his lack of consciousness.

2. Turn on the defibrillator and set the discharge energy at its maximal level (400 watt-seconds); make certain the synchronizer is "OFF."

3. Apply a generous amount of electrode paste to the defibrillator paddles and position the paddles on the chest wall in the positions shown in Fig. 12.

*Fig. 12*

4. Hold the paddles tightly against the chest; the energy is then discharged with the trigger.

5. In most instances precordial shock delivered with a proper technique will terminate fibrillation instantly. If the arrhythmia persists, a second shock should be given immediately.

It is of utmost importance that defibrillation be accomplished as soon as the arrhythmia is detected and that no time be spent in starting oxygen or performing external cardiac massage. These latter measures, while valuable outside an intensive care facility, represent a tragic waste of time in a setting where defibrillation can be accomplished immediately.

6. After normal sinus rhythm has been restored by defibrillation, the nurse has many duties and responsibilities relative to the subsequent management of the patient. Of most importance is her role in the prevention of recurrence of this lethal arrhythmia. She must be vigilant and seek electrocardiographic warnings indicative of the threat of recurrence.

***Cardiogenic shock.*** As noted in the preceding discussion of cardiogenic shock, the results of treatment are very poor or hopeless when shock of this type is in an advanced stage. The earlier shock is detected and treated the greater the chance for survival.

By recognizing comparative changes in the heart rate, blood pressure, and electrocardiogram, the development of shock may sometimes be noted in an early stage. The nurse should not merely take vital signs and record them, but she should always compare these with previous recordings in a thoughtful way to identify any trend.

Once shock is fully apparent, only the combined integrated action of the physician-nurse team offers hope for maintaining the patient's life. The specific nursing duties at this point are related to the treatment program being used. These duties and actions are described in detail in the chapter on shock and are not repeated here.

*Congestive heart failure.* The nursing role in the treatment of left ventricular failure is considered in the following chapter, "Circulatory Emergencies."

Although acute left ventricular failure (pulmonary edema) may develop with apparent suddenness, there are usually prodromal warnings to suggest that this complication of acute myocardial infarction is developing.

The likelihood of detecting such failure before it becomes overt can be greatly increased by repeated and planned observation of the patient at the bedside. The nurse should be particularly aware of the early symptoms that may precede overt left ventricular failure. These include mild dyspnea, orthopnea ("Could you raise the head of the bed a little?"), cough, restlessness, and insomnia.

During her nursing care the nurse can often detect the presence of distended neck veins (with the bed positioned at a 45° angle), which are one of the earliest signs of the failing heart. Thus, the keystone of the nursing role revolves about careful observation.

*Thromboembolism.* The problem, treatment, and nursing role of pulmonary and systemic thromboembolic complications are specifically considered in the following chapter. It is, nevertheless, worthwhile to mention briefly certain aspects of the nursing role as they particularly relate to acute myocardial infarction.

*Bed rest as a source of thromboembolism.* There is little doubt that the customary practice of treating patients with acute myocardial infarction with "complete bed rest" contributes to the high incidence of thromboembolism. Many physicians have relaxed the strict programs, used in earlier years, for this reason. It is important that the physician-nurse team interpret "complete bed rest" similarly so that consistency in management can be achieved. While bed rest may ultimately prove to be of great importance (a fact not clearly proved thus far), it seems unreasonable that *all patients* would require the identical type of bed rest. Ideally, bed rest should be individualized and based upon the clinical picture, including the presence or absence of chest pain, fatigue, arrhythmias, and heart failure. There has been a tendency to liberalize patient activity and to permit the patient to sit in a bedside chair. The nurse should observe the response to this activity and take careful note of the development of arrhythmias during this period. The extent of subsequent activity can be gauged in this way.

*Straining at stool as a source of embolism.* The occurrence of pulmonary embolism during defecation is sufficiently common to merit attention. Presumably, the increase in venous pressure created by straining at stool is the precipitating factor in the development of embolic phenomena. There is good evidence to show that the use of the bedside commode is associated with less straining and less expenditure of energy than is the use of the bedpan.

**Ventricular Rupture.** Rupture of the left ventricular wall in almost all instances results in sudden death. The major nursing duty is to make certain that the sudden loss of consciousness, heartbeat, and blood pressure are not due to treatable and reversible causes such as ventricular fibrillation and standstill.

If the rupture occurs in the interventricular wall, death may not be abrupt. The sudden onset of right ventricular failure in conjunction with decreased left ventricular performance should create suspicion that interventricular septal rupture may have occurred.

## Bibliography

*Texts*

BELAND, I. S.: *Clinical Nursing.* Macmillan Co., New York, 1965.

BELLET, S.: *Clinical Disorders of the Heartbeat,* ed. 2. Lea and Febiger, Philadelphia, 1963.

BREST, A. N., and MOYER, J. H.: *Cardiovascular Drug Therapy.* Grune and Stratton, New York and London, 1965.

BURCH, G., and WINSOR, T.: *A Primer of Electrocardiography,* ed. 4. Lea and Febiger, Philadelphia, 1960.

CECIL, R. L., and LOEB, R. F.: *A Textbook of Medicine,* ed. 11. Benson and McDermott (eds), W. B. Saunders Co., Philadelphia, 1963.

*Coronary Care Units—Specialized Intensive Care Units for Acute Myocardial Infarction Patients.* U.S. Department of Health, Education and Welfare: Public Health Service Publication No. 1250: Division of Chronic Diseases, Heart Disease Control Program, Washington, D.C. 1964.

FOWLER, N.: *Physical Diagnosis of Heart Disease.* Macmillan Co., New York, 1962.

FRIEDBERG, C. K.: *Diseases of the Heart.* ed 3. W. B. Saunders Co., Philadelphia, 1966.

GOODMAN, L. S., and GILMAN, A.: *The Pharmacological Basis of Therapeutics,* ed 2. The Macmillan Co., New York, 1955.

GORDON, A. S. (ed): *Cardiopulmonary Resuscitation Conference Proceedings,* Conducted by the Ad Hoc Committee on Cardiopulmonary Resuscitation, Division of Medical Sciences of the National Research Council; Washington, D.C. Printing and Publishing Office of National Academy of Sciences, 23 May 1966.

HARRISON, T. R., and REEVES, T. J.: *Principles and Problems of Ischemic Heart Disease.* Year Book Med. Pub., Inc., Chicago, 1968.

HURST, J. W. and LOGUE, R. B.: *The Heart, Arteries and Veins.* McGraw-Hill, New York, 1966.

MELTZER, L. E., PINNEO, R., and KITCHELL, J. R.: *Intensive Coronary Care—A Manual for Nurses.* The Charles Press, Philadelphia, 1965.

MELTZER, L. E., KITCHELL, J. R., KILLIP, T., LOWN, B., GAZES, P., UNGER, P.: *The Current Status of Intensive Coronary Care.* The Charles Press, Philadelphia, 1966.

MELTZER, L. E., KITCHELL, J. R. (ed.) et al.: *Cardiac Pacing and Cardioversion.* The Charles Press, Philadelphia, 1967.

MODELL, W. et al.: *Handbook of Cardiology for Nurses,* ed. 5. Springer Pub. Co., New York, 1966.

WEIL, M. H., and SHUBIN, H.: *Diagnosis and Treatment of Shock.* Williams and Wilkins Co., Baltimore, 1967.

WHEELER, DOROTHY (ed.) et al.: *Aggressive Nursing Management of Acute Myocardial Infarction.* The Charles Press, Philadelphia, 1968.

*Periodicals*

ABREU, X.: An Experience in the Nursing Care of Selected Patients on Electronic Monitors. Monograph 5, *A.N.A.* 1962 Clinical Sessions, pp. 18–36.

BAKER, P. A.: Myocardial Infarction Accompanied by Cardiogenic Shock. *Nurs. Times* 63:338, 17 Mar. 1967.

BEAN, M. et al.: Monitoring Patients Through Electronics. *Amer. J. Nurs.* 63:65–69, Apr. 1963.

BERNSTEIN, H.: Drug Treatment of Cardiac Arrhythmias. *Amer. J. Nurs.* 64:118–120, Jul. 1964.

BRAUNWALD, E.: The Pathogenesis and Treatment of Shock in Myocardial Infarction. *Johns Hopkins Med. J.* 121:421, Dec. 1967.

BRUCE, T. A. and BING, R. J.: Clinical Management of Myocardial Infarction. *J.A.M.A.* 191:124–126, 11 Jan. 1965.

CAMPBELL, E. J.: Methods of Oxygen Administration in Respiratory Failure. *Ann. N.Y. Acad. Sci.* 121:861–870, 24 Mar. 1965.

COHEN, D. B., DOCTOR, L., and PICK, A.: The Significance of Atrioventricular Block Complicating Acute Myocardial Infarction. *Amer. Heart J.,* 55:215–219, Feb. 1958.

COHN, J. N.: Myocardial Infarction Shock Revisited. *Amer. Heart J.* 74:1, Jul. 1967.

COODLEY, E. L.: Current Status of Enzyme Diagnosis in Cardiovascular Disease. *Amer. J. Med. Sci.* 252:633, Dec. 1966.

CRAWLEY, M.: Care of the Patient with Myocardial Infarction. *Amer. J. Nurs.* 61:68–70, Feb. 1961.

DAY, H. W.: Effectiveness of an Intensive Coronary Care Area. *Amer. J. Cardiol.* 15:51–54, Jan. 1965.

DENBOROUGH, M. A. et al.: Arrhythmias and Late Sudden Death After Myocardial Infarction. *Lancet* 1:386, 24 Feb. 1968.

FAULK, E. A., Jr. and HURST, J. W.: Clinical Problems of Cardioversion. *Amer. Heart J.* 70:248–274, Aug. 1965.

FOWLER, N. O.: Physical Signs in Acute Myocardial Infarction and Its Complications. *Progr. Cardiovasc. Dis.* 10:287, Jan. 1968 (41 ref.).

GEDDES, J. S., et al.: Prognosis After Recovery from Ventricular Fibrillation Complicating Ischemic Heart Disease, *Lancet* 2:273, 5 Aug. 1967.

GROSSMAN, J. I. et al.: Lidocaine in Cardiac Arrhythmias. *Arch. Int. Med.* (Chicago) 121:396, May 1968.

HARRIS, A. et al.: Treatment of Slow Heart Rates Following Acute Myocardial Infarction. *Brit. Heart J.* 28:631, Sep. 1966.

HARRISON, T. R.: Psychological Management of Patients with Cardiac Disease. *Amer. Heart J.* 70:136, 1965.

HURWITZ, M. and ELIOT, R. S.: Arrhythmias in Acute Myocardial Infarction, *Dis. of the Chest* 45:616–626, June 1964.

JEWITT, D. E. et al.: Incidence and Management of Supraventricular Arrhythmias After Acute Myocardial Infarction. *Lancet* 2:734, 7 Oct. 1967.

JUDE, J. R., KOUWENHAVEN, W. B., and KNICKERBOCKER, C. G.: Cardiac Arrest: Report of Application of External Cardiac Massage on 118 Patients. *J.A.M.A.* 178:1063–1070, 16 Dec. 1961.

JULIAN, D. G. et al.: Disturbances of Rate, Rhythm and Conduction in Acute Myocardial Infarction: A Prospective Study of 100 Consecutive Unselected Patients with the Aid of Electrocardiographic Monitoring. *Amer. J. Med.* 37:915, Dec. 1964.

KANNEL, W. B. et al.: Epidemiology of Coronary Heart Disease. *Geriatrics* 17:675–689. Oct. 1962.

KILLIP, T.: Treatment of Myocardial Infarction in a Coronary Care Unit. *A. J. Cardiol.* 20:457, Oct. 1967.

KILLIP, T. and KIMBALL, J. R.: A Simple Bedside Method for Transvenous Intracardiac Pacing. *Amer. Heart J.* 70:35–39, Jul. 1965.

KILLIP, T.: Synchronized DC Precordial Shock for Arrhythmias. *J.A.M.A.* 186:1–7, 5 Oct. 1963.

LEW, E.: Survivorship After Myocardial Infarction. *Amer. J. Pub. Health* 57:118, Jan. 1967.

LOWN, B.: The Coronary Care Unit, New Perspectives and Directions. *J.A.M.A.* 199:188, 16 Jan. 1967.

LOWN, B.: "Cardioversion" of Arrhythmias, I. *Mod. Concepts Cardiovasc. Dis.* 33:869–873, Aug. 1964.

LOWN, B. et al.: "Cardioversion" of Atrial Fibrillation. *N.E.J.M.* 269:325–331, 15 Aug. 1963.

LYON, A. F., and DeGRAFF, A. C.: Antiarrhythmic Drugs. Part II. Clinical Use of Quinidine. *Amer. Heart J.* 69:834–837, Jun. 1965.

McCALLUM, H. P.: The Nurse and the Respirator. *Nurs. Clinics N. Amer.* 1(4):597, Dec. 1966.

MELTZER, L. E. and KITCHELL, J. R.: The Incidence of Arrhythmias Associated with Acute Myocardial Infarction. *Prog. Cardiovasc. Dis.* 9(1):50–63, 1966.

MELTZER, L. E.: Coronary Care, Electrocardiography and the Nurse. *Amer. J. Nurs.* 65 (12):63–67 Dec. 1965.

MELTZER, L. E.: Concept and System for Intensive Coronary Care. *Acad. Med. of N.J. Bull.* 10 (4):304–311, Dec. 1964.

MELTZER, L. E. et al.: Prothrombin Levels and Fatality Rates in Acute Myocardial Infarction. *J.A.M.A.* 187:986–993, 1964.

MINOGUE, W. F., SMESSART, A. A., and GRACE, W. J.: External Cardiac Massage for Cardiac Arrest Due to Myocardial Infarction. *Amer. J. Cardiol.* 13:25–29, Jan. 1964.

MOWER, M. M., MILLER, D. J., and NACHLAS, M. M.: Clinical Features Relative to Possible Resuscitation in Death After Acute Myocardial Infarction. *Amer. Heart J.* 67:437–444, Apr. 1964.

NACHLAS, M. M., and MILLER, D. J.: Closed Chest Cardiac Resuscitation in Patients with Acute Myocardial Infarction. *Amer. Heart J.* 69:448–459, Apr. 1965.

PANTRIDGE, J. F.: Cardiac Arrest After Myocardial Infarction. *Lancet* 1:807, Apr. 1966.

PARKER, D. L. et al.: Delirium in a Coronary Care Unit. *J.A.M.A.* 201: 702, 28 Aug. 1967.

PEEL, A. A. F. et al.: A Coronary Prognostic Index for Grading Severity of Infarction. *Brit. Heart J.* 24:745, Nov. 1962.

PINNEO, R.: Nursing in a Coronary Unit. *Amer. J. Nurs.* 65(2):76–79, Feb. 1965.

RESTIEAUX, N. et al.: 150 Patients with Myocardial Infarction—Treated in the Coronary Care Unit. *Lancet* 1:1285, 17 Jun. 1967.

REYNOLDS, E. W.: The Use of Potassium in the Treatment of Heart Disease. *Amer. Heart J.* 70:1–5, Jul. 1965.

ROSENBERG, B., DOBKIN, G., and RUBIN, R.: The Intravenous Use of Ethacrynic Acid in the Management of Acute Pulmonary Edema. *Amer. Heart J.* 70:333–336, Sep. 1965.

ROTHFIELD, E. L. et al.: Idioventricular Rhythm in Acute Myocardial Infarction. *Circ.* 3:203, Feb. 1968.

SAFAR, P. et al.: Resuscitative Principles for Sudden Cardio-Pulmonary Collapse. *Dis. Chest* 43:34–49, Jan. 1963.

SAMPSON, J. J. et al.: Heart Failure in Myocardial Infarction. *Prog. Cardiovasc. Dis.* 10:1–29, Jul. 1967 (112 ref).

SHUBIN, H. et al.: The Treatment of Shock Complicating Acute Myocardial Infarction. *Progr. Cardiov. Dis.* 10:30, Jul. 1967 (182 ref).

SLOMAN, G. et al.: Coronary Care Unit: A Review of 300 Patients Monitored Since 1963. *Amer. Heart J.* 75:140, Jan. 1968.

SOWTON, E.: Cardiac Pacemakers and Pacing. *Mod. Concepts Cardiovasc. Dis.* 36:31, Jun. 1967.

SPANN, J. F. et al.: Arrhythmias in Acute Myocardial Infarction. *N.E.J.M.* 271:427–431, 27 Aug. 1964.

STEINBERG, J. S. and HURST, J. W.: The New Role of the Nurse in Cardiac Arrest. *Nurs. Clin. of N. Amer.* 2:245, 2 Jun. 1967.

WOLFF, I. S. et al.: The Patient with Myocardial Infarction. Spec. Supp., *Amer. J. Nurs.* 64:(11), C 1–32, Nov. 1964.

ZOLL, P. M.: Sudden Cardiac Death, A Review of Its Pathophysiology and a Discussion of Cardiac Monitoring. *J.A.M.A.* 186:34–36, Nov. 1963.

ZOLL, P. M. et al.: Ventricular Fibrillation: Treatment and Prevention by External Electric Currents. *N.E.J.M.* 262:105–112, 21 Jan. 1960.

# Chapter III

# Circulatory Emergencies

JOHN T. KIMBALL, M.D.
MARY T. BIELSKI, R.N., M.S.
JOHN E. LEE, M.D.
MARILYN ABRAHAM, R.N., M.S.

PART I

## *The Stroke Syndrome*

### THE PROBLEM

It is hardly an exaggeration to say that the purpose of all medical care is to preserve brain function. Surgical restoration of a defective heart valve, renal dialysis, treatment of shock, insulin therapy, and fluid and electrolyte replacement all have the common goal of preventing brain damage and restoring intellectual function. In an intensive care unit this goal is especially evident, for the nervous system is directly threatened by the entire spectrum of severe illness. It is important to recognize these threats and to prevent their consequences. This section deals specifically with failure of circulation to the brain. The pertinence of this discussion to intensive care is not only the management of the patient with a stroke, but also the prevention of brain damage in any patient whose circulatory and metabolic regulation is precarious.

Anyone caring for severely ill patients should be aware of the extreme vulnerability of the brain and of its rigid requirements for constant supplies of oxygen and glucose via the circulating blood. Though it contributes less than 3% of total body weight, the human brain consumes 25% of the oxygen used by the body at rest and receives 15% of cardiac output. It utilizes more than 80% of the glucose secreted by the liver at rest. These are strict demands and must be met constantly if the brain is to function properly. The brain has no storage capability for oxygen or glucose and is entirely dependent on its blood supply. If the cerebral blood supply is cut off, consciousness is lost within ten seconds, and within two to three minutes irreparable brain damage begins. Beyond this point no degree of medical skill and no intensity of nursing care can restore or replace lost neurons.

Stroke refers to the rapid or sudden impairment of cerebral circulation with resultant disturbance of neurologic function. It includes cerebral infarction, which is destruction of brain tissue due to arterial thrombosis or embolism, and intracranial hemorrhage either into brain tissue or into the subarachnoid space surrounding the brain.

**Cerebral infarction.** Cerebral infarction implies necrosis of brain tissue and is the final result of arterial insufficiency or ischemia. Its usual cause is atherosclerotic narrowing or occlusion of the larger arteries in the neck or near the base of the brain, with thrombus formation at the narrowed site. Prolonged hypertension also leads to arterial narrowing, but affects smaller arteries more than does atherosclerosis and often causes multiple focal infarctions within the brain. These may appear over a period of many months as a series of small strokes. Diabetes is accompanied by narrowing of both large and small arteries, and is associated particularly with strokes in the young and middle aged.

Cerebral infarction may also result from embolism. Chronic atrial fibrillation, myocardial infarction, mitral stenosis, and bacterial endocarditis are the heart disorders most likely to produce cerebral embolism. Fat embolism may follow large bone fractures or severe crushing injuries. One of the hazards of cardiac surgery is cerebral embolism produced by air or fragments of clot or tissue.

**Intracranial hemorrhage.** Intracranial hemorrhage causes brain damage primarily by direct destruction of tissue. Blood may escape from a ruptured artery under high pressure and form a hematoma within the brain which displaces surrounding structures. Cerebral hemorrhage is most often the result of hypertension. Hemorrhage from an arterial aneurysm can be directed entirely into the subarachnoid space, but usually enters brain tissue as well. Subarachnoid hemorrhage alone is not necessarily associated with neurologic deficit, but the irritant nature of the blood breakdown products may cause arterial spasm and subsequent ischemia.

**Precipitating factors.** There are several factors which may precipitate strokes, particularly when the cerebral circulation is already compromised by atherosclerosis. It is important that each of these factors be controlled if strokes are to be prevented:

1. Decreased cardiac output: myocardial ischemia or infarction, congestive heart failure.
2. Hypotension: acute blood or fluid loss, peripheral vasodilation (fever, septicemia, postural hypotension.
3. Anemia: hemoglobin less than 10 grams.
4. Hypoglycemia.
5. Hypoxia.
6. Polycythemia: hematocrit over 55%.

Any of these factors alone can cause brain damage, but their danger is increased when there is underlying atherosclerotic narrowing of carotid, vertebral, or intracranial arteries.


## ASSESSMENT OF THE PROBLEM

### The Clinical Picture

**Cerebral infarction.** The symptoms of cerebrovascular disease are those of focal neurological disorder of abrupt onset. The specific symptoms depend on which arterial system is involved and which area of the brain is deprived of normal circulation. This localization can be made on the basis of history and neurologic examination, and usually is specific enough to determine at least whether the carotid or the vertebral-basilar arterial system is affected. The symptoms described below are those involving infarction of a large part of the area supplied by the specific arteries; however, less typical cases are found more frequently because of variation in the degree of arterial insufficiency and collateral circulation.

*Carotid artery system.* Carotid artery occlusion characteristically results in hemiplegia, sensory loss, and visual field defect on the *opposite* side of the body. Frequently, weakness is greatest in the hand. If the dominant hemisphere (usually the left) is involved, disturbances of speech and comprehension may be prominent. With non-dominant hemispheric damage, a peculiar indifference to the opposite side of the patient's own body and his environment is often noted.

A similar picture results from occlusion of the middle cerebral artery, and cannot be distinguished with certainty from carotid occlusion. Loss of consciousness does not often occur with the onset of carotid or middle cerebral occlusion.

*Vertebral-basilar system.* Vertebral or basilar artery occlusion is more likely to produce a bilateral neurological deficit. In addition to weakness and sensory loss on one or both sides, dizziness, double vision, and difficult swallowing are common. The mechanical act of speech is impaired, rather than the comprehension of language. Visual field defects are less common. Sudden or rapid loss of consciousness results when the brain stem is severely damaged by basilar artery thrombosis or hemorrhage.

**Cerebral hemorrhage.** Cerebral hemorrhage can occur in the distribution of any artery, but most commonly is deep within one hemisphere or in the vital areas of the brain stem. Headaches and loss of consciousness are frequent with the onset of hemorrhage, and the patient usually is hypertensive.

**Cerebral embolism.** Cerebral embolism can strike any area, but is most frequent in the carotid-middle cerebral distribution. Evidence of heart disease and emboli elsewhere in the body would be expected.

**Classification of strokes.** The temporal profile of onset of cerebral ischemia and infarction is important for both treatment and prognosis of stroke patients and is the basis for the following classification:

1. The impending stroke or transient ischemic attack (TIA).
2. The stroke in evolution or progressive stroke.
3. The completed stroke.

***Transient ischemic attack.*** The TIA is a brief episode of neurologic symptoms lasting usually from a few seconds to about 30 minutes and caused by temporary, reversible insufficiency of blood supply to focal brain areas. The specific symptoms depend on the area of brain involved, but they often can be recognized as belonging to the carotid or the basilar system. Transient weakness, numbness, speech disturbance, blurred vision, dizziness, and confusion occur singly or in combination. The great importance of recognizing these attacks is that they may precede cerebral thrombosis as a warning and provide the opportunity for prevention of permanent brain damage.

The basic pathology of the TIA is a narrowed artery supplying the area affected, but it is not always apparent what transient change in hemodynamics causes the temporary symptoms. Hypotension, cardiac irregularity, minute emboli, smoking, hypoglycemia, anemia, and polycythemia are among the factors which have been associated with these attacks, but often no cause can be found. If the attacks recur repeatedly, complete recovery of function becomes less likely, and permanent neurologic deficit gradually appears.

***Stroke in evolution.*** The stroke in evolution is the progressive development of neurologic deficit due to an increasing degree of cerebral ischemia and infarction. The process may require hours or days for completion, and may be step-wise or gradually progressive. There is no way to determine at any point in the evolution how much further damage will occur. Neurologic symptoms will be slight at first and gradually increase in severity and in the variety of disturbed functions. The pathologic process causing the stroke is thought to be extension of a thrombus, which occludes the artery in which it originated or extends to additional arteries.

***Completed stroke.*** The majority of strokes are complete before the patient reaches medical care. The onset of stroke is usually abrupt, and often occurs during sleep or shortly after arising;

maximum damage is reached within minutes, and the patient is aware of a sudden catastrophe which has deprived him of strength, sensation, speech, or vision. Unconsciousness rarely accompanies acute cerebral infarction unless it involves a large portion of a cerebral hemisphere or the brain stem.

**Physical examination.** The extent and progress of brain disease from stroke are assessed by the neurologic examination. Among patients in whom complete neurologic evaluation is not possible or feasible, much valuable information can be obtained by a few careful observations. Neurologic function can deteriorate rapidly, but changes can be detected if serial observations have been made with accuracy and recorded for reference. The most informative measures of neurologic function are:

1. State of consciousness.
2. Respiration.
3. Eyes.
4. Motor activity.

*State of consciousness.* State of consciousness can vary from normally alert to comatose. A normally alert patient is clearly oriented to time, place, and person, can discuss the circumstances of his hospitalization in reasonable detail, can do simple calculations, and responds appropriately to his environment. Specific questions should be asked to determine each of these points, and the answers recorded. Casual social conversation is inadequate for evaluating mental status and provides no basis for future reference. The mental status of the patient who has lost language function can be evaluated (although less precisely) by noting his interest in his environment and his ability to carry out motor tasks. Deterioration of mental status means progression of brain dysfunction, and must be detected in its early stages if therapy is to be effective. Such deterioration may not always be quietly progressive. The irritable, irascible patient, the patient who is inappropriately facetious (especially toward nurses), or the one who is simply inattentive may be displaying symptoms of organically disturbed mentation.

*Respiration.* Disease of the central nervous system causes three main patterns of abnormal breathing, according to the location of brain damage:

1. CHEYNE-STOKES RESPIRATION is characterized by a regular, waxing and waning pattern, each cycle gradually alternating between hyperventilation and apnea. It indicates the presence of bilateral brain disease resulting from either structural damage or anoxia. Since Cheyne-Stokes breathing is often accompanied by decreased alertness, its onset is an important visible and audible clue to a change in neurologic status. It first becomes apparent when the patient is asleep.

2. NEUROGENIC HYPERVENTILATION is a deep, forceful, regular breathing which accompanies damage to the pontine area of the brain stem. Patients with this respiratory pattern are unconscious. A change from Cheyne-Stokes to sustained hyperventilation represents an extension of brain damage, probably to irreparable levels.

3. ATAXIC BREATHING is completely irregular in rate and amplitude, and is the usual pattern just preceding total respiratory failure in progressive brain stem lesions. It may occur, however, even in alert patients with low brain stem disorders, but is always a danger signal indicating that artificial respiration may be required at any moment.

It is important to consider non-neurological disturbances of respiration in assessing the breathing pattern of patients with stroke. The incidence of pneumonia, congestive heart failure, and pulmonary embolism is high in these patients and these problems must be distinguished from neurological disorders of respiration.

*Eyes.* The pupils and extraocular movements are important features to be noted by repeated examinations. Normally, the pupils are equal in size and constrict briskly in response to bright light. The resting position of the eyes is straight ahead (or slightly divergent during sleep), and the two eyes should move smoothly and in parallel through their full range of motion. Eye movements can be tested by voluntary fixation of gaze or by following a moving object. Inequality of the pupils or a sluggish or absent light reflex may be the only signs of increased intracranial pressure. Loss of full extraocular movements and deviation of resting eye position are further signs of intracranial hypertension.

*Motor activity.* Valuable information about the motor system can be obtained by simply observing the patient. Awake or asleep, normal patients usually move all four extremities when changing posture and position. Persistence of a single posture or paucity of movement in an extremity suggests weakness. An externally rotated foot suggests loss of normal tone in the leg. Prolonged or spasmodic rigid extension of both legs (or of all the extremities) is a sign of severe disturbance of the upper brain stem (decerebrate rigidity). In a conscious patient, motor strength can be tested simply by having him hold both arms elevated at 45 degrees; this can be timed to the point of fatigue for easy quantitation. Patients with stroke occasionally have motor seizures. Careful observation of the location of onset and spread of seizure activity can lead to specific localization of the site of brain injury.

**Diagnostic procedures.**

*Lumbar Puncture.* Lumbar puncture (spinal tap) is performed to measure intracranial pressure and to obtain a specimen of cerebrospinal fluid (CSF). Spinal tap is warranted when there is serious doubt as to diagnosis (e.g., cerebral infarction vs. intracranial hemorrhage). However, the practical value of the information to be obtained must outweigh the risk. While this risk is generally negligible, in the presence of increased intracranial pressure the procedure can be disastrous, since rapid changes in intracranial fluid dynamics may cause the brain to shift and be compressed against the unyielding skull or meninges. It is prudent policy to examine the optic fundi and skull x-rays for evidence of intracranial hypertension immediately before performing a spinal tap. When a spinal tap is attempted, if the opening pressure is above 300 mm, the needle should be withdrawn at once; with lesser pressures an appropriate amount of CSF should be collected for laboratory tests. CSF is observed for color and clarity by comparing it with water against a white background; normal CSF is sparkling clear and colorless. A specimen is examined promptly for cells, and another specimen is sent to the laboratory for determination of protein and sugar content and for serologic testing. Cultures for pyogenic bacteria, tubercle bacilli, and fungi, as well as cytologic exam for tumor cells, can be performed when indicated. It is not necessary for a patient to lie in bed for any specific time following spinal tap. If headache ensues, it may be relieved by having the patient lie flat in bed.

*Arteriography.* The cerebral arteriogram is an x-ray of the brain's vascular system obtained by injecting a radiopaque solution into the carotid artery by means of catheters, or high pressure injections into brachial, femoral, or axillary arteries. A complete arteriographic study requires a combination of these techniques for visualization of both carotid, and both vertebral, arteries. The purposes of arteriography are to confirm the diagnosis, to locate the site of arterial stricture or obstruction, and to outline any surgically treatable arterial lesions. Although local anesthesia is usually employed, the procedure remains uncomfortable and, for some patients, frightening. The patient should be in the fasting state for arteriography. There is a small but definite risk that arteriography will at least temporarily worsen the patient's neurologic condition. Part of the risk is from hematoma at the arterial puncture site and can be minimized by applying firm pressure to the site for at least ten minutes immediately on removing the needle, followed by an ice pack for 30–60 minutes and repeated observation of the puncture site and the pulse in the affected artery.

*Electroencephalography.* The electroencephalogram (EEG) is a record of the location of disturbed cerebral function. The electrodes are either small metal discs (applied with paste) or thin needles which are inserted into the scalp. The procedure entails no significant discomfort, risk, or special precautions.

*Echoencephalography.* This test measures the reflection of sound waves from midline structures of the brain and serves to detect displacement of brain tissue by intracranial mass lesions. High frequency sound waves are directed through the intact scalp, and their echo is recorded photographically, all without danger or discomfort.


## PRINCIPLES OF TREATMENT

### Immediate management of cerebral ischemia

At the onset a transient ischemic attack cannot be distinguished from cerebral infarction. In either case the same immediate steps are taken as soon as symptoms of cerebral ischemia are recognized. These steps are often diagnostic as well as therapeutic.

1. The patient is kept initially in the supine position to enhance cerebral blood flow. (This position should not be maintained for prolonged periods.

2. Blood pressure is supported with vasopressors if the diastolic pressure is below 60 mm Hg.

3. As soon as a blood sample is drawn for sugar determination, 25 grams of glucose should be given by mouth or by vein as a 50% solution.

4. Oxygen by nasal catheter with a flow of 6 liters per minute should be started. Even with fully saturated hemoglobin the small increment of oxygen dissolved in plasma may be beneficial. Carbon dioxide inhalation (5% $CO_2$ with oxygen rather than paperbag rebreathing, which leads to hypoxia) has been advocated to dilate cerebral arteries and increase blood flow. The value of this has not been established, since there is no evidence that the blood flow is increased to the ischemic brain area by this means.

5. An electrocardiogram should be taken to ascertain any arrhythmias or the presence of acute myocardial infarction. It is not uncommon for the stroke syndrome to accompany acute myocardial infarction (by embolization or cerebral ischemia). All patients with stroke should have an electrocardiogram promptly after admission.

6. If there is evidence of cardiac failure, rapid digitalization is indicated to improve the circulation.

7. Procaine block of the stellate ganglion to remove sympathetic vasoconstriction may increase cerebral blood flow in some patients, but there is no assurance that the added flow is being shared by areas of ischemia.

It will have become apparent by the time these measures have been undertaken whether the ischemic symptoms were those of a self-limited transient attack or were the beginning of an evolving cerebral infarct. At this point additional diagnostic and therapeutic measures must be considered.

### Definitive therapeutic approaches

**Anticoagulation.** The value of anticoagulation has been established for the treatment of transient ischemic attacks, cerebral embolism, and stroke in evolution. The two anticoagulents most widely used are warfarin and heparin. Each has its specific uses and advantages.

*Warfarin (Coumadin, Panwarfin).* The initial dose of warfarin is 20–35 mgm followed the next day by 10–15 mgm. Thereafter maintenance doses of 2.5 mgm to 10 mgm daily are usual, but must be carefully regulated in accordance with the prothrombin time. By the commonly used Quick method, prothrombin time is reported in seconds and in per cent of normal prothrombin activity. For optimum anticoagulant therapy, the prothrombin time is maintained at approximately $2\frac{1}{2}$ times the control value in seconds, or 15–20% of normal. The usual procedure is to draw a blood specimen for prothrombin time in the morning and to give warfarin in the evening after the laboratory result is known.

Anticoagulation can be continued indefinitely by this method, though daily prothrombin times are unnecessary after stable levels have been maintained for 7–10 days.

*Heparin.* Rapid anticoagulation with heparin is used to impede the progress of evolving stroke and to prevent recurrence of cerebral emboli. Effective anticoagulation can be attained within ten minutes by the use of heparin sodium intravenously. Heparin may be given by intermittent injections or by continuous intravenous drip. An effective intermittent method is to give 5,000–10,000 USP units intravenously every four hours. About one hour before the next scheduled injection, a whole blood coagulation time (Lee-White method) is determined. Clotting time should be nearly normal (6–10 minutes) before the next dose of heparin is given to prevent cumulative effects which would increase the risk of bleeding. Once regulation is obtained, less frequent clotting times are required. Even though this method produces peaks and troughs of anticoagulant level, it appears to be effective and relatively safe.

Continuous intravenous heparin is given in dilution of 1,000 USP units per 100 ml physiologic saline (or 5% dextrose in water) at such a rate as to increase clotting time to two to three times normal. Usually, this requires 15–25 drops per minute, but the response is quite variable, and clotting times must be repeated every 30–60 minutes until stability is reached.

Since heparin anticoagulation requires such meticulous care, it is used only until adequate control with warfarin can be achieved. Warfarin may be started concomitantly with heparin therapy and regulated according to prothrombin times as usual, with one important exception. Heparin may prolong the pro-thrombin time, so that the prothrombin time must be checked when the effect of heparin is least, i.e., within an hour before the next heparin injection.

COMPLICATIONS OF ANTICOAGULANT THERAPY

The major complication of anticoagulant therapy is bleeding. Minor bleeding is usually manifested by easy bruising or mild hematomas, and requires only that the level of anticoagulation be reduced temporarily. Small hematomas around injection sites are fairly common, and the fact that they are to be anticipated should be considered in planning drug therapy for anticoagulated pa-tients. Severe hemorrhage is more likely in hypertensive patients or in those with a previous history of peptic ulcer disease. If this problem develops, rapid reversal of anticoagulation with antidotes and replacement of blood loss are mandatory.

Vitamin K is the most effective antidote for oral anticoagu-lants. Minor bleeding or an excessively prolonged prothrombin time can be controlled by 2.5 to 10 mgm Vitamin K, but severe bleeding may require up to 200 mgm. The drug can be given orally as 5 mgm tablets or slowly intravenously as a 10 mgm/ml solution in saline. Ordinarily, prothrombin time will return to normal limits in 6–8 hours.

The duration of the anticoagulant effect produced by heparin administration is so short that minor bleeding can be controlled simply by omitting the next dose. As an antidote, the slow intra-venous injection of 50 mgm protamine sulfate will usually return the clotting time to normal within five minutes. Also, if necessary, the effect of heparin can be counteracted by transfusion with 250 to 500 cc of fresh whole blood.

The principal contraindications to anticoagulant therapy are signs of bleeding, bloody or xanthochromic cerebrospinal fluid, peptic ulcer, hepatic disease, pregnancy, recent treatment with large doses of salicylate or steroids, and hypertension. Except for active bleeding, the remaining factors are only relative contraindi-cations, and the risk must be weighed against the potential benefit of anticoagulation therapy for the particular patient. In patients with stroke, a spinal tap should always be performed before anti-coagulation therapy is initiated. Blood pressure over 180/110 should be carefully reduced by appropriate drugs concomitantly with the administration of anticoagulant medication.

Anticoagulation therapy must usually be discontinued for surgical procedures, though even complex cardiac and vascular surgery can be performed safely with prothrombin times at 25% levels. To interrupt warfarin therapy for surgery, the previous day's dose is omitted; administration of the drug can be resumed the evening following surgery.

A more difficult problem regarding anticoagulant therapy is posed by the appearance of symptoms of cerebral ischemia following arteriography or surgery. To begin heparin therapy promptly in this circumstance is to risk bleeding, but to delay may mean the risk of permanent brain damage. If possible, heparin should be withheld for 12 hours after arteriography or surgery.

**Vascular surgery.** Surgical treatment of stroke has proved effective in many cases and can be expected to be used more widely in the future. Intracranial aneurysms can be clamped off directly, or the pressure within them reduced by carotid compression or ligation. Atherosclerotic plaques can be removed from vertebral and common carotid arteries (at their origins) and from carotid arteries in the neck. Even an occluding thrombus can be removed from the carotid if surgery is performed within a few hours. The entire cervico-cranial circulation must be clearly demonstrated by arteriography prior to surgery. If surgical treatment of acute strokes is planned, it is necessary to have the clinical examination, arteriography, and vascular surgery so smoothly coordinated that the entire procedure can be completed in a few hours at any time of day or night. Otherwise, surgery must be limited to prophylaxis of stroke after stenosis of an appropriate artery has been demonstrated.

**Fibrinolytic therapy.** Enzymatic agents capable of dissolving fibrin thrombi within blood vessels have been used in experimental and clinical situations with some success. At present, however, the usefulness of fibrinolytic enzymes for the treatment of cerebrovascular disease has not been clearly demonstrated.

**Therapy for cerebral edema.** Cerebral ischemia and infarction are followed by edema of the damaged area and surrounding brain tissue. This edema may threaten further brain injury from compression. This is a common phenomenon following cerebral infarction and accounts for the clinical deterioration often observed 24 hours or so after a stroke seems to have stabilized. The symptoms of cerebral edema are those of increasing diffuse cerebral damage and brain stem compression: obtundation, increasing motor deficit, periodic breathing, and abnormalities of pupils and eye movement.

Treatment of cerebral edema following infarction has not yet proved to be very effective. Hypertonic urea and mannitol which cross the blood-brain barrier only slowly may provide temporary relief by their osmotic "drying" effect.

Mannitol is preferable to urea because it is associated with less rebound of intracranial pressure. Furthermore, urea cannot be used in patients with severe renal damage. A 20% solution of mannitol in water is infused by vein in dosages of 1–1.5 grams per kilogram body weight over a period of about 30 minutes. This will reduce intracranial pressure for two to four hours and may be repeated if urine volume is copious. Unless the urinary volume is replaced, dehydration will result.

Glucocorticoids, as well as urea and mannitol, have been more effective in reducing edema of brain tumors than edema of stroke. Dexamethasone is given in an initial dose of 10 mgm intravenously, followed by 4 mgm every 6 hours intramuscularly.

### Prevention of complications

Once a completed stroke has developed, there is little that medical care can do to hasten the restoration of damaged neural tissue. The patient's course at this time is dependent primarily on the presence or absence of complications and specifically on the quality of his medical and nursing care.

The likelihood of complications is markedly increased in the unconscious patient. The principal *complications* among patients in coma are:

*1. Obstruction of airway and aspiration of secretions.* The unconscious patient cannot swallow or cough voluntarily and may have lost swallowing and coughing reflexes. Therefore, some form of artificial airway must be established which can be kept clean, allow easy access to suctioning, and permit adequate airflow. Ideally, the airway should also prevent aspiration. All these requirements are met by the cuffed tracheostomy tube, #6 size or larger. However, tracheostomy should be avoided, if possible, and a cuffed endotracheal tube used unless coma is prolonged. The management of tracheostomy has been considered in detail in Chapter I, "Respiratory Insufficiency and Failure."

**2. *Pneumonia.*** Patients with impaired cough should be kept semi-prone and turned from side to side every two hours. Occasional lung inflation by a positive pressure apparatus helps prevent atelectasis and promotes drainage; but positive pressure can also drive mucus plugs deeper into the lungs unless preceded by thorough suctioning.

Pulmonary infection should be treated with appropriate antibiotics after culture and sensitivity studies have been made. Antibiotics may kill bacteria, but they do not keep an airway clean.

One of the complications of tracheostomy procedure is aspiration of blood. Since blood provides an excellent culture medium in the lung and, in addition, can produce chemical pneumonitis, alveolar-capillary block, and anoxia, bleeding around a tracheostomy site must be detected and stopped promptly.

The likelihood of vomiting and the danger of aspiration are especially great following intracranial hemorrhage or brain-stem infarction.

**3. *Urinary tract infection.*** Shortly after a stroke, many patients develop urinary retention which causes considerable discomfort or agitation. Later, incontinence is a common problem. Either situation requires catheterization; the attendant risk of infection must be recognized. This complication is difficult to avoid, but can be ameliorated by the use of strict sterile technique, condom catheters, when possible, and 3,000 cc fluid intake daily to increase urine flow. Once infection is suspected, cultures and sensitivity tests should be employed to determine appropriate antibiotic therapy.

**4. *Decubitus ulcers.*** Decubitus ulcers of the skin invariably result when patients remain immobile for more than a few hours.

The earliest change in the skin is seen as a fairly well outlined area of redness, followed by edema, blister formation, and then skin breakdown. Decubiti can always be prevented, but cannot always be healed. The basic rule to prevent decubiti is to turn the patient frequently (at least every two hours) and to keep the skin clean and dry. Skin creams with lanolin or mineral oil are sometimes useful. Two of the most effective methods of preventing decubiti are the alternating-pressure mattress and a sheepskin beneath the patient with the fleece side next to his skin.

*5. Limb mobility.* From the very onset of paralysis, it is important to keep the joints freely movable. Movement through a full range of motion several times a day is an essential part of stroke care. To prevent stiff joint and muscle contractures, physical therapy is as much a part of intensive care of stroke patients as any other measure.

*6. Emotional factors.* One of the most devastating effects of a stroke is its emotional impact on the patient, on his family, and on medical personnel caring for him. Initially, everyone tends to despair. The patient one day is alert, active, productive; the next day he is crippled, helpless, dependent. He is afraid of this incapacity, of losing his mind, and of death—all reasonable fears and each terribly difficult to deal with. For example, he may be aphasic and agonizingly frustrated in his ability to communicate. The family shares all these feelings plus the prospect of being burdened with medical costs and the care of an invalid and possibly the loss of family income. They, too, feel helpless, afraid, and often ambivalent in their hopes for the patient's recovery. Medical personnel, who frequently enjoy the ability to offer definitive relief for illness, are exasperated by their inability to do anything about a patient with completed stroke. They become indifferent and perhaps antagonistic toward the patient and his family.

Although it is not easy, it is exceedingly important for physicians and nurses caring for stroke patients to keep in mind the fact that their attitude and manner may be the only clues a patient has as to his condition or prognosis. In the acute stage, the patient needs reassurance; learning to live with disability can come later. The attitude of medical personnel is important, too, with patients who seem to be unaware of their surroundings. They may be able to hear and understand what is said even without any means of responding. Special care is required not to surprise anxious patients with painful or complex procedures. Each procedure should be explained to the patient, conscious or unconscious, and to his family. Some patients may be indifferent to one side of their environment or may have lost one-half of their field of vision, and should be approached from their intact side to avoid confusing them. These small points of medical care are those touches of humanity especially necessary in caring for patients with disease of the brain which, after all, is the prime human organ.

## THE NURSING ROLE

Little differentiation should be made between the roles of the nurse and the physician if ideal care is to be given to the patient with stroke. There are, however, certain primary independent responsibilties of the nurse which relate to the prevention of complications. These include the following duties and actions.

A. **Maintenance of airway through proper positioning and adequate suctioning.**

   *Methods.*

   1. The patient should be placed in a side-lying position without a pillow. A turning-sheet should be placed under the hips and thorax to assist in turning him from side to side at least once in each two-hour period. If possible, more frequent turning should be done in order to promote satisfactory pulmonary ventilation.

   2. The supine position should be avoided to prevent aspiration of secretions and obstruction of the airway.

   3. The prone position should be used for short periods of time. This may be combined with twenty-minute intervals of postural drainage. A convenient method of postural drainage involves positioning the patient with his head at the foot of the bed and tilting the bed by use of the foot gatch. It is helpful to support the rib cage and shoulder of each side (alternately) with a firm pillow in order to insure drainage of each lobe.

   4. Oral, pharyngeal, and tracheal suctioning should be done with a #14 whistle-tip catheter attached to a suction apparatus

by way of a Y-tube. This facilitates non-traumatic suctioning during the withdrawal of the catheter (see Chapter I, "Respiratory Insufficiency and Failure").

5. Observation of the quantity and consistency of secretions should be noted in order to assist in the ultimate decision regarding tracheostomy.

**B. Observation of vital signs—to determine degree of cerebral involvement.**

*Methods.*

1. Blood pressure, pulse, and respiration should be observed at least every hour until stable. The quality of respiration, in addition to rate and rhythm, should be noted in order to determine early signs of respiratory involvement and/or obstruction.

2. Pupillary response to light (an ordinary flashlight) should be evaluated at regular intervals. Eye care should be done at this time; methyl cellulose eye drops will help to prevent corneal irritation and local infection.

3. The level of consciousness (response to verbal, touch, and painful stimuli) should be noted each hour until a consistent reaction is obtained.

**C. Prevention of complications of immobilization.**

*Muscle stretching or contracture.* By a conscientious effort to provide proper position, support, and range of motion of major muscle groups, muscle contracture or stretching can be prevented. This program must begin during the immediate hospitalization period to avoid extended "rehabilitation" time, effort, and expense.

*Methods.*

1. Selection of bed: the patient should be placed on a bed with a firm mattress and a footboard with a wooden block to keep the mattress away from the footboard. This permits proper foot alignment when the patient is prone and prevents pressure on the heel when the patient is side-lying.

2. Position and support during side-lying: the upper extremity should be supported by a firm, doubled pillow to maintain abduction at a right angle to the forearm, which is placed in external rotation to a 45 degree angle. The wrist and fingers should be kept in partial extension by the use of a roll around the wrist and hand. The leg should be flexed at the hip and knee and supported from the knee to the foot by firm pillows or bolsters; the foot should be kept in dorsiflexion with a firm bolster (which, in turn, is kept firm by the footboard). The lower leg (the one on which the patient is lying), should be hyperextended and flat on the bed with the foot in dorsiflexion firmly against the footboard. The back should be kept straight with the weight evenly distributed on the shoulder, side, and hip. There is need for a pillow at the back to maintain this position. The lower arm should be abducted and flexed at the elbow, the hand placed parallel with the head.

3. Positioning when prone: internal rotation of the shoulder should be prevented by placing firm, small bolsters under each shoulder. The epigastric area should be kept free of pressure by means of a small pillow under one side of the pelvis to allow easier abdominal breathing. (An oversized pillow at this site would promote flexion of the hips.) The feet should be kept in firm dorsiflexion against the footboard.

4. Range-of-motion activities should be done passively by the nurse during the immediate post-stroke period. Aiming to maintain the range present at the time of the stroke, passive exercises should be given immediately upon admission to the hospital, unless specifically contraindicated. The movements should be carried to full range (or until the point of resistance), and held to the count of five. The movement should be performed smoothly and gradually and never rapidly. Because muscles are likely to be flaccid rather than spastic in the immediate post-stroke period, proper support must be given during these activities to avoid muscle stretching. The limb should be held at the joint and not at the muscle body.

5. As soon as the patient can comprehend direction, he should be instructed in quadriceps setting to maintain tone in the quadricep muscles of the unaffected leg.

6. Ambulation should begin at the earliest possible moment —when vital signs stabilize.

 a. The patient should be brought to a sitting position for 15 minutes every two hours with legs and feet dangling over the bedside (but supported on a chair).

 b. Attention to signs of postural hypotension (increase in pulse rate, diaphoresis, pallor) is important throughout the interval of initial ambulation. Application of Ace bandages (or elastic stockings) prior to ambulation activities is helpful in reducing postural hypotension due to venous stasis (particularly in the affected side). Range-of-motion activities of the lower extremities prior to and following the sitting position also discourages venous stasis.

***Bowel and bladder function.*** The prevention of bowel impaction and irregularity require a planned, consistent course of action in which communication between team members is fundamental.

***Methods.***

1. Rectal suppositories are useful. They should be given at the same time each day in accordance with the pre-stroke bowel habit of the patient. Initially, best results are obtained by placing the patient on his side (well supported and protected) during the bowel movement. (Use of a bedpan is not necessary, and at times seems to impede adequate fecal evacuation.) As soon as practicable, a bedside commode should be utilized further to encourage normal evacuation. Adequate intake of bulk and fluid will avoid the need for "fecal softeners" or laxative. Enemas should not be used to encourage regularity.

2. Bladder function in the initial post-stroke period is nearly always abnormal either in the form of retention and/or incontinence. If at all possible, the use of the Foley catheter should be avoided. With incontinence, the condom catheter is often beneficial. This catheter should be changed daily. It may be removed at night and replaced with a plastic bag (e.g., shower cap), filled with an absorbable material (cotton/gauze squares). Continuous wearing of the condom catheter predisposes to local irritation and tissue breakdown. If a Foley catheter becomes necessary,

measures should be taken to prevent and detect infection: strict sterile technique during placement, daily urinary pH determinations, taping of the catheter to the upper thigh to prevent pressure from pull, and thorough cleansing of the external urinary meatus at least every six hours. The collection bag should be placed below the bladder level to prevent backflow. In the presence of adequate urinary flow, irrigation of the catheter becomes unnecessary.

**D. Combating mental confusion and despair**
   *Methods.*
   1. Explanation of "what has happened" to clarify the sudden dependent position in which the patient finds himself.
   2. Explanation of what is being done to the patient, and why and how.
   3. Identification, by name and role, of personnel who enter into his environment and care.
   4. Reassurance that family members have been notified of his hospitalization (or are present), and of the cause for it.
   5. Early efforts to permit him to share in the decisions being made regarding his care; initially this may involve explanation only.
   6. Emphasis of positive aspects of his condition and incorporation of these into his care; e.g., permit him to hold the glass, assist with turning, etc.

**E. Evaluation of need for referral to paramedical services**
   *Speech:* the nurse should evaluate the patient's ability to perceive and to utilize speech as his means of communication. She should attempt, at these early stages, to avoid the formation of poor habits of communication: for instance, gestures rather than speech (when speech is possible); encouragement of signals (grasp, blink when speech is not possible).
   *Social Service:* the nurse should evaluate, through observation of behavior and the content of voiced concern, the need of the patient and his family for the assistance of the medical social worker. The nurse should make this referral in order to provide those involved with this additional source of aid in their attempts to understand and to accept what has occurred, as well as in planning for future care.

PART II

# Acute Congestive Heart Failure
# (Pulmonary Edema)

## THE PROBLEM

The term "acute congestive heart failure" misleadingly implies that the heart has failed abruptly; in fact, the onset of congestive failure is insidious in most cases. It is the seeming suddenness of overt left ventricular failure, in the form of acute pulmonary edema, that has created the impression of an abrupt change. Such severe cardiac decompensation is life threatening and demands prompt investigation to determine precipitating causes and to permit rapid, effective therapy. Acute pulmonary edema is most often associated with acute myocardial infarction or paroxysmal arrhythmias with a rapid ventricular rate.

Acute infection or the overadministration of fluids may precipitate pulmonary edema in patients whose cardiac reserve is reduced. Less common etiologies of acute pulmonary edema are: hypertensive crisis, acute rheumatic or viral carditis, valvular perforation, idiopathic cardiomyopathy, or hyperkinetic heart disease secondary to anemia or thyrotoxicosis.

In acute pulmonary edema, the basic physiologic abnormality is pulmonary congestion with accumulation of plasma-like fluid in the alveolar and intra-alveolar lung spaces. This state results from hemodynamic abnormalities associated with left ventricular failure. Specifically, decreased cardiac output with elevation of the end diastolic left ventricular pressure and volume leads to left atrial and pulmonary venous hypertension. Pulmonary congestion develops rapidly under these circumstances, and acute pulmonary edema ensues.

Because of poor oxygen diffusion across the edematous alveolar membranes, arterial oxygen unsaturation may occur and exaggerate the problem. Hypotension, cardiac arrhythmias, and a progressive deterioration in myocardial function may result when the fall in arterial oxygen saturation is severe. (This problem was considered in Chapter I, "Respiratory Insufficiency and Failure").

## ASSESSMENT OF THE PROBLEM

### Symptoms

*Dyspnea.* The cardinal symptom of acute pulmonary edema is severe dyspnea. The onset of respiratory distress may be dramatically sudden or may develop over a period of several hours. Lying down accentuates the patient's dyspnea, and he finds breathing more comfortable in the upright position. In its most advanced form a paroxysmal cough productive of white to pink foamy sputum is typical, and respirations are generally of a wheezing quality. Pulmonary edema secondary to acute myocardial infarction is usually associated with chest pain.

*Severe agitation.* Severe agitation due to reduced cerebral blood flow is common, and stark fear is usually evident during the acute phase.

*Syncope.* Lightheadedness and syncope are sometimes seen during acute pulmonary edema, particularly in patients with preexisting cerebrovascular atherosclerosis.

### Signs

1. Obvious respiratory distress with tachypnea.

2. Tachycardia which is unrelated to blood pressure. The blood pressure may be at normal, hypotensive, or hypertensive levels.

3. Diaphoresis in the presence of cutaneous vasoconstriction (cold, clammy skin).

4. Cutaneous (peripheral) cyanosis is common, but central cyanosis is seen only in the most severe cases.

5. Pulmonary auscultation reveals diffuse wheezes and (usually) moist, bubbling rales throughout the chest.

6. A gallop rhythm is often present on cardiac auscultation.

7. Distended, pulsating neck veins are often observed (with the patient sitting at a 45° angle).

8. An enlarged liver, hepatic tenderness, and peripheral edema may be present if there is concomitant right-sided heart failure. (In patients with acute myocardial infarction presenting

with pulmonary edema, the left heart usually fails independently of the right heart, and these latter signs are absent.)

**Studies**

1. Chest x-rays reveal pulmonary congestion in the form of alveolar edema or as pleural effusions.

2. The electrocardiogram may show sinus tachycardia with non-specific ST segment and T wave changes. When pulmonary edema is secondary to acute myocardial infarction, hypertension, or mitral stenosis, typical patterns suggesting these primary entities may be present.

3. Arterial blood oxygen analysis may show varying degrees of arterial unsaturation.

4. Leucocytosis is usually present and urinalysis may show albumin.

## PRINCIPLES OF TREATMENT

The primary aims of treatment of acute congestive heart failure are to improve pulmonary ventilation and oxygen saturation, to reduce pulmonary venous congestion and blood volume, and to improve myocardial contractility and work performance.

**Methods for improving pulmonary ventilation and oxygen saturation**

a. *Oxygen inhalation therapy.* Because of decreased arterial saturation, oxygen therapy is of vital importance. Oxygen can be administered in any of the following ways. (These methods were considered in detail in Chapter I, "Respiratory Failure and Insufficiency.")

1. Nasal catheters may be used to deliver 30%–40% concentrations of oxygen at flow rates of 4–6 liters per minute.

2. Face masks theoretically allow the administration of 100% oxygen (when used with an airtight mask and a non-rebreathing bag). Masks may be attached to positive-pressure breathing devices if assisted ventilation is desired, and will deliver 40%–100% oxygen saturation, depending on the air-oxygen setting.

3. Intermittent positive-pressure ventilation with either a volume or pressure cycle machine may be used. (Positive-pressure

ventilators should *not* be used in *hypotensive* patients, since the resulting positive intrathoracic pressure will impede venous return to the right heart and cause a more marked fall in cardiac output.)

Regardless of the mode of oxygen administration, the gas should be humidified prior to inhalation. This can be accomplished by bubbling it through water or with nebulizer devices. A 30% solution of ethyl alcohol in water is an effective humidifying agent, with the added advantage of reducing pulmonary secretions by its anti-foaming action.

**b. *Bronchodilators.*** Since bronchospasm may complicate acute pulmonary edema, the administration of bronchodilators is generally indicated. The agents commonly used are:

1. *Aminophylline.* 250–500 mgm of this drug may be administered either intravenously or as a rectal suppository. In addition to its bronchodilator effect, aminophylline increases cardiac output, as secondary to a direct myocardial stimulating action, and may have a dilator effect on the coronary arteries. When given intravenously, the dose should be diluted to 50 cc and then injected slowly over a 15–20 minute period. The blood pressure and pulse rate should be monitored during this period to detect the development of arrhythmias or hypotension.

2. *Epinephrine and isoproterenol (Isuprel).* 1 cc of a 1:100 solution of either drug (diluted in 5 cc of saline) may be administered by a nebulizer to relieve bronchospasm. These drugs must be used cautiously to avoid drug-induced arrhythmias.

3. *Morphine.* The parenteral administration of opiates, particularly 12–15 mgm of morphine sulfate, may produce impressive relief of dyspnea in acute pulmonary edema. Part of the beneficial effect may be due to allaying anxiety and decreasing the work of breathing as a result of reduced venous return. It has been shown that morphine causes packing of blood in peripheral vascular beds, thereby producing a type of internal phlebotomy.

### Methods for reducing pulmonary venous congestion and blood volume

**a. *Rotating tourniquets.*** Rubber tourniquets or blood pressure cuffs are applied proximally to three or four extremities at a pressure (between the systolic and diastolic levels) designed to obstruct venous return without interfering with arterial inflow to the limb. The tourniquets result in pooling of blood in the affected extremities and a decrease in the volume of blood returning to the overburdened heart. When pulmonary congestion has resolved, the tourniquets are released, one at a time, at 20–30 minute intervals. Simultaneous removal of all tourniquets is poor practice, because of the possibility of recurrence of pulmonary congestion resulting from the sudden increase in venous return from the extremities.

Automatic rotating tourniquet devices are available and are very useful as a time-saving measure.

b. *Diuretic therapy.* Although the specific actions of the different classes of diuretics vary widely, the common effect of all diuretics is to increase sodium and water excretion via the kidneys. This loss of water and sodium tends to decrease the blood volume (toward normal levels) and in turn reduces pulmonary congestion. There is no evidence that these drugs have a beneficial effect on the heart itself, and their therapeutic value is secondary to the renal action.

The most effective diuretics in current use are, in decreasing potency:

1. ethacrynic acid (Edecrin) and furosemide (Lasix),
2. mercurials (Mercuhydrin, Thiomerin),
3. benzothiadiazides (Chlorothiazide, Hydrochlorothiazide, etc.),
4. aldosterone antagonists (Aldactone A), and
5. carbonic anhydrase inhibitors (Diamox).

Selection of a diuretic should be based on the speed and magnitude of the diuresis desired. With full-blown pulmonary edema, the intravenous administration of ethacrynic acid or furosemide has become the treatment of choice and can be expected to produce a rapid and impressive diuresis. Unless the clinical situation is critical, overzealous administration of these drugs should be avoided, because rapid shifts in fluid volume and electrolyte concentrations may produce life-threatening side effects. In addition to the desired loss of sodium and water, all of these diuretics result in the excretion of potassium and bicarbonate in varying ratios. Excessive losses of potassium and chloride ions, particularly those occasioned by the use of the more potent agents, may cause a metabolic alkalosis. Paradoxically, the aldosterone antagonists may actually produce hyperkalemia. The combined administration of diuretics may result in a progressive rise in blood urea nitrogen. A thorough familiarity with the individual and combined actions of diuretic drugs is essential if the toxic effects of electrolyte disturbances and azotemia are to be avoided.

c. *Fluid and sodium restriction.* Every attempt should be made to restrict intravenous and oral fluid intake for at least the first 24 hours following an episode of acute pulmonary edema. No more than 1000 to 1200 cc of fluids should be administered during this period. Sodium chloride intake should also be severely restricted, at least until acute congestive heart failure is well controlled.

d. *Phlebotomy.* This method of rapidly decreasing the blood volume should be reserved for patients with intractable pulmonary edema who do not exhibit hypotension. 250–500 cc of blood is removed, using a standard blood donor set. (This blood can be sent to the blood bank for storage, or the red blood cells may be packed and reinfused.)

**Methods for improving myocardial contractility and work performance.** The administration of a digitalis preparation is the specific treatment for acute left ventricular failure. This drug improves myocardial contractility (inotropic action) and thereby increases cardiac output. The resultant effect is a fall in left ventricular end diastolic pressure and volume, with a secondary decrease in pulmonary congestion.

The particular digitalis preparation used will depend on the urgency of the situation. In severe pulmonary edema, rapidly acting parenteral preparations, such as Ouabain or deslanoside may be life saving. If the degree of pulmonary edema improves significantly before digitalization is begun (on the basis of the above program), a less rapid-acting cardiac glycoside can be used.

**Major complications of acute pulmonary edema**

There are three complications of acute pulmonary edema which may lead, directly or indirectly, to death:

1. A progressive deterioration of cardiac and pulmonary function despite therapy. Certain patients show no response to treatment and die of *power failure* of the heart.

2. Serious cardiac arrhythmias are common sequelae of heart failure and may result in death. Drug or electrical treatment of arrhythmias are often ineffective in the presence of advanced left ventricular failure.

3. Complications of therapy include electrolyte imbalance, opiate overdosage, and digitalis toxicity, and overadministration of oxygen may lead to irreversible cardiac, respiratory, or nervous system depression.

## THE NURSING ROLE

**A. Assessment of the patient's clinical status.** The nurse should carefully obtain and record the following information in a planned manner at regular intervals:

1, blood pressure;
2, pulse: rate, quality, rhythm;
3, skin, lip or nailbed cyanosis (presence or absence);
4, mental state;
5, rate and type of respirations;
6, character of pulmonary secretions; and
7, urinary output and fluid intake.

**B. Cardiac Monitoring.** All patients in pulmonary edema should have continuous monitoring of the electrocardiogram to detect arrhythmias at their onset. This monitoring should be a nursing duty. (See Chapter II, "Acute Myocardial Infarction".)

**C. Oxygen administration.** In order that oxygen be administered safely and efficiently to the patient with acute pulmonary edema, the following points must be considered:

1. Support the patient in the most efficient position for ven-

tilation by raising the head of the bed and using pillows to permit full chest expansion. At times it may be worthwhile to place the patient in a lounge-type chair rather than his bed.

2. Maintain a clear airway. If the patient cannot expectorate his secretions, nasopharyngeal suctioning should be performed at appropriate intervals.

3. The *system* of oxygen administration should be checked frequently as follows:

    a. Position of cannulas and fit of face masks. It is wise to reassure the patient that the face mask will not impede respirations.

    b. Humidifying device.

    c. Air oxygen mixture and rate of administration.

4. Observe the patient for signs of hypoxia or decreased respiratory rate and depth. Special attention must be given to patients with chronic lung disease, since oxygen may depress the respirations with resultant hypoventilation, hypoxia, and hypoxemia. Therefore, in addition to observing the rate and depth of respirations, signs of increasing confusion, depression, or other mental alterations should be noted and reported to the physician immediately. The oxygen flow for patients with chronic lung disease is usually set at a low level, and all personnel must be instructed not to increase it to levels customarily used.

5. When positive pressure assisted ventilation is used:

    a. Explain the proper use of equipment to the patient and give assistance as needed.

    b. Before positive pressure oxygen is administered, the patient should attempt to clear his airway. If this is unsuccessful, suctioning should be employed to prevent mucus plugs from being forced further into the bronchi.

    c. Check that face mask fits properly—i.e., no "leaking of air."

    d. Verify correct machine settings and function.

    e. Maintain proper fluid level in nebulizer.

    f. Observe cardiac monitor for arrhythmias during nebulization of epinephrine or Isuprel.

    g. Determine blood pressure to rule out hypotension during the administration of intermittent positive pressure breathing assistance.

**D. Diuretic therapy.** Urinary output and fluid intake should be carefully measured at frequent intervals (every hour or less if a catheter is in place) from the time of the patient's admission to the end of the critical period.

The nurse should be alert for side effects of diuretic therapy, particularly those due to electrolyte imbalance.

1. Excessive loss of potassium may result in muscle weakness and abdominal distension. Hypokalemia is also associated with increased sensitivity to digitalis, and the cardiac rate and rhythm should be carefully monitored in those patients who receive diuretic therapy and digitalis concomitantly.

2. The combination of sodium loss induced by diuretics and the decreased intake of salt in the diet may result in excessively low serum sodium levels (hyponatremia). In this situation, patients are usually drowsy and lethargic and may complain of muscle cramps (see Chapter VII, "Water and Electrolyte Imbalances"). Hyponatremia can also result from excessive fluid intake, which causes a dilution of serum sodium. In this instance the fluid intake must be restricted to 600–800 cc per day.

3. Thiazide diuretics have a tendency to increase both blood glucose and uric acid levels. Therefore, the urine of diabetic patients should be checked for sugar and acetone while these drugs are being administered. Attacks of gout are not uncommon.

**E. Rotating tourniquets**

1. Place tourniquet around upper segment of extremity.

2. Check peripheral pulses periodically to make certain that arterial blood flow has not been obstructed.

3. Rotate one tourniquet to a free limb every fifteen to twenty minutes in the established manner. Placing the tourniquets over pajama sleeves and trousers or over a hand towel will protect the skin from being pinched.

4. When therapy is discontinued, remove tourniquets one at a time at 20–30 minute intervals.

5. Determine blood pressure for hypotension.

**F. Phlebotomy**

1. Have blood donor sets available.

2. Collect the blood carefully and dispatch it to the blood bank for proper storage and handling.

3. Check blood pressure for hypotension during phlebotomy.

**G. Administration of opiates**

1. Observe for secondary respiratory depression.

2. Keep morphine antagonists, such as Nalorphine or Levallorphan tartrate, available for immediate use.

3. Be alert for signs of nausea and vomiting and position patient to avoid aspiration if vomiting occurs.

4. Remain at bedside or nearby until apprehension and restlessness are controlled.

**H. Digitalis therapy.** Since there is only a narrow range between the effective and toxic dosage of digitalis, it is important that the nurse be keenly aware of the signs and symptoms of digitalis overdosage:

1. The pulse rate and cardiac rhythm should be checked immediately before digitalis administration. Whenever the heart rate is below 60, the physician should be notified before the drug is given. Similar discretion should be used if frequent premature ventricular contractions, bigeminy or paroxysmal atrial tachycardia or heart block is noted on the monitor.

2. Digitalis overdosage may also be suspected if the patient complains of anorexia, nausea, or vomiting, drowsiness, diarrhea, abdominal pain or mental confusion. Consult the physician whenever there is doubt about symptoms suggesting digitalis toxicity.

3. Drugs to combat digitalis toxicity should be on hand and available for immediate use. The most commonly used drugs for this purpose are potassium chloride, EDTA, diphenylhydantoin (Dilantin), and propranolol hydrochloride (Inderal).

**I. To provide rest for the patient**

1. As the patient's activities will be limited as the result of his cardiac dysfunction, physical assistance must be given when he is ambulating or resting in bed or chair.

2. Proper positioning should provide comfort, help prevent complications of bedrest, and allow for effective pulmonary ventilation. Fowler's position is most effective and comfortable for the

patient with dyspnea secondary to pulmonary congestion. Elevating the head of the bed, either mechanically or on blocks, rather than merely raising the gatch of the bed allows for a better and more restful alignment of the patient. Pillows are helpful in supporting the patient as his position is changed. A foot block or firm foot roll is helpful in preventing the patient's sliding down in bed.

3. In order to conserve the patient's energy, the activities involved in physical care and management should be carried out in an unhurried manner and be spaced throughout the day, with provision for frequent, undisturbed rest periods.

4. Large meals should be avoided, both to conserve energy and to prevent the diversion of large amounts of blood to the visceral area. Smaller meals can also be helpful in achieving weight reduction in obese patients, since this will reduce the cardiac work load. Visceral congestion may cause anorexia, nausea, and vomiting; thus, attention to the patient's actual food intake is important.

5. Another energy-saving measure is prevention of constipation and straining at stool. Stool softeners and cathartics should be administered as indicated.

6. Often the patient's concern regarding his condition and other personal worries interferes with his ability to rest. The nurse should be alert for these problems and consult with other members of the health team regarding the assistance of the patient with his difficulties. In addition to emotional support by the health team, many patients will require some sedation to help them rest. Plans for more detailed health teaching and counseling should be postponed until the patient's condition improves.

**J. Dietary management.** Reduction of sodium intake is an essential therapeutic aim for the patient with congestive heart failure. The restriction of sodium may vary from 200 mg to 3000 mg daily, depending on the severity of the patient's illness and other factors. This restriction is difficult for many patients to tolerate. Providing flavorings such as lemon juice, vinegar, and vanilla, and spices such as thyme and garlic powder (not salt), in place of sodium chloride is quite helpful. Commercially prepared salt substitutes should not be used until their contents have been reviewed and approved by the physician. This is particularly important in patients with associated renal disease, since many of these preparations contain potassium in amounts capable of causing hyperkalemia in this situation.

Whenever possible, the patient should be given an opportunity to choose his food within his limitation. This involves him in his care and also provides an excellent opportunity for teaching him about diet.

PART III

# Hypertensive Crisis

## THE PROBLEM

When the diastolic blood pressure is greatly elevated (usually more than 140 mm Hg), a dangerously high degree of stress is placed on the heart and the peripheral, cerebral, and renal arterial vasculature. Acute, severe hypertension may rapidly produce congestive heart failure with pulmonary edema, hypertensive encephalopathy, intracranial hemorrhage, and acceleration of renal failure. In the strictest sense, hypertensive crisis is associated with one or more of these complications. It is a frank medical emergency requiring immediate recognition and effective treatment of both the elevated blood pressure and its secondary complications.

Hypertensive crisis is most often the result of one of the following abnormalities:

1. **Malignant hypertension.** Briefly, the available data suggest that the associated blood pressure elevation is the result of interreacting abnormalities of peripheral vasomotor receptors, renal release of angiotensin II precursors, increased adrenal cortical production of aldosterone (with secondary sodium and water retention), and hyperactive hypothalamic discharge with increased peripheral arteriolar vasoconstriction.

2. **Head trauma.** Associated hypertension is presumably due to a

secondary derangement in intracerebral regulation of peripheral vasomotor activity.

**3. Pheochromocytoma.** Concomitant blood pressure elevation is due to the increased production and release of catecholamines by the tumor.

**4. Toxemia of pregnancy.** Although the basic cause of this syndrome is not known, important associated abnormalities are excessive sodium and water retention plus severe generalized vasoconstriction, resulting in a disproportionate increase in diastolic blood pressure.

**5. Acute glomerulonephritis.** Hypertension associated with this disease is due to increased renal release of renin, with a secondary increase in circulating blood levels of the potent vasoconstrictor substance angiotensin II, and a related increase in adrenal cortical production of aldosterone with resultant sodium and water retention.

## ASSESSMENT OF THE PROBLEM

The onset of hypertensive crisis is usually heralded by the rather rapid development of hypertensive encephalopathy, intracranial hemorrhage, or acute congestive heart failure with pulmonary edema. Physical examination usually reveals the presence of a diastolic blood pressure elevation to levels greater than 140 mm Hg, in association with one of the following syndromes:

**Hypertensive encephalopathy.** Clinical findings include severe generalized headache, mental confusion, somnolence, nausea, vomiting, generalized convulsions, coma, hyperreflexia, papilledema, plus retinal hemorrhages and exudates. Lumbar puncture may be hazardous in view of almost certain elevation of cerebral spinal fluid pressure.

**Intracranial hemorrhage.** When a cerebral vessel ruptures, central nervous system dysfunction usually parallels the magnitude of the hemorrhagic process. If bleeding is localized, there may be focal signs; if bleeding has been extensive, massive irreversible defects may exist. Xanthochromic or frankly bloody cerebrospinal fluid negates the need for a more extensive diagnostic evaluation, unless surgical intervention is planned.

**Acute congestive heart failure with pulmonary edema.** The clinical manifestations of this syndrome have been described previously in Part II of this chapter.

## PRINCIPLES OF TREATMENT

The basic therapeutic aim is rapidly to reduce the markedly elevated diastolic blood pressure. In patients with minimal renal disease and no significant coronary artery or cerebrovascular atherosclerosis, this can be done with reasonable safety. When a rapid fall in blood pressure is likely to exacerbate existing renal, myocardial, or cerebral ischemia, clinical judgment must be used in weighing these risks against those of a therapeutic regimen designed to produce a less rapid and more modest decrease in the diastolic pressure level.

Methods for decreasing the blood pressure:

**Drug therapy**

### A. *Modes of administration*

1. INTRAMUSCULAR ROUTE
Drugs administered in this manner have a longer onset of action and require repeated administration every 3–5 hours.

2. INTERMITTENT INTRAVENOUS THERAPY
The drug dosage is diluted with 20–50 cc of 5% dextrose in water in a syringe and is then injected into the intravenous infusion tubing at a rate of 1 cc per minute until there is a fall in blood pressure. During injection of the drug, blood pressure should be monitored every 15–30 seconds. Once the blood pressure is controlled, readings should be rechecked every 15–30 minutes. Additional doses of drug should be administered in an identical fashion when the blood pressure begins to rise above the desired level.

3. CONTINUOUS INTRAVENOUS THERAPY
Although this mode of drug administration is consistently effective and allows blood pressure control with the least variation, *constant supervision by trained personnel is required*. The infusion must be repeatedly adjusted to prevent either hypotension

or a return of the hypertension. The selected drug is diluted in 1000 cc of 5% dextrose in water and is administered preferably with "microdrip" techniques. This solution is connected in "piggyback" fashion to a constant flow infusion of plain 5% dextrose in water. This permits the operator to stop and start administration of the dilute drug solution without the risk of plugging at the venipuncture site. The blood pressure should be monitored every 30–60 seconds until a rate of infusion is reached that consistently controls the blood pressure at the desired level. Thereafter the rate of drug infusion and blood pressure must be checked every 15–30 minutes.

### B. *Specific types of drug therapy*

1. RESERPINE (SERPASIL)
Two mgm to 10 mgm may be given intramuscularly every 4–8 hours. Although generally effective, its disadvantages are:

      a. a relatively slow onset of action (2–4 hours),

      b. unpredictable magnitudes of hypotensive effect, and

      c. central nervous system depression with occasional Parkinson-like motor activity.

2. HYDRALAZINE (APRESOLINE)
This agent is particularly effective in treating hypertensive crisis associated with acute glomerulonephritis or toxemia of pregnancy. It is contraindicated in patients with acute left ventricular failure. Dosages are 20–60 mgm intramuscularly, 20–40 mgm intermittently intravenously, or 50–100 mgm in 1000 cc of 5% dextrose in water via continuous intravenous infusion.

3. GANGLIONIC BLOCKING AGENTS
These drugs produce profound hypotension unless carefully administered, and they often cause urinary retention and/or paralytic ileus. The head of the bed should be elevated for full orthostatic effect.

a. *Trimethaphan (Arfonad)*
This drug is rapidly and consistently effective. It has a short duration of action which requires a minute-to-minute regulation

of the infusion rate. The usual dosage is 1 gram in 1000 cc of 5% dextrose in water via continuous intravenous drip.

b. *Pentolinium (Ansolysen)*

The usual dosage is 5–50 mgm intramuscularly, 5 mgm intermittently intravenously, or 50–150 mgm in 1000 cc of dextrose in water.

### 4. DIAZOXIDE

The drug consistently and effectively lowers blood pressure associated with toxemia of pregnancy. 200–400 mgm is administered intermittently and intravenously.

### 5. METHYLDOPATE HYDROCHLORIDE (ALDOMET)

This agent is usually effective in lowering blood pressure while causing the least decrease in cardiac output and renal blood flow. Its main disadvantage is a relatively slow onset of action (2–4 hours). Dosage may vary from 250 to 1000 mgm in 1000 cc of 5% dextrose in water intravenously every 6–8 hours.

### 6. PHENOXYBENZAMINE (DIBENZYLINE)

A potent alpha-adrenergic blocking agent effective in the diagnosis and treatment of catecholamine-secreting tumors such as pheochromocytoma. A 10 mgm/Kg dose is diluted in 250–500 cc of 5% dextrose in water and infused slowly over at least one hour. Duration of action is 12–24 hours.

### 7. PHENTOLAMINE (REGITINE)

This agent is not as effective as phenoxybenzamine in controlling hypertensive crisis secondary to pheochromocytoma. Intermittent doses of 2.5–5 mgm intravenously will often give only partial blood pressure control.

### C. *Other considerations of drug therapy*

1. A decrease in diastolic blood pressure to 100–110 mm Hg is usually sufficient to allow control of hypertensive crisis complications with a minimal risk of renal, myocardial, or cerebral ischemia.

2. A dilute solution of norepinephrine (4 ampoules of Lev-

ophed in 500 cc of 5% dextrose in water) or other vasopressor agents should be kept in constant readiness should serious hypotension develop from excessive drug effect.

3. Specific treatment should be started for the complications of hypertensive crisis concurrent with the administration of antihypertensive therapy (e.g., acute pulmonary edema).

4. Once parenteral drug therapy has brought the blood pressure under control, consideration should be given to initiating long-term antihypertensive therapy.

### D. *Complications of hypertensive crisis therapy*
1. Obviously, if a patient presents one complication (e.g., hypertensive encephalopathy) every effort must be made to prevent other complications inherent to the fullblown syndrome (acute pulmonary edema or intracranial hemorrhage).

2. The induction of hypotension during treatment of hypertension. Unless this complication of treatment is promptly controlled by vasopressor therapy, additional damage in the form of cardiovascular, cerebrovascular, or renovascular ischemia or infarction may result.

3. Since convulsions are common, care should be taken to prevent the patient from injuring himself.

## THE NURSING ROLE

**A. Blood pressure recording.** Whenever a patient's blood pressure is taken, it should be compared with previous readings. Where there is a difference, more frequent observations should be made to determine whether a trend is evident. Significant changes should be reported immediately, since a progressive rise in the blood pressure may cause further insult.

**B. Central Nervous System Complications.** Signs of disorientation, confusion, irritability, lethargy, complaints of headache, difficulty with vision, or vomiting should also be sought. Since convulsions may occur, the patient should be protected from injury by padded siderails. A mouth gag to protect the tongue and a plastic airway should be kept at the bedside. A parenteral preparation of an anticonvulsant medication such as diphenylhydantoin (Dilantin) or sodium amobarbital (Amytal) should also be on hand. The environment should be kept as quiet as possible.

## C. Additional Considerations.

1. Signs and symptoms of acute heart failure should be recognized and reported immediately. Materials and medications necessary to deal with this situation should be readily available.

2. Instructions regarding drug dosage and maintenance of blood pressure range must be clear, completely understood, and meticulously followed.

3. If the medication is to be administered intravenously, make certain that the infusion bottles are clearly labeled as to their contents. A labeled tab should be placed near the clamp of the infusion tubing to further identify the solution being administered. This is especially helpful when the rate of flow requires frequent alteration.

4. When recording the patient's blood pressure, it is important also to note the rate and quality of the pulse and respirations, as well as the rate (microdrops per minute) of the antihypertensive drug infusion. Careful observations regarding the patient's appearance, behavior, complaints, and comments are valuable in assessing the clinical course and should be recorded by the nurse.

5. A careful record of fluid intake and urinary output is essential.

6. One of the most serious hazards of hypertensive crisis therapy is hypotension secondary to overtreatment. It is imperative that instructions regarding the administration of antihypertensive medication be carried out with precise exactness. In addition, early signs of shock or inadequate arterial circulation must be recognized and reported promptly.

If hypotension develops during therapy, drug administration should be discontinued immediately by the nurse and the responsible physician notified. Vasopressor agents should be available and ready for use.

Part IV

# *Pulmonary Embolism*

## THE PROBLEM

Pulmonary embolism, with or without pulmonary infarction, is much more common than is suspected clinically. Autopsy studies indicate that pulmonary embolism may be a major cause of death in as high as 15% of hospital fatalities. It most often occurs in the elderly, debilitated cardiac patient and in patients with traumatic fractures of the hip or pelvis. In less than 50% of cases is the correct diagnosis suspected prior to death.

There are several factors predisposing to pulmonary embolism:

a. Prolonged immobilization with peripheral venous stasis, phlebothrombosis, and/or thrombophlebitis.

b. Chronic congestive failure with stasis of blood in the heart and systemic veins.

c. Increased viscosity of blood (polycythemias or dehydration).

d. Increased blood coagulability (e.g., polycythemia vera).

e. Damage of the vascular endothelium secondary to trauma or inflammation, as in phlebitis, arthritis, or fracture of hip or pelvis.

According to autopsy studies, emboli may reach the lungs from one or more of the following thrombolic sites:

| *Thrombolic Site* | *Approximate Incidences (various studies)* |
|---|---|
| right ventricle | 4% |
| pelvic veins | 16% |
| inferior vena cava | 19% |
| right atrium | 23% |
| leg veins | 46% |
| origin unknown | 21% |

Emboli from these sites are characteristically multiple and most often involve the lower lobe arteries. Only 10% of pulmonary emboli produce infarction of living tissue; most go unnoticed. Pulmonary embolism causes an increase in airway resistance. This is due to terminal bronchial constriction with secondary atelectasis and decreased pulmonary compliance.

The usual cardiopulmonary responses to the embolic episode are:

1. Decreased tidal volume.

2. Increased pulmonary artery pressure and resistance. This effect is noticed only with massive pulmonary embolism where there is a 50% decrease in the cross-sectional area of the main pulmonary artery or occlusion of 5 of the 8 lobar arteries.

3. Decreased cardiac output resulting in hypotension or shock.

4. Decreased oxygen saturation not corrected with 100% oxygen (only with the circumstances described in #2).

5. Decreased carbon dioxide due to hyperventilation.

## ASSESSMENT OF THE PROBLEM

As suggested, pulmonary embolism may produce no symptoms; on the other hand, it may result in shock, cardiac arrest, and death. Between these extremes is a so-called "typical" clinical pattern.

### Symptoms

1. Dyspnea, tachycardia, and tachypnea are almost invariably present.

2. Cough with pleuritic chest pain is present in about 50% of cases.

3. Hemoptysis is reported in 25% of instances.

### Physical findings

1. Tachycardia and tachypnea in 75%–90% of cases
2. Accentuated pulmonic second sound—95%
3. Fever—55%
4. Pulmonary rales—55%
5. Thrombophlebitis—35%
6. Pleural friction rub—20%
7. Cyanosis—15%

8. Pallor, mental confusion, and signs of pulmonary consolidation or effusion may also be present.               .

**Laboratory and diagnostic studies**
   *Blood*
   1. Leucocytosis—W.B.C. is greater than 10,000 in 50% of cases.
   2. Increased total bilirubin—about 70% of cases.
   3. Serum enzyme elevation. The lactic dehydrogenase (LDH) is usually elevated, while transaminase levels (SGOT, SGPT) are normal.
   *Electrocardiogram.* Ectopic supraventricular tachycardias with non-specific S-T segment and T wave changes are most commonly seen. Transient evidence of right atrial enlargement (P— Pulmonale), right axis deviation, or right bundle branch block are present much less frequently (less than 25% of cases).
   *Chest x-ray.* Most commonly noted abnormalities are semispherical or half-spindle shaped infiltrates along a pleural surface often associated with a pleural effusion. Plate-like atelectasis with diaphragmatic elevation on the affected side is less often seen. If a major pulmonary artery is obstructed, a decrease in vascularity on the involved side with vascular congestion in the opposite lung field may be present. (It should be appreciated that a chest film is of minimal diagnostic help in the immediate postembolic period and that a normal chest film offers no assurance that embolization has not occurred).
   *Intravenous angiocardiography.* This is probably the most rapid and reliable diagnostic study that will document the presence of pulmonary embolism; however, false negative studies are common when only small terminal pulmonary arterioles are occluded.
   *Lung Scanning.* The use of radioactively tagged I[131] macroaggregates of albumin followed by scanning techniques has proved to be an effective method for detection of pulmonary emboli.


**PRINCIPLES OF TREATMENT**

**Therapeutic approach.** The therapeutic approach will, of course, depend on the severity of the attack and the degree of cardiovascular involvement accompanying the pulmonary vessel obstruction. In those instances in which shock, pulmonary edema, or life-threatening arrhythmias occur, the treatment program is obviously directed toward life-saving measures, as described in Chapter II; "Acute Myocardial Infarction."

When cardiovascular function is not seriously compromised and life is not immediately threatened, the following program may be employed:

**A.** *Oxygen.* Oxygen administration is indicated in the presence of either dyspnea or cyanosis. This can be given via a nasal catheter; however, intermittent positive pressure ventilation with the nebulization of bronchodilators may be of greater value to assure adequate pulmonary ventilation and relieve bronchospasm with atelectasis if such exists.

**B.** *Anticoagulation therapy.* Heparin should be started promptly if the diagnosis of pulmonary embolism is strongly suspected (assuming the absence of contraindications to its use). The drug should be continued for seven to ten days following the acute embolic episode and should be discontinued only if severe secondary complications supervene. Oral anticoagulants such as warfarin or Dicumarol should be started during the period of heparin therapy and continued for 6–8 weeks following the acute embolic episode.

**C.** *Fibrolytic therapy.* At the present time, agents (e.g., Fibrinolysin) capable of lysing clots have not become standard therapy in pulmonary embolism. There is considerable interest in urokinase for this purpose; however, the evidence is still experimental.

**D.** *Pulmonary artery embolectomy.* Since perhaps 50% of patients dying of pulmonary embolism live at least one hour following the acute episode, pulmonary embolectomy is theoretically practicable. In those patients not likely to survive with conservative management alone, this procedure may be contemplated. Although at least 50 patients are reported to have undergone successful pulmonary thromboembolectomy using cardiopulmonary bypass techniques, this method of treatment cannot be seriously considered unless a surgical team with proper facilities for bypass and angiography is available immediately.

**Complications of pulmonary embolism.** In patients sustaining the more massive forms of embolism who do not die promptly, additional complications are usually the result of associated low cardiac output and include:

1. Cerebrovascular occlusion.
2. Acute myocardial infarction.
3. Acute renal failure with oliguria.
4. Intractable cardiac arrhythmias.
5. Hepatic congestion and necrosis.
6. Ischemic infarcts of the gastrointestinal tract.

In less severe pulmonary embolism, complications are more likely to be the result of the localized process or its treatment. These may include:

1. Bronchopneumonia secondary to poor pulmonary ventilation, atelectasis, and stasis of secretions.
2. Pulmonary abscess at the site of infarction. This occurs infrequently.
3. Bleeding into the skin, central nervous system, gastrointestinal and/or genitourinary tract as a complication of anticoagulation therapy.
4. Recurrent embolism. This, unfortunately, occurs all too frequently in spite of the best medical management, particularly where the underlying cause or predisposing factors are uncontrolled.

## THE NURSING ROLE

**A. Repeated bedside observations.** Frequent planned observations are especially important for the patient who is predisposed to developing a pulmonary embolism, since immediate recognition of complications and subsequent treatment may be life-saving. These observations should include signs of sudden dyspnea, tachycardia, pleuritic chest pain, apprehension, and agitation.

**B. Determination of the vital signs.** The vital signs, including blood pressure, pulse, and respiration should be measured frequently to detect signs of circulatory failure at its inception. The patient's skin and mucous membranes are noted for signs of cyanosis and pallor. Mental confusion must be recognized and protective measures must be designed to prevent accidents and injury.

**C. Oxygen.** Oxygen therapy and its attendant problems are discussed in Chapter I, "Respiratory Insufficiency and Failure."

**D. Intravenous therapy.** An infusion of 5% dextrose in water should be started in anticipation of the need for emergency intravenous drug therapy to combat cardiovascular catastrophes.

**E. Sedation.** Particular care must be taken with the use of morphine or meperidine HCl in patients with pulmonary embolism. Hypoventilation is a common undesirable side effect and is to be avoided.

**F. Cardiac monitoring.** All patients with pulmonary emboli should have continuous cardiac monitoring.

**G. Prevention of additional embolism.**

1. When chest x-rays are performed, the patient should be moved in an unhurried, gentle manner to avoid straining which may in turn dislodge additional thrombi. The same precautions are necessary with intravenous angiography.

2. Stool softeners are useful in preventing straining at stool.

3. Conscientious nursing care is essential to prevent those conditions that predispose to venous stasis and further thrombus formation. A high percentage of thrombi that later become pulmonary emboli originate in the legs; therefore, special attention must be given to the extremities. Patients confined to bed should be maintained in proper body alignment. The legs should be observed for signs of thrombophlebitis. Warm, reddened sensitive areas in the calf should be reported immediately. Note should also be made if a patient experiences pain in his calf upon dorsiflexion of the foot.

The continuous use of blanket rolls, pillows, etc., placed under the knees must be avoided. This dangerous practice may result in sufficient pressure at the popliteal area to obstruct venous return from below. Raising the knee gatch of the bed is a similarly poor practice, because it permits pooling of blood in the pelvic veins. Any device used to provide flexion of the knees should be used only periodically.

To enhance venous return, the muscles of the feet and legs should be exercised regularly, either passively or actively, according to the clinical situation. A footboard or firm roll placed to maintain the feet in dorsiflexion is very helpful. This not only provides for good foot alignment, but also serves as a resistance against which the patient may exert pressure to exercise the muscles of the feet and legs. Quadriceps and gluteal muscle-tightening exercises should also be carried out several times each hour by the patient. Further to encourage venous return, elastic stockings are helpful. These should be removed at least every eight hours to inspect the skin and to prevent breakdown from uneven pressure and/or excessive drying of the skin.

Every attempt should be made to encourage adequate fluid intake, thereby avoiding dehydration with hemoconcentration.

PART V

# Systemic Arterial Embolism

## THE PROBLEM

With rare exceptions, a systemic arterial embolism results from thrombi originating in the left atrium or ventricle which break loose and become lodged in the peripheral arterial circuit. Thrombi from the right atrium or venous system may reach the left heart and arterial circulation via a patent foramen ovale or atrial septal defect, but this is uncommon. Systemic arterial embolism occurs much less frequently than does pulmonary embolism.

The common predisposing causes of systemic embolization are:

**1. Rheumatic heart disease with mitral valve dysfunction.** Autopsy studies have shown that approximately 45% of patients dying with rheumatic heart disease and mitral stenosis have left atrial thrombi, presumably as the result of chronic blood stasis with endothelial damage in this chamber. In 250 patients with mitral stenosis followed for at least 10 years without surgical intervention, an incidence of systemic embolism of 16% has been reported. This complication was the cause of death in 19% of patients dying during the observation period.

**2. Acute myocardial infarction.** The associated damage to the endothelial surface of the left ventricle allows the formation of a mural thrombus, parts of which may subsequently become emboli. Mural thrombi in the left ventricle were noted in 37% of patients dying of myocardial infarction in one series; acute systemic emboli were found in 25% of these subjects. Thrombus may also be found in the left auricular appendage, but much less often. In decreasing frequency, the organs most often involved by emboli are the kidneys, brain, spleen, extremities, and intestinal tract. Central nervous system infarction causes the largest number of deaths in those patients having symbolic embolism. Prior to the availability of anticoagulants, systemic embolism was recognized clinically in approximately 11% of patients with acute myocardial infarction. Numerous studies have shown that associated thrombo-embolic complications can be significantly reduced by the use of anticoagulants during the acute and convalescent phases of myocardial infarction.

**3. Chronic congesitve heart failure.** Chronic congestive heart failure, per se, may result in the formation of thrombi within the left atrium or ventricle, due to the stasis of blood in these chambers.

**4. Arterial endothelial damage.** Arterial endothelial damage due to trauma or inflammation may be associated with local thrombus formation, embolism, and arterial occlusion.

**5. Septic emboli.** Non-specific valvular inflammation, viral myocarditis, or bacterial endocarditis may result in embolism.

The pathophysiological changes associated with arterial embolism are the result of ischemic infarction of the affected organ or organs. The cessation of blood flow distal to the obstruction may result in vasospasm that further compromises perfusion of the involved organ or extremity.

## ASSESSMENT OF THE PROBLEM

The clinical picture seen with acute arterial embolism varies with the part of the arterial tree and associated organ system affected.

**Cerebrovascular system.** In most cases, the onset of symptoms is sudden. The carotid system either at the bifurcation of the common vessel or, more often, the smaller internal carotid branches are most frequently involved. Occlusion at these sites produces a stroke type syndrome (see Part I of this chapter), the magnitude and severity of which is dependent on the amount of cerebral tissue becoming ischemic or infarcted. Changes in mental status may vary from slight transient confusion with dysarthria and aphasia to sudden syncope and coma. Motor function impairment may range from weakness of short duration to complete, persistent paralysis. Spinal tap may yield clear to slightly xanthochromic fluid with a slight leucocytosis and protein content increase. If the embolus is septic, the cell count and protein level may be strikingly abnormal. Cerebrovascular arteriography may be helpful in differentiating large vessel embolism from cerebrovascular hemorrhage, aneurysm, or thrombosis (secondary to an atherosclerotic process). Although angiography carries a definite risk in this setting, it should be performed if embolism to a surgically accessible carotid vessel seems likely.

**Coronary artery.** Coronary artery embolism is uncommon; it most often follows cardiac surgery where fragments of thrombus, fibrin, calcium, or air bubbles occlude a coronary vessel. The effects of anesthesia or incisional pain may mask the usual symptoms of acute myocardial infarction, making diagnosis on this basis difficult. The diagnosis usually depends on the development of acute electrocardiographic changes typical of myocardial infarction, since the WBC, sedimentation rate, and serum enzymes are commonly elevated from cardiac surgery itself.

Coronary artery occlusion from emboli may occur with rheumatic heart disease, with atrial thrombi, or bacterial endocarditis. The associated syndrome may be indistinguishable from atherosclerotic coronary occulsion.

**Renal embolism.** The acute onset of flank pain with local tenderness, fever, and hematuria are the classic signs of renal arterial embolism; sudden hypertension may also occur. Leucocytosis and albuminuria are common. Intravenous pyelography may reveal poor or absent renal function on the involved side if a major renal artery is obstructed. If a large or medium-sized renal vessel is occluded, selective renal arteriography will usually demonstrate the obstruction.

**Mesenteric artery embolism.** This complication is often dramatically sudden in onset. It is characterized by severe, constant, generalized abdominal pain, fever, nausea, and vomiting, with either bloody diarrhea or constipation. If not recognized and treated promptly, septic or hypovolemic shock may result in death, often within 12–18 hours of the first symptoms. On physical examination the abdominal findings initially may include mild to moderate distention with diffuse tenderness and hyperactive bowel sounds. Later the abdomen may become rigid and silent. Leucocytosis and progressively rising hematocrit due to intra-abdominal plasma volume sequestration are often observed. Plain x-rays of the abdomen may show distended loops of fluid-filled bowel, or there may be a ground-glass appearance. Although aortography may be diagnostic in cases where infarction is extensive, a rapid deterioration in the patient's condition usually necessitates prompt surgical exploration.

**Splenic embolism.** This complication is usually associated with the sudden onset of sharp stabbing pain in the left upper quadrant of the abdomen. The pain is often increased by deep breathing and may radiate into the left infrascapular area posteriorly. Splinting of the abdomen and diaphragm are common, as are localized left upper quadrant signs of peritoneal inflammation. Differentiation between splenic and renal infarction may be difficult. Splenic rupture is rare. Radiographic examination of the chest may reveal elevation of the left diaphragm with plate-like pulmonary atelectasis or a small pleural effusion.

**Extremity arterial embolism.** Emboli originating from the heart may lodge at the bifurcation of the abdominal aorta (saddle embolus) or in the arterial tree of the upper and lower extremities. Arterial embolization distal to the brachial or subclavian vessels may go unrecognized because of the excellent circulation beyond these points. Complete or partial occlusion of the aortic bifurcation or the major arteries to the lower extremities almost always produces significant symptomatology. Initially, there may be a sudden onset of pallor, coldness, numbness, and tingling in the involved extremity. Within minutes, pain (often severe in degree), with decreased sensation and weakness or even complete paralysis, may develop. Pallor may change to blotchy cyanosis. On examination, the extent of these changes will roughly indicate the site of vessel occlusion. Absent arterial pulsation, hypothermia, anesthesia, and diminished or absent tendon reflexes confirm the diagnosis on physical examination. Bilateral lower extremity dysfunction indicates probable occlusion at the aorta bifurcation. Unilateral demarcation of findings is usually associated with common iliac or femoral artery obstruction, while foot and calf abnormalities are most often the result of occlusion at the popliteal artery level. Arteriography provides the most accurate method of demonstrating the site of obstruction and is important to the vascular surgeon planning embolectomy.

## PRINCIPLES OF TREATMENT

The primary aims of treatment of thromboembolism are directed toward salvage and return of function of the involved organ or extremity and prevention of recurrent thromboembolism.

**Methods**

**A. Surgery.** Early surgical intervention with thromboembolectomy is the treatment of choice in patients with major vessel occlusion. Thromboembolism to the upper extremities, the spleen, or lower extremities distal to the popliteal area less frequently produces dysfunction of a sufficient magnitude to warrant surgery. It is important to assess the hazards of surgical intervention (particularly in those cardiac patients who are already critically ill) compared with the possible threat to life or organ system function without surgery. As a general rule, the earlier operation is carried out the higher the percentage of success. If thromboembolism involves the extremities, operability should be based on a clinical assessment of limb viability, rather than elapsed time alone.

**B. Anticoagulation therapy.** The purpose of anticoagulation therapy is the prevention of propagation both at the site of embolus origin and the point of arterial occlusion. Unless surgical intervention is imminent, rapid anticoagulation should be begun as soon as the clinical diagnosis seems reasonably well established. This is accomplished as follows:

1. Continuous intravenous heparin drip 200–250 mgm of heparin diluted in 500 cc of 5% dextrose in water is administered intravenously at a rate to achieve and maintain a venous clotting time of 2–3 times normal control. This method is the most rapid and effective way of anticoagulating patients with acute thrombo-embolism; however, the technique demands careful and frequent observations on the reliability of the intravenous infusion and the blood-clotting times. If these observations cannot be made with complete reliability, other methods of heparin administration should be used.

2. Intermittent intravenous heparin administration. 50–100 mgm of heparin is given intravenously every 4–6 hours, depend-ing on the individual patient's blood-clotting time dose-response curve (again aiming for a clotting time 2–3 times the control level just prior to the next heparin dose).

3. Intermittent deep subcutaneous heparin administration. 50–100 mgm of heparin is given subcutaneously (usually in the posterior hip area) every 4–6 hours, according to blood-clotting time response. This method of heparin administration may be the least reliable and predictable. Unless each dose is properly in-jected deeply into the subcutaneous tissues (not intramuscularly), drug absorption and subsequent blood-clotting times may vary widely. Subcutaneous administration does offer the advantage of requiring less constant supervision and avoids multiple veni-punctures. Heparin therapy should be continued for 5–7 days following the acute embolic episode. Before heparin is discon-tinued oral anticoagulant therapy (warfarin or Dicumarol) should be started and optimal control achieved.

**C. Sympathectomy.** Although surgical lumbar sympathec-tomy is not generally recommended as a definitive therapy for pa-tients with acute lower extremity thromboembolism, "pharma-cologic" sympathectomy via caudal or epidural block has been suggested as adjunctive therapy by some clinicians. Since this tech-nique is most often used in association with other conservative, nonsurgical treatment of distal lower or upper extremity throm-boembolism, its definitive value is difficult to assess.

Stellate ganglion block has not been shown to be of value in the conservative management of acute cerebrovascular arterial em-bolism.

**D.** *Fibrinolysins.* As noted, available fibrinolytic agents have not been demonstrated as being wholly safe for general use, and cannot be recommended. The development of hemorrhage into what were initially ischemic cerebral infarcts has been reported following fibrinolysin infusion, and their administration would seem to be contraindicated in this setting.

## THE NURSING ROLE

**A. Observation of patient.** Because the element of time is so crucial, nurses caring for patients susceptible to arterial embolism must be constantly alert for signs and symptoms of arterial occlusion.

The nurse should listen very carefully to the complaints of her patients, since they may suggest the need for immediate medical evaluation. If a patient with a cardiac disorder complains of severe pain in the chest, abdomen, extremities, or flank area, the physician should be notified immediately regarding the nature of the patient's complaints as well as the nurse's observation of the patient, including his blood pressure, temperature, pulse, and respirations. If possible, appropriate specimens of urine, stool, or vomitus should be described and stored for examination.

Medication for relief of pain should be withheld until the physician has an opportunity to examine the patient. Patients exhibiting signs of central nervous system dysfunction such as confusion, impairment of motor function, syncope, or coma should be protected from injury.

**B. Anticoagulant therapy.** Extreme care must be taken when anticoagulant therapy, particularly intravenous heparin, is employed. Constant checks must be made on the rate of dilute heparin solution administration (see previous discussion in Part I of this chapter).

**C. Methods to prevent lower extremity arterial occlusion.** If the patient complains of discomfort in an extremity, it should be gently examined for temperature, color, sensation, motion, and presence or absence of arterial pulse. The extent of symptoms is noted, as is the presence or absence of an area of demarcation of symptoms. If occlusion is suspected, the following steps should be taken:

1. Carefully wrap the limb in a cotton blanket, since trauma from striking the siderails, brushing against the bed linen, striking the opposite limb, or unnecessary handling by the staff may cause additional damage.

2. Place a padded bed "cradle" over the limb for protection.

3. If the area requires bathing with water, its temperature must not exceed body temperature.

4. Prevent exposure of the affected area to heat. Remove hot water bottles, heating pads, heat lamps, etc., from the patient's unit.

5. Inspect the area periodically. Note the color, temperature, absence or presence of arterial pulse, sensation and strength of the extremity. Report changes promptly.

6. If the patient is moved for diagnostic studies and/or surgery, the moving should be done in a smooth, careful manner, making sure that all personnel are aware of which limb is involved and the need for caution.

## Bibliography

BELAND, L. IRENE: *Clinical Nursing.* The Macmillan Co., New York, 1965.

CECIL, R. L. and LOEB, R. F.: *A Textbook of Medicine.* 11th Edition, W. B. Saunders Co., Philadelphia, 1963.

COLES, CATHERINE H., et al.: *A Procedure for Passive Range of Motion and Self-Assistive Exercises.* (Rehabilitative Nursing Techniques —3). Kenny Rehabilitation Foundation, Minneapolis, 1964.

COVALT, NILA K.: Preventive Techniques of Rehabilitation for Hemiplegic Patients. *G.P.,* Vol. XVII, No. 3, March 1958.

FISHER, C. M., DALAL, P. M., and ADAMS, R. D.: Cerebrovascular Disease and the Stroke Syndrome. *Principles of Internal Medicine,* Harrison, T. R., ed., 4th edition. McGraw-Hill, New York, pp. 1747–1795, 1962.

GIFFORD, R. W.: Management of Hypertensive Emergencies. *Postgraduate Medicine.* Vol. 34, pp. 145–149.

GOODMAN, L. S. and GILMAN, A.: *The Pharmacological Basis of Therapeutics. 3 Edition.* The Macmillan Co., New York, 1965.

LORENGE, E. F., et al.: Urologic Problems in Rehabilitation of Hemiplegic Patients. *Journal of the American Medical Association,* 169:1042–1046, March 7, 1959.

MARSHALL, JOHN: *The Management of Cerebrovascular Disease.* Little, Brown, and Co., Boston, 1965.

McDOWELL, F. H., ed.: Treatment of Stroke. *Modern Treatment,* 2:13–114, 1965.

SASAHARA, A. A. and STEIN, M.: *Pulmonary Embolic Disease.* Crane & Shatton, 1965.

SMITH, GENEVIEVE W.: *Care of the Patient with a Stroke: A Handbook for Patients, Family and the Nurse.* Springer Pub. Co., New York, 1959.

TAYLOR, MARTHA and MARKS, MORTON: *Aphasia Rehabilitation Manual and Therapy Kit.* McGraw-Hill Book Co., New York, 1955.

WHITEHOUSE, FREDERICK A.: Psychosocial Problems of the Stroke Patient and Family. Presented at Graduate Nursing Course, New Orleans, Louisiana, June 17, 1963. (Available from the Amer. Heart Association.)

CHAPTER IV

# Shock

LUCY BRAND, R.N., M.S.
ALAN P. THAL, M.D.

## THE PROBLEM

The fundamental problem in shock, regardless of its etiology, is a marked reduction in blood flow through tissues. This inadequacy of tissue perfusion results, initially, in cellular hypoxia and ultimately, in tissue asphyxia. The body attempts to control the metabolic consequences of impaired tissue perfusion, but at a certain point such control is lost and shock becomes irreversible. The primary aim in the treatment of shock is to increase tissue perfusion. Unless this is accomplished early after onset, subsequent therapeutic measures are of no avail and death can be anticipated. Because of the short interval between the onset of shock and the point of irreversibility, it is essential that the etiology of the problem be identified promptly and that a planned therapeutic program be initiated by expert personnel at the earliest possible moment.

At the present time it is customary to classify the shock syndrome in the following generalized categories according to etiology:

**1. Hypovolemic shock.** Because of excessive blood loss, either from spontaneous causes (gastrointestinal bleeding from varices or ulcer disease) or as a result of surgical procedures or trauma, circulating volumes become inadequate to meet the body's demands of tissue oxygenation and the shock state ensues. Similar depletion of circulating volume may occur as the result of fluid loss either through the gastrointestinal tract (profound diarrhea, vomiting, fistulous loss, etc.) or from the body surfaces (extensive burns).

**2. Bacteremic or septic shock.** Profound circulatory collapse may result as a complication when certain bacteria invade the blood stream. This circumstance is most common in the presence of gram-negative infections, including those due to coliform bacilli, meningococci, proteus, and salmonella organisms. It is believed that these bacterial infections result in production of certain lethal toxins which ultimately affect vascular integrity and lead to a decreased tissue perfusion (endotoxic shock). This type of shock is especially common in elderly men following genitourinary tract instrumentation or surgery.

**3. Cardiogenic shock.** Primarily as a consequence of acute myocardial infarction, the left ventricle fails to pump enough to supply blood (and oxygen) to peripheral tissues. Because of either extensive structural damage to the ventricle, or as a result of metabolic changes secondary to myocardial hypoxia, the strength and force of left ventricular contraction are reduced. (This subject is considered in further detail in Chapter II, "Acute Myocardial Infarction.")

**4. Other forms of shock, including anaphylactic shock and shock related to acute metabolic disturbances.** The injection of a foreign protein (e.g., horse serum and various penicillin preparations) into a person sensitized to it by a previous administration may result in an anaphylactic reaction—sudden vascular collapse. This form of shock, distinguished by its rapid onset, appears related to an antigen-antibody reaction in the tissues from which histamine is liberated with resulting constriction of various arteriolar beds.

It is increasingly clear that the clinical course (and the treatment) of each of these entities is quite different and that the only common factor is the failure of tissue perfusion. In view of the lack of further understanding of the precise pathophysiology that interrelates these forms of shock, this chapter will consider only the general picture and treatment of decreased tissue perfusion.

## ASSESSMENT OF THE PROBLEM

Because of the diverse etiologies of the shock syndrome, a categorical description of its clinical course cannot be made.

Nevertheless, certain clinical features are similar regardless of the cause of the shock state.

The major manifestations of decreased tissue perfusion are as follows:

**1. Skin.** An early sign which may suggest shock is increased activity of the sympathetic nervous system. This is reflected in part by sweating and coolness of the skin due to constriction of the peripheral vessels. Therefore, when shock exists the skin is usually described as "cold and clammy"; however, warm, dry skin may exist, especially in septic shock.

**2. Level of consciousness.** In its early stages, shock is usually associated with obvious anxiety (again due to sympathetic nervous system hyperactivity with increased secretion of adrenalin). As the perfusion to the brain becomes lessened, the level of consciousness declines and confusion, agitation, and restlessness all develop. Ultimately, coma supervenes.

**3. Oliguria.** Decreased blood flow to the kidneys is a constant finding in shock. This effect is reflected by a decreased output of urine. Under normal conditions the kidneys should be able to excrete 1 cc of urine per minute (60 cc/hour). In the presence of shock the volume of urine is substantially reduced below this level and in many instances the output of urine ceases completely.

**4. Hypotension.** The characteristic effect of shock is a decrease in systolic blood pressure with a lesser reduction in diastolic pressure.

It is important to realize that hypotension, by itself, is not shock, and that unless other clinical manifestations are present, a low systolic pressure should not be construed as shock. In many instances a systolic pressure of only 70 or 80 mm of mercury may be of sufficient magnitude to permit adequate tissue perfusion in vasodilated patients.

**5. Pulse rate.** As part of the response to increased sympathetic stimulation, the pulse rate increases. The rate is further elevated by compensatory mechanisms of the body (particularly in hypovolemic or cardiogenic shock), which attempt to preserve adequate circulation by increasing the number of beats per minute when the circulating volume is insufficient. In the terminal phases of shock the pulse rate may become very slow.

**6. Respiration.** Usually breathing is rapid and of shallow quality.

Many believe that the ultimate cause of death in shock is related to the disturbance in pulmonary circulation which is reflected in the rate and volume of respiration.

**7. Metabolic acidosis.** Because of the inadequacy of circulation and the stasis of blood, metabolic products of cellular metabolism accumulate and produce a state of acidosis. The body attempts to compensate for this acidosis by using its multiple buffer systems. These compensatory mechanisms may fail and overt acidosis develops.

In addition to the preceding major manifestations of shock, there are many lesser findings that comprise the total picture. These factors vary according to the etiology and are not present in all patients. They include peripheral cyanosis, elevated, or reduced body temperature, collapsed peripheral veins, and, in cardiogenic shock, distended neck veins.

At the present time precise methods for assessing the degree of shock (that is, the exact reduction in tissue perfusion) or for detecting its earliest manifestations are for the most part available only in research units. The usual approach to the clinical problem is as follows:

**1. Repeated, planned recording of clinical signs.** Such observation of the patient remains the basic guide for assessment. By seeking and detecting the earliest manifestations of sympathetic nervous system activity (rapid pulse; cool, sweaty skin; pale, anxious face), the imminent development of shock may be suspected early enough to allow preventive therapy.

**2. Measurement of urinary volume.** By means of catheter drainage, urinary volume must be measured at frequent intervals in precise fashion.

**3. Central venous pressure (CVP).** Knowledge of the CVP is particularly valuable as a guide to fluid replacement in hypovolemic shock and is also useful in assessing the venous return in other forms of shock. By itself the CVP can be misleading and the measurement should always be interpreted in conjunction with other clinical and hemodynamic data. Because the capacity of the circulatory system is in a constant state of change, estimation of the amount of fluid needed in the treatment of shock cannot be made on a rule-of-thumb basis; CVP measurement is mandatory in this situation. By noting the response of CVP to fluid infusion, a dynamic gauge becomes available for measuring the replacement volume required in some forms of shock.

**4. Measurement of degree of blood lactic acidosis.** By determining the pH, $pCO_2$, and standard bicarbonate levels, the extent of acid-base derangement accompanying shock can be estimated. Metabolic acidosis is reflected by a low pH and a low standard bicarbonate.

**5. Measurement of cardiac output.** Cardiac output measurement is a valuable technique in assessing the clinical course of cardiogenic shock. However, there are no simple methods for performing these determinations, and the study must still be considered an experimental tool.

**6. Measurement of blood volume.** In hypovolemic shock, particularly, it is helpful to know the actual blood volume. This measurement can be obtained with isotope techniques rapidly and without great difficulty.

**7. Constant monitoring of arterial blood pressure.** A simple, but effective, method for monitoring arterial blood pressure is as follows:*

*Materials required*

  1. an intravenous pole

  2. adhesive tape, 65–70″ in length, 1½″ wide

  3. extension tubing (Bardic #1750), 30″ long with a capacity of 5.8 cc (4 tubes)

  4. 3-way stopcock

  5. an arterial catheter

  6. venesection tray

  7. an empty sterile bottle

  8. a 500 cc flask (containing saline with heparin) along with intravenous tubing for flush purposes (flush solution)

*Procedure* (See Fig. 1)

  1. Extend the intravenous pole to its maximum height.

  2. The adhesive tape is marked at successive intervals of 5.4″. The bottom line is labeled as zero and each successive interval as 10, 20, 30, etc. Since each 5.4″ represents 10 mm Hg, a reading scale for pressure measurement is available.

---

\* This method was devised by Robert F. Wilson, M.D., Assistant Professor of Surgery, Wayne State University, College of Medicine.

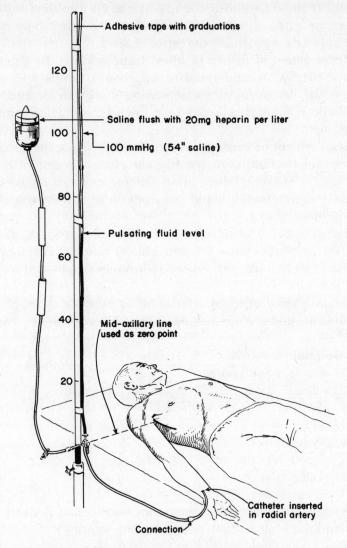

Adhesive tape with graduations

120

Saline flush with 20mg heparin per liter

100

100 mmHg (54" saline)

80

Pulsating fluid level

60

40

Mid-axillary line used as zero point

20

Catheter inserted in radial artery

Connection

*Fig. 1. Direct arterial blood pressure measurement*

3. Secure the calibrated adhesive tape to the length of the intravenous pole with the zero point at the level of the patient's midaxillary line.

4. Connect three extension tubes together and fasten adjoining tubing to the intravenous pole so that one end extends over the top and into an empty sterile bottle and the other end (the

male tip) extends free below the zero point for subsequent attachment.

5. The free end of the extension tube and the end of the intravenous tubing from the flush bottle are connected to two of the arms of a 3-way stopcock.

6. The fourth extension tube is attached to the third arm of the stopcock.

7. The entire system is filled with flush solution (the sterile bottle at the top of the tubing will catch the overflow when filling and washing out the tubing).

8. The fourth extension tube (Step 6) is then connected to an arterial catheter that has been placed in the radial artery.

9. The stopcock is turned so that the fluid in the extension tube on the intravenous pole is in continuity with the arterial system.

10. The level of fluid in the long extension tube represents the *mean* arterial blood pressure.

11. When the system is functioning correctly, the fluid level in the extension tube should fluctuate with each heart beat. If this does not occur, the arterial line is partially occluded and flushing is required.

## PRINCIPLES OF TREATMENT

The fundamental aims of treatment in shock are to increase tissue perfusion and to preserve adequate respiration. Other objectives are to prevent complications and to protect the patient from environmental stresses.

**1. Methods for increasing tissue perfusion.** The first step in improving tissue perfusion is to ascertain the etiology of shock. Obviously, the treatment of hemorrhagic (hypovolemic) shock must be directed to replacing the inadequate circulating blood volume, whereas in cardiogenic shock volume replacement is of minimal concern compared to the need for increasing the force of myocardial contraction to combat the low output.

The differential diagnosis is not usually very difficult. Thus, the patient with severe chest pain and ECG findings of acute myocardial infarction would be likely to have cardiogenic shock, and the patient with massive bleeding from esophageal varices would be a candidate for hypovolemic shock. The diagnosis of septic shock is perhaps the least obvious and requires astute clinical suspicion which is later confirmed by laboratory identification of the bacterial agent. However, in advanced states special forms of shock may exist concomitantly, and establishing the diagnosis is far more difficult.

The methods for treating inadequate perfusion vary according to the etiology. The following are general rules for therapy.

**Fluid replacement.** Hypovolemic shock is treated primarily by expanding the vascular volume. Fluid lost by frank hemorrhage, vomiting, diarrhea, or burns must be adequately replaced with appropriate fluids as rapidly as possible. The types of fluid replacement are dependent on the amount and kind of fluid lost.

TYPES OF FLUID USED FOR REPLACEMENT

a. *Blood.* Where hemorrhage is the major cause of shock, replacement of whole blood is essential. Large volumes are sometimes necessary and must be administered rapidly. Unless the blood is warmed to body temperature, it can act as a hypothermic agent. In shock this effect can be dangerous because reduction of the body temperature below 32° C may result in cardiac slowing, with decreased output or the development of ventricular fibrillation.

The use of "old" blood (collected more than 21 days before its intended use) can be hazardous to patients in shock. The breakdown of red blood cells during prolonged storage results in the transfer of intracellular potassium to the serum. This increased concentration of serum potassium, along with acidosis (that develops in vitro while the blood is standing) are distinctly dangerous in aggravating the very biochemical abnormalties found in the shock state itself.

Another danger accompanying the use of rapid large infusions of blood is the binding of calcium in the bloodstream by the citrate solution (used to prevent clotting of the stored blood). This decrease in serum calcium may lead to cardiac arrest. To prevent this threat, calcium gluconate should be given intravenously after every second or third unit of blood.

b. *Ringer's lactate solution.* The intravenous infusion of this solution is commonly used for rapid expansion of the vascular volume.

c. *5% dextrose in water.* In those instances in which the loss of free water is great (e.g., burns), fluid replacement with dextrose solution is preferable to salt solutions to avoid electrolyte overloading.

d. *Normal saline solution with sodium bicarbonate added.* This solution is used primarily to correct the metabolic acidosis accompanying shock. The bicarbonate, acting as an alkali, assists the buffer mechanism in controlling acidosis.

e. *Concentrated albumin.* When there is excessive loss of protein (e.g., in burns, pancreatitis, or peritonitis), concentrated albumin is used to increase the colloidal osmotic pressure. In this way fluid escape from the vascular tree (because of protein depletion) can be controlled.

f. *Dextran.* Both regular and low-molecular weight (LMW) dextran have been recommended as a means of expanding the plasma volume rapidly. At the present time LMW dextran is waning in popularity, because it is less effective as a volume expander than regular dextran or hydroxy-ethyl starch.

METHOD OF FLUID REPLACEMENT

As stated, the fluid replacement volume is best gauged on the basis of the response of the central venous pressure. Maintenance of effective atrial filling is the aim of optimum fluid therapy. A rapid rise in CVP (or right atrial pressure) may indicate that the vascular tree is loaded to capacity. On the other hand, an increase in blood pressure without a significant rise in CVP suggests that hypovolemia still exists. This cardiovascular response to a fluid load is the single most important measurement that can be made in hypovolemic shock.

For this measurement to be of diagnostic or therapeutic significance, the tip of the CVP catheter must be in the superior vena cava or the right atrium. Pressures recorded from the lesser venous channels may have little meaning because of the influence of venous constriction and intervening venous valves in the peripheral veins.

The method for placement of a central venous catheter is described on page 293. In addition to the use of a saline manometer, CVP can be recorded and monitored by electronic equipment. The major advantage of these latter devices is that they display the values continuously and permit simple, unequivocal readings. Disadvantages are the expense and the need for frequent flushing of the system to ensure continuous monitoring. The amounts of fluid required for this latter purpose may be of sufficient volume to contribute to the overload of an already filled vascular tree.

**2. Methods for preserving adequate respiration.** The prevention of respiratory failure is essential to survival in shock. An underlying problem in maintaining respiratory efficiency is the presence of metabolic acidosis. This acidosis results from accumulation of hydrogen ions secondary to inadequate tissue perfusion. In metabolic acidosis, excess hydrogen ions stimulate the respiratory center to increase pulmonary ventilation in an effort to rid the body of carbon dioxide and thus maintain the hydrogen ion concentration within the homeostatic range. As a result of this respiratory center stimulation, the breathing becomes rapid and deep (hyperventilation). This response consumes a considerable amount of energy, and unless the acidosis is controlled by effective therapy, fatigue and failure of the compensatory mechanism will ultimately occur. The process is insidious and demands constant close observation to detect minor deviations in the respiratory pattern.

Measurement of the $pCO_2$ indicates the effectiveness of this compensatory respiratory mechanism to combat metabolic acidosis. A low $pCO_2$ in the presence of low pH and bicarbonate levels (metabolic acidosis) indicates that the respiratory buffer system is compensating. However, a rising $pCO_2$ in the face of a persistently low pH should be recognized as a warning that the compensatory mechanism is failing and that respiratory assistance will be needed. Clinical symptoms that suggest this latter complication are a decrease in the rate and depth of respiration and the onset of cyanosis. The administration of oxygen in this particular setting is valueless, and removal of accumulated carbon dioxide can be achieved only by means of assisted ventilation with a respirator.

In the earliest stages of this particular problem the need for adequate respiration may be met by the use of a pressure-controlled respirator (such as a Bird respirator), which is triggered by patient demand. In more advanced cases, where the $pCO_2$ levels are very high and where obvious clinical signs of respiratory failure exist, the piston type, volume displacement respirator (Engstrom, Emerson, or Morch) is indicated. The piston type respirator is so powerful that it can convert the problem of respiratory acidosis to one of respiratory alkalosis within 10–30 minutes. Frequent arterial gas studies, including oxygen saturation, pH, and $pCO_2$ (for which blood samples must be collected in a heparinized syringe) are essential for regulation of the piston type machine, as well as for determining the efficacy of treatment. Because of the changing need for pressure-controlled and piston-type respirators, it is recommended that both be available for treatment of patients in shock.

To obtain adequate mechanical ventilation, a tracheostomy is usually required. Prior to this surgical intervention, ventilation is accomplished through a cuffed endotracheal tube attached to a respirator or controlled manually. This preparation permits an elective tracheostomy to be performed without the hazards of hypoxia or hypercarbia.

The selection of the tracheostomy tube is very important, because maximal ventilation is dependent upon a "Lo-leak" system in the pressure-controlled respirator, as well as some piston-type respirators. The double-cuffed rubber tracheostomy tube is the tube currently preferred in our unit. Because the pressure areas on the trachea can be altered by means of the two cuffs, this tube produces less tissue necrosis and minimizes the potential hazard of tracheal erosion. Furthermore, it is safer than the double-cannula metal tube with its applied endotracheal tube cuff (there is the hazard of these cuffs slipping down and occluding the tracheostomy tube opening). On the other hand, the double-cuffed rubber tube has the theoretical disadvantage of being more difficult to keep clean (because it lacks an inner cannula and must be changed every 24 hours). This problem does not appear to be significant in an intensive care unit.

A further discussion of the treatment of respiratory insufficiency is found in Chapter I.

### 3. Drug therapy.

*Vasodilators.* After many years during which the administration of vasopressors remained the keystone of shock treatment, the concept was developed that this therapy was misdirected and that the basic approach should be to *dilate* the peripheral vessels rather than to attempt to constrict them. The use of vasodilators was advocated on the basis that the peripheral vessels were maximally constricted because of the large outpouring of norepinephrine (as part of the body's response to shock) and that significant redistribution of blood would occur by inhibiting this constriction. In principle, by relaxing arteries and veins with blocking agents such as phentolamine (Regitine) or phenoxybenzamine (Dibenzyline), the vascular volume could be increased and blood trapped peripherally could be made available for tissue perfusion. This practice has been enthusiastically accepted by some investigators, but its ultimate value remains uncertain. It is clear that the use of these alpha receptor blocking agents should be employed only in those situations where increasing the vascular space might be beneficial. In the presence of hypovolemic shock, provision must be made for adequate (and rapid) fluid replacement when these agents are used.

*Digitalis.* The realization that decreased cardiac output is a common factor in hypovolemic and cardiogenic shock has made it evident that drugs which will improve myocardial contraction should be a fundamental part of the treatment program for shock. Most clinicians employ digitalis for this purpose. The most rapidly acting digitalis preparations (particularly Ouabain and deslanoside) are usually given intravenously early in the course of shock. The usual initial dose of Ouabain is .30 to .50 mgm which may be repeated in small increments within an hour. Deslanoside (Cedilanid D) is usually administered in a dose of 0.8 mgm, with subsequent increments of 0.4 mgm. These drugs should not be given to patients who are digitalized already. In cardiogenic shock, digitalization appears especially valuable.

*Isoproterenol.* This drug is used for the same reason as digitalis, namely, to increase the force of myocardial contraction and thus improve cardiac output. Isoproterenol (Isuprel) is the strongest inotropic agent known and is more effective than digitalis for this one purpose. The usual dosage is 1 mgm isoproterenol diluted in 500 cc of fluid. The drug must be administered intra-venously by microdrip technique while the patient is under con-stant electrocardiographic monitoring. In addition to its pro-pensity for inducing ventricular arrhythmias, isoproterenol may also result in inspissation of bronchial secretions. For these rea-sons, the drug must be used cautiously.

*Antibiotics.* Antibiotic therapy is important primarily in the treatment of bacteremic shock. When this form of shock is sus-pected, blood cultures should be drawn immediately and anti-biotics started, even though the responsible organism is unknown at the moment. In this particular situation, recognizing that most instances of septic shock are the result of gram-negative enteric bacteria, a combination of Ampicillin, Polymixin, and Keflin may be used until cultures and sensitivities are available.

*Steroid Therapy.* The use of huge amounts of corticosteroids has been recommended as an adjunctive therapy in shock. The precise role of steroids in this situation is by no means clear and there is some evidence to indicate that they may be of no value, or even harmful. Nevertheless, they are often used and some in-vestigators remain enthusiastic about their value.

There is agreement that when steroids are employed their dosages should not be merely in the replacement range, but should be in pharmacologic quantities. Some advocate using at least 3000 mgm of hydrocortisone each day. Furthermore, the drug should be given early in the course of shock, rather than as a final desperate effort after other drugs have failed.

There are several theoretical dangers associated with steroid therapy in this high dosage range. These include inhibition of the antibody response, permitting uncontrollable infection; the ag-gravation of diabetes; and acute gastrointestinal bleeding.

*Mannitol.* Acute renal tubular necrosis (lower nephron nephrosis, discussed in Chapter XIII, "Renal Dialysis") is a common complication of severe trauma which produces shock (e.g., burns) or of prolonged hypotension. To prevent this acute renal damage, osmotic diuretics, including urea and mannitol, have been used.

Mannitol is thought to increase renal blood flow by decreasing resistance in the renal vascular system. For this reason it may be of use in the patient who has persistent oliguria despite adequate fluid replacement. The usual method of administration of mannitol involves an intravenous injection of 100 cc of 20% mannitol within 15 minutes. If effective, an increase in urine flow is apparent within 30 to 40 minutes. If the urinary output does not increase within this time interval, it may be assumed that renal damage has already occurred (providing that adequate hydration exists at the time).

Caution must be used with mannitol, particularly among patients with existing left ventricular failure, because the blood volume usually expands prior to diuresis and pulmonary edema may ensue. Because mannitol administration may result in decreased serum sodium, serum sodium levels should be determined.

*Vasopressors.* The basic principle in using vasopressors is to achieve and maintain a mean blood pressure of 70 to 80 mm of Hg (mean blood pressure $= \frac{\text{systolic} + \text{diastolic}}{2}$). Attempting to increase the blood pressure beyond these levels is a poor practice, because the agents increase the oxygen demand of the heart at the same time and, as a result, may cause serious (death-producing) arrhythmias.

A variety of vasopressor agents are available, the most popular of which are levarterenol (Levophed), metaraminol (Aramine), and mephentermine (Wyamine). Because the vasopressor drugs must be diluted in rather large volumes of fluid prior to administration, the problem of overloading the vascular system is not uncommon. One solution to this difficulty is utilization of an infusion pump, which permits the delivery of controlled minute amounts of the undiluted drug. Vasopressor therapy is discussed additionally in Chapter II, "Acute Myocardial Infarction."

## THE NURSING ROLE

**Pre-admission preparation.** Because the reversibility of shock is clearly related to the rapidity with which tissue perfusion is increased, it is essential that treatment be instituted as soon as the diagnosis is established. To accomplish this essential aim, expert personnel must be mobilized and equipment and material made ready for immediate use. These activities must begin prior to the anticipated arrival of the patient in the intensive care unit.

The following equipment and supplies should be assembled and prepared by the nurse:

*Equipment.*
    a. respirators: pressure cycled and volume controlled
    b. cardiac monitor
    c. oxygen and suction apparatus, if not available from central source
    d. hypothermia unit with telethermometer and rectal probe
    e. bed scale and gram scale
    f. blood warmer

*Supplies.*
    a. tracheostomy set with cuffed tracheostomy tubes
    b. venesection trays
    c. venus catheter: polyethylene 35–42″ in length; radiopaque; diameter p.e. 180–280
    d. Foley catheter and tray
    e. urimeter
    f. arterial cannulae
    g. equipment for direct arterial blood pressure measurement
    h. Levine tube and other suction catheters
    i. endotracheal tubes and laryngoscope
    j. central venous pressure measurement apparatus
*Intravenous Fluids.*
    a. Ringer's solution
    b. 5% dextrose in normal saline
    c. 5% dextrose in water
    d. normal saline solution
    e. dextran

**Patient care and comfort.** Patient comfort is essential to patient survival. The nursing role in achieving such comfort is unique. Unless preventive measures are employed, serious complications can develop from prolonged discomfort.

The patient in shock often must be in the same position, flat on the back, for several hours. This enforced immobilization may result in additional complications. For example, it has been shown experimentally that this type of recumbency and inactivity can depress respiration. This factor, in conjunction with dehydration, often leads to atelectasis and pulmonary infection (which contribute to pulmonary shunting) that might have been prevented. The nurse should change the patient's position as frequently as possible by a simple means, such as elevating the head slightly and/or slipping a pillow under one side. During the treatment period deep breathing and coughing should be encouraged.

Another complication of this total inactivity is the reduction of adequate venous return resulting from the loss of tone of voluntary muscles. In addition, the prolonged pressure on the legs from lying in bed without movement can lead to peripheral thrombosis. Again, the nurse can contribute to the total care by utilizing preventive measures. Simple exercises such as wiggling the toes or flexion and extension of the ankles can be very effective in this regard. In the unresponsive patient, the nurse should initiate passive exercises at propitious times during the course of treatment.

The control of pain is of course essential to physical comfort. It should be remembered that analgesics or narcotics should be given intravenously in shock patients. Hypodermic administration is ill-advised because of the delay in drug absorption secondary to impaired circulation. The usual intravenous dosage of analgesics or narcotics is one-half to two-thirds of the customary hypodermic dosage.

The emotional impact from the shock state is profound. Everywhere the patient looks there are bottles, tubes, machines, and people. One machine is forcing air down his throat; another is "beeping" continuously. Tubes are coming from his bladder, nose, arms, and throat. His whole body image is distorted. Nurses and doctors are scurrying about, hanging up bottles, taking others down, adjusting machines. The sensory input is enormous. All of this is superimposed on an already confused mental state engendered by the shock syndrome. The nurse can do much to help the patient maintain some equilibrium at this awesome time. All of the following are worthwhile practices:

1. Explain each procedure before it is done and reiterate its need while the treatment is in progress.

2. Identify and explain the equipment surrounding the patient.

4. Initiate a quiet, organized plan for personnel activities. Sudden movement or noise can be very detrimental to the patient's physical status in this setting.

5. Protect the patient from unnecessary exposure.

If the patient is to adapt to this extraordinary stress and survive, the combined efforts of a doctor-nurse team are mandatory. The constant presence of a nurse qualified to make decisions is essential.

"Provide emotional support and relieve patients' apprehension," are common jargon in the nursing world today. One interpretation of this concept might be to provide an atmosphere that permits the patient to feel he is receiving the best care possible. A physician-nurse team possessing self-confidence and organized direction makes the patient feel secure. While there is no evidence that this type of planning will decrease the patient's apprehensiveness, we can at least be certain that it does not add to it.

## Specific Nursing Duties in the Treatment Program

*Fluid replacement.* Fluid replacement is determined by the amount and type of fluid lost. Therefore, accurate measurement of various forms of fluid loss is essential to planning proper therapy. The nursing role in this regard is of paramount importance. Assessing fluid loss accurately and completely includes the following considerations.

1. An indwelling Foley catheter is essential to determine urine volume. Because the quantities of urine excreted are likely to be very small during the shock state, an accurate, calibrated urine collector is mandatory. In our institution the urimeter collector is preferred to the more complex electric urinometer for several reasons: it is easier to read and easier to clean; it hangs on the bed away from the feet of attending personnel; and it is less expensive.

Changes in the urinary volume represent perhaps the most

meaningful index of the success or failure of therapy. The nurse should check the output every few minutes and measure it at least every half-hour.

2. Accurate measurement of emesis, liquid stools, chest drainage, and gastrointestinal drainage are easily obtained by customary methods. However, measurement of draining wounds and incontinence presents a challenge to the nurse's ingenuity. One recommended method for measuring wound drainage involves actual weighing of dressings. A gram scale (diabetic type) with a small cake pan attached to the weighing platform can be used effectively for this purpose. The difference between the total weight of the wet dressings and the total weight of similar dry dressings accurately indicates the amount of drainage lost. A list of the weight of each kind of dressing should be attached to the scale for convenient reference. The weight of drainage fluid, in grams, is converted to milliliters on a one-to-one basis and is recorded.

Fluid loss on bed linen can be estimated in similar fashion; however, since the dry weight of individual linens varies considerably, it is necessary to weigh each piece and tag it before use. A kilogram scale is required for this purpose.

One guide for estimation of this loss involves regular measurement of the total body weight with stretcher or bed scales. A bed scale which permits continuous recording of the body weight is particularly effective. Changes of only a few grams in either direction can be recognized immediately and changes in therapy instituted.

3. Not all fluid is lost externally, and the fluid extravasated from the vascular space into a "third" compartment (e.g., peritoneal cavity or chest cavity) must also be considered in replacement therapy. This type of fluid loss is just as critical as external loss, because it is useless in terms of circulatory function. This internal loss is difficult to measure.

When the internal loss is localized to a measurable site (e.g., the peritoneal cavity), the size of this "third" compartment can be identified simply by the use of a tape measure. In this situation the nurse should measure the abdominal girth every eight hours to obtain a picture of the amount of fluid lost into this cavity. Additional material regarding fluid loss is found in Chapter VII, "Water and Electrolyte Imbalances."

## Preservation of Adequate Respiration

1. The rate and depth of respiration must be observed almost continuously to permit the detection of early respiratory failure. Slowing of the rate in the presence of an elevated $pCO_2$ suggests failure of the respiratory compensatory mechanism and indicates the need for assisted respiration.

2. The nursing role regarding the care of tracheostomy and the use of respirators has been described in detail in Chapter I, "Respiratory Insufficiency and Failure."

### Drug Therapy

VASODILATORS

1. The increase in vascular space effected by vasodilators is accompanied by a sudden reduction in blood pressure; therefore, the blood pressure must be monitored regularly and carefully when such therapy is initiated. The nurse should stop the administration of the drug and increase fluids in the event of abrupt and profound hypotension. However, a mean BP of 70 is usually acceptable.

2. The central venous pressure (CVP) should be monitored whenever these blocking agents are used. The decrease in peripheral resistance results in a substantial drop in the CVP. The volume of fluid needed to fill the suddenly enlarged vascular space is gauged by the CVP. The nurse should adjust the rate of fluid replacement to maintain a reasonably normal CVP, in accordance with the physician's instructions. A continuous fall in CVP, despite fluid replacement, indicates a dangerous situation and implies that the rate and volume of replacement are inadequate.

3. Careful assessment of the clinical state, including skin temperature, color, and the state of cardiac function should be noted and recorded as a means of estimating the effectiveness of treatment.

4. Make certain that the patient is kept in a flat position while these drugs are being administered. Elevating the head could prove disastrous in view of the orthostatic hypotension which may be produced.

DIGITALIS

1. The nursing role during digitalis therapy has been described in the chapter on circulatory emergencies. In this acute situation, particularly where very rapidly acting and potent agents are used, the nurse should be aware of the pulse rate at all times.

2. Because digitalis toxicity may occur in this setting, continuous ECG monitor observation is essential.

ISOPROTERENOL

1. Because of its extreme potency and the threat of inducing fatal arrhythmias by overly rapid infusion, isoproterenol must be given with extreme caution. In addition to using a microdrip system, the infusion bottle should be "piggybacked" to an existing intravenous line, but not to a CVP catheter. (A CVP catheter frequently requires irrigation to maintain patency for accurate reading. When increasing the drip rate for this purpose, the rate of the piggyback line may be affected, leading to disastrous results when either Isuprel or vasopressors are incorporated in the piggyback fluid.) In the event of an arrhythmia induced by the drug, administration can be stopped instantly without closing an essential conduit.

2. Once an isoproterenol infusion is started, the patient must be constantly attended by a nurse. If premature ventricular contractions or ventricular tachycardia are noted on the ECG monitor (see chapter on acute myocardial infarction), the infusion must either be slowed down or stopped. A defibrillator must be at the bedside.

3. Accurate measurement of urinary volume and blood pressure should be made about every 20 minutes in order to assess the effectiveness of therapy.

ANTIBIOTICS

Whenever septic shock is suspected, blood for culture should be drawn promptly. Additional samples of urine, sputum, and fluid from draining wounds or sinuses should be taken at the same time for culture to identify the infective organism.

STEROID THERAPY

1. Patients who receive huge amounts of steroids are predisposed to serious infection. In shock, where pneumonia, wound infection, and bacteremia are common sequelae, the threat of overwhelming infection must be guarded against. The patient should be protected against obvious sources of infection from environment and personnel, family, and visitors.

2. Careful examination of urinary and fecal excretions, as well as vomitus, should be made to ascertain the onset of bleeding induced by steroids.

MANNITOL

1. When mannitol is employed, the nurse should carefully verify the patency of urinary catheter drainage prior to the injection.

2. The urinary output should be measured and recorded every 15 minutes for two hours following mannitol injection.

3. If urinary output does not increase after mannitol, infusion of additional fluid must be restricted.

4. The nurse should carefully observe the patient for possible signs of left ventricular failure. The onset of dyspnea, tachypnea, or the detection of distended neck veins is cause for concern that the cardiovascular system has been overloaded by volume expansion.

VASOPRESSORS

1. Careful monitoring of the blood pressure is absolutely essential whenever vasopressors are being administered. As indicated in the section on treatment, the goal is to maintain a blood pressure level sufficient to insure perfusion, but not to attain normal pressures.

2. Because of the propensity for ventricular arrhythmias to develop during infusion of pressor substances, ECG monitoring should be employed, and if frequent premature ventricular contractions are observed, the nurse should notify the physician.

3. In the event of tissue infiltration, particularly with levarterenol bitartrate (Levophed), the intravenous drip must be

stopped immediately because of the threat of tissue ischemia and necrosis developing from localized vasoconstriction in the immediate area.

4. The nurse should be alert for early signs of left ventricular decompensation or the sudden onset of pulmonary edema when vasopressors are being used. The rise in blood pressure caused by vasopressors is the result of peripheral vessel constriction. This diverts blood from peripheral areas to the central circulation and creates the threat of overloading the pulmonary circuit.

If such failure occurs, the nurse should immediately decrease the intravenous flow to a minimum, and notify the physician. The head of the bed should be elevated to combat respiratory distress when pulmonary edema develops.

## Bibliography

HARDAWAY, ROBERT M. III: *Syndromes of Disseminated Intravascular Coagulation.* Charles Thomas, Springfield, Ill., 1966.

HEWER, C. L.: The Physiology and Complications of the Trendelenberg Position. *Canadian Med. Assoc. J.,* 74:285, 1956.

McMICHAEL, J. and McGIBBON, J. P.: "Postural Changes in Lung Volume." *Clinical Science.* 4:175–183, December 1939.

MILLS, LEWIS C., ed.: *Shock and Hypertension.* Grune and Stratton, New York.

MOYER, CARL: Burns. *Archives of Surgery.*

POWERS, SAMUEL R., KILEY, JOHN E., BOBA, ANTONIO: Renal Failure in Surgical Patients. *Current Problems in Surgery,* November 1965.

STRAVITZ, JOESEPH G. and GROSSBLATT, NORMAN, eds.: *Septic Shock.* National Academy of Sciences National Research Council, Proceedings of a Workshop, September 11–12, 1964.

THAL, ALAN P., WILSON, ROBERT F.: Shock. *Current Problems in Surgery,* Year Book Medical Publishers, Inc., September 1965.

WARD, R. O.: Postoperative Paralysis in the Upper Extremity. *Lancet,* 1:423, 1950.

WEIL, MAX H., WHIGHAM, HOWARD: Head-Down (Trendelenberg) Position for Treatment of Irreversible Hemorrhagic Shock. *Annals of Surgery,* 162:905–909, November 1965.

WEIL, MAX H., SHUBIN, H., and BIDDLE M.: Shock Caused by Gram-Negative Microorganisms: Analysis of 169 Cases. *Annals Internal Medicine.* 60:384, 1964.

ZIMMERMAN, BERNARD: Postoperative Management of Fluid Volumes and Electrolytes. *Current Problems in Surgery,* Year Book Medical Publishers, Inc., December 1965.

ZWEIFACH, B. W.: Etiology of the Shock Syndrome. *The Heart Bulletin,* 14:26 March–April 1965.

CHAPTER V

# Hepatic Failure

WILLIAM V. MCDERMOTT, JR., M.D.
ANNA SUPPLE, R.N., B.S.N.

## THE PROBLEM

Hepatic failure, frequently referred to by the rather indefinite and inaccurate term of "hepatic coma," is usually characterized by varying degrees of encephalopathy. While not a simple clinical entity, the problem can be divided into two general categories: exogenous and endogenous hepatic failure.

**Exogenous Hepatic Failure.** Exogenous hepatic failure is associated with portal hypertension and results primarily from the shunting of portal blood around the liver. In this way, metabolic components from the gastrointestinal tract, which normally would be altered during the passage of portal blood through the liver, are enabled to enter directly into the systemic circulation. The clinical picture of hepatic failure develops secondarily to this metabolic disturbance. These circumstances typically occur in patients with liver cirrhosis in whom the portal bed is obstructed and collateral vessels develop which bypass the liver.

Of the metabolites shunted around the liver, ammonia appears to be the major factor involved in causing the syndrome of exogenous hepatic failure. Under normal conditions, ammonia is produced by the action of micro-organisms on proteins in the gastrointestinal tract and is found in high concentrations in the portal blood returning from the bowel to the liver. Within the liver ammonia is metabolized to urea through the Krebs-Henseleit cycle, and thus does not enter the systemic circulation.

When collateral channels develop, however, as a result of portal bed block within the liver, the absorbed ammonia can then bypass the liver and reach high levels in the peripheral blood, particularly in the presence of a large nitrogenous load in the gastrointestinal tract. The major bypass to the systemic circulation occurs via a network of esophageal veins (varices).

When patients with hepatic cirrhosis and portal hypertension (as evidenced by esophageal varices) develop bleeding from varices, the blood in the bowel constitutes an enormous nitrogenous load producing high ammonia concentrations. In addition to this insult, there is decreased hepatic blood flow (an almost invariable sequela of cirrhosis), which reduces the ability of the liver to clear the ammonia that has already reached the systemic circulation. As a result of the increased concentration of ammonia within the systemic circulation, the central nervous system is affected and in some unknown manner encephalopathy develops. It should be realized that hepatic function itself may be reasonably intact even though encephalopathy exists and that the syndrome may result from massive ammonia overloading alone. The clinical picture is not always one of coma, and for this reason the term encephalopathy is preferable to "hepatic coma."

**Endogenous Hepatic Failure.** Endogenous hepatic failure refers to liver failure resulting from actual parenchymal tissue destruction and involves the loss of normal hepatic functions. Obviously, this type of hepatic failure is more serious and complicated than exogenous portal systemic encephalopathy, since it involves loss or impairment of multiple liver functions. In addition to hyperammonemia (which may, in fact, not be an important part of this syndrome), there are defects in carbohydrate, fat, and protein metabolism. Additionally, disturbances occur in blood coagulation, fluid and electrolyte balance, detoxification mechanisms, and renal function (in an unexplained manner), which are all the result of liver destruction.

These two forms of hepatic failure do not necessarily occur independently; most often they coexist in varying proportions. As noted, some patients with reasonably adequate liver function may bleed massively from esophageal varices and develop encephalopathy purely from hyperammonemia; others may develop the same clinical picture without preexisting portal hypertension as a result of acute yellow atrophy caused by viral hepatitis or hepatotoxins. Between these extremes there may be a combination of endogenous and exogenous hepatic encephalopathy.

## ASSESSMENT OF THE PROBLEM

**History.** The patient's history is particularly significant in determining the type of hepatic failure and its subsequent treatment. In many cases, because of encephalopathy, the patient is unable to give a coherent history; in others, the problem is further complicated by acute alcoholism, and it is necessary in these instances to question friends and relatives carefully.

Inquiry should be made about alcoholic intake, occupation, exposure to hepatotoxins, contact with viral hepatitis, and injections. A history of previous gastrointestinal symptoms should be sought to avoid the erroneous conclusion that all episodes of bleeding in patients with cirrhosis are due to esophageal varices. Many of these patients have peptic ulcers, and it is obviously imperative to rule out this source of gastrointestinal hemorrhage. The possibility of an unrelated bleeding diathesis should also be considered. A history of bleeding episodes following dental treatment, minor lacerations, or the development of ecchymotic areas are cause for suspicion; a bleeding or coagulation defect or a past history of transient confusion or disorientation may offer a clue to the presence of long standing, but intermittent, portal-systemic encephalopathy.

**Physical examination** The physical examination, although complete, should concentrate on specific evidences of liver disease in the form of hepatosplenomegaly, ascites, jaundice, testicular atrophy, alterations of hair distribution, clubbing of fingers, Dupuytren's contractures, and parotid swelling. Associated vascular changes related to liver disease are arterial spiders located on the head, neck, upper thorax, and shoulders; large superficial veins in the periumbilical areas, as well as the chest and abdomen; and palmar erythema. Advanced signs of liver disease are manifest by flapping tremors and a sickish, sweetish breath odor called "fetor hepaticus."

**Diagnostic methods.** As previously discussed, it is important to determine whether hepatic failure is the result of hyperammonemia from portal shunting or is due to advanced parenchymal destruction. Several diagnostic methods are utilized for this purpose:

1. *Needle biopsy of liver.* A small plug of liver tissue is obtained by insertion of a Vim-Silverman needle into the liver substance. The usual site for this biopsy is between the anterior and posterior axillary lines in the 8th or 9th intercostal space. The procedure is fundamentally simple and can be performed at the bedside with very little discomfort to the patient and without general anesthesia. The ease and success of the biopsy depend, to a large degree, upon complete cooperation of the patient. To this end, it is essential that the nurse explain the procedure and rehearse the patient in the proper method of inhaling, exhaling, and breath-holding at the end of expiration, so that his full cooperation can be obtained.

The biopsy is performed with the patient supine, and with his head turned to the left. The patient's right arm is elevated and adducted so that his right hand grasps the opposite side of the bed at the level of his left shoulder. Following the biopsy, the patient should be instructed to remain on his right side with the right arm flexed under the hypochondrium. Bed rest is essential for 24 hours after the biopsy, because it is in this period that hemorrhage is likely to occur.

Contraindications to needle biopsy of the liver include an uncooperative patient, decreased prothrombin time, peritonitis, ascites, and extrahepatic obstructive jaundice. Complications which may arise as a result of the procedure are pain at the site of insertion of the needle with radiation to the right shoulder; epigastric pain or discomfort; hemorrhage into the peritoneum due to the accidental penetration of an intercostal vessel or the diaphragm; bile peritonitis, as a result of puncture of a bile duct; and shock. A reaction to local anesthesia, which also may occur, can be prevented if a skin test is performed the night before the procedure with the anesthetic that is to be used. Emergency equipment should be available at the bedside during and after the biopsy procedure.

2. *Esophagogram and upper GI series.* These radiographic examinations are performed primarily to determine the source of bleeding causing hematemesis. The finding of esophageal varices is clear evidence of the development of a large collateral circula-

tion and can account for hyperammonemia. To avoid the possibility of intestinal obstruction following barium administration, it is important that both a laxative and an enema be used after the examination.

3. *Esophagoscopy.* The esophagoscope is inserted into the esophagus for direct visualization of the source of esophageal bleeding. This procedure permits an immediate diagnosis as well as specific identification of the bleeding site. The danger of esophageal perforation and the possibility of traumatic rupture of the varices have discouraged use of this type of instrumentation except between bleeding periods.

The night before examination, the patient is skin tested with cocaine, the usual topical anesthetic employed in esophagoscopy. Since this anesthetic diminishes the gag reflex for about a four-hour period, it is extremely important that the nurse recognize the need to withhold fluids and food during this period. For the same reason, it is necessary to maintain the patient on his side with the head of the bed elevated. An airway should be available at the bedside for emergency purposes. If the patient, as well as the nurse, is cognizant of the absence of the gag reflex, the possibility of aspiration will be minimized.

4. *Splenic portography and splenic pulp manometry.* By the injection of a contrast medium such as Hypaque into the splenic pulp, it is possible to visualize the venous inflow tract of the liver on x-ray examination. This procedure, portography, is an important diagnostic method in the establishment of a diagnosis of portal hypertension. Splenic pulp manometry is used to measure the actual portal vein pressure, which, of course, reflects the degree of portal hypertension.

Contraindications of this test include bleeding tendency, sensitivity to the dye, severe debility, and anemia. Some of the complications which may result are allergic reaction to the dye, pain in the left upper quadrant, and splenic lacerations. Dye reactions are not infrequent and, for this reason, it is imperative that a careful history of possible allergies be obtained prior to initiating the procedure. In the event that such a reaction occurs, the patient should be kept motionless. The possibility of an allergic reaction can be reduced by using a test dose of 1 cc of Hypaque intravenously. Some clinicians prefer to use antihistamines pro-

phylactically in all patients given these dyes. Obviously, epinephrine and other emergency drugs should be on hand at all times
when this dye is administered. Lesser reactions to the procedure
are burning sensation at the injection site, a feeling of abdominal
pressure, warmth and facial flushing, and a metallic taste.

As with liver biopsy, these tests require patient cooperation,
and coaching in breath-holding is advised prior to the procedure.
Other preparations for these tests should include the use of
Neomycin by mouth for 24 hours before, as well as a Neomycin
enema the morning of the procedure. Prothrombin, bleeding, and
clotting times should be known before attempting this test. In the
event that splenic pulp manometry is contraindicated because of a
bleeding tendency, hepatic vein catheterization is sometimes performed.

5. *Hepatic vein catheterization (wedge hepatic pressure).*
A radiopaque catheter is inserted as far as it will go into the right
or left hepatic vein to occlude the flow of blood into the hepatic
vein. This process results in the transfer of pressure from the
sinusoidal bed to the head of the catheter. The purposes of this
test are measurement of the hepatic vein pressure, estimation of
the hepatic blood flow, and visualization of the outflow tract of the
liver. Contraindications are an uncooperative patient, sepsis, or
history of pulmonary embolization.

6. *Laboratory tests.* To assess hepatocellular function, a
battery of tests are performed. The normal values for these tests
are shown in Table 1.

Those tests concerned with bilirubin metabolism are used to
evaluate the degree of jaundice and to help to distinguish between
intrahepatic and extrahepatic causes of the jaundice.

Determination of the serum proteins gives valuable informa-
iton regarding severity of liver dysfunction. The albumin-globulin
ratio and the electrophoretic pattern of the various proteins are
particularly significant in this regard.

Blood ammonia levels are of great value in assessing the extent of portal systemic shunting; however, blood ammonia levels
are also increased with hepatocellular damage. To distinguish the
particular source of hyperammonemia, blood urea nitrogen determinations should be made concurrently with the ammonia levels.
Blood urea nitrogen is frequently extremely low when the hyper-

## Table 1

NORMAL VALUES FOR LABORATORY TESTS IN LIVER DISEASE

| | | |
|---|---|---|
| *Bilirubin:* | direct | 0.1–0.4 mgm/ml |
| | total | 0.3–0.8 mgm/ml |
| *BSP Retention:* | 30 minute retention | 0–12% |
| | 45 minute retention | 0–5% |
| | % disappearance rate | 11–15 mgm/minute |
| *Serum Alkaline Phosphatase* | | 2–5 (Bodansky) |
| *Total Serum Cholesterol* | | 180–250 mgm/100 ml |
| *Proteins:* | total serum protein | 6.3–8.0 gm/100 ml |
| | albumin | 3.5–5.5 gm/100 ml or 63–69% |
| | globulin | 1.4–3.4 gm/100 ml or 3.9–7.3% |
| *Prothrombin Time* | | 10–20 seconds (Quick) |
| *Coagulation Time* | | 6–10 minutes (Lee & White) |
| | | 10–30 minutes (Howell) |
| *Cephalin Flocculation* | | 0–1 + |
| *Serum Glutamic Pyruvic Transaminase* | | (SGPT) 10–40 units |
| *Serum Glutamic Oxalacetic Transaminase* | | (SGOT) 10–40 units |
| *Arterial Blood Ammonia* | | 20–50 ug/ml |
| *Bleeding Time* | | 1–3 minutes (Duke) |
| | | 2–4 minutes (Ivy) |
| *Icteric Index* | | 3–8 units |
| *Thymol Turbidity* | | 0–5 units |
| *Fibrinogen* | | 150–300 mgm/100 ml |
| *Non-Protein Nitrogen* | | 25–30 mgm/100 ml |
| *Urea* | | 20–40 mgm/100 ml |
| *Urea Nitrogen* | | 10–20 mgm/100 ml |
| *Urobilinogen,* urine | | 0–4 mgm/24 hours |
| feces | | 40–280 mgm/24 hours |
| *Platelets* | | 200,000–500,000/cu mm |

ammonemia is the result of hepatocellular function rather than of portal shunting.

Many other laboratory studies which delineate specific aspects of liver function can be performed. The composite profile obtained from these tests offers information regarding the severity and progress of this disease.

## PRINCIPLES OF TREATMENT

**Control of hemorrhage.** Hemorrhage is the major life-threatening complication of cirrhosis of the liver. There are many methods of controlling bleeding, but perhaps the most frequently used technique is balloon tamponade. In order to control esophageal bleeding, the most frequent locus of bleeding, tubes with attached balloons are inserted to compress the large veins in the distal esophagus.

Little purpose would be served in describing each of these balloons in detail, since their general design and use are similar. The most commonly used system is that described by Sengstaken and Blakemore, which involves a triple lumen rubber tube with two latex balloon attachments. One lumen functions as a naso-gastric suction tube, and a second communicates with a round balloon which resides in the stomach. The third lumen connects to an elliptical balloon (situated above the gastric balloon), which is used for direct compression of the esophageal varices. The tube is inserted through the nose into the stomach. The round gastric balloon attached to lumen #2 is inflated with 250 to 300 cc of air and the lumen clamped. The main tube is then withdrawn slowly until the distended balloon is tight against the cardioesophageal junction. It is then secured in this position by placing a piece of foam rubber under the tubing at the nostril area. This padding provides traction on the tubing to maintain the balloon at the cardioesophageal junction and also protects against the threat of pressure ulceration at the nares. The esophageal lumen (#3), is connected by a Y tube to a manometer, and the elliptical balloon is inflated to a pressure between 35 and 40 mm Hg with a bulb syringe. To insure control of esophageal bleeding, this pressure must be carefully maintained. The nasogastric suction lumen (#1), is attached to an ordinary intermittent gastric suction machine. Maintenance of this nasogastric suction serves two purposes: it enables the physician to assess whether or not the balloon mechanism has been effective to control bleeding, and it permits the stomach to be kept empty.

**Tracheostomy.** Because of the likelihood of aspiration in a coma-tose patient with this type of gastrointestinal hemorrhage, trache-ostomy is often performed as a prophylactic measure. Methods of preventing infection at the tracheostomy site are scrupulous care of the surgical wound, frequent changes of the tracheostomy tube, removal of secretions in and around the tube so as to prevent crusting around the tube with resultant occlusion, and mainte-nance of intermittent positive pressure breathing in order to sup-port cardiorespiratory functions and adequate oxygenation.

**Drug therapy.** Because of the inability of the diseased liver to detoxify certain drugs, the use of medications poses a particular danger in these patients. Extreme caution must be exercised in the administration of sedatives, analgesics, and hypnotics. Under some circumstances (particularly great agitation), and regardless of the possible development of hepatic coma, these medications must be used. Unfavorable reactions can be reduced by limiting the dose and frequency of administration.

If sedation is absolutely necessary, Librium, barbital, and phenobarbital are usually the drugs of choice. All of these are excreted by the kidney rather than the liver. The dosage of analgesics or hypnotics should be less than the amounts customarily given patients without liver damage.

**Parenteral therapy.** Patients with hepatic failure invariably require a constant venous conduit because of the need for large quantities of blood, plasma, and fluids. An inlying catheter placed either percutaneously or by direct cutdown on a large vein is the method of choice. Type and amount of parenteral fluids will change from hour to hour, because of extreme fluctuations in the patient's requirements, and a standardized program of fluid administration is ill-advised. Large amounts of blood (usually fresh) are required, as are large volumes of human serum albumin and plasma to combat ascites. Fluid orders must be carefully and frequently re-evaluated in accordance with rapid alterations in the patient's clinical state.

If replacement of fluid is excessive for the body's need, hypervolemia can develop. The cardiovascular system cannot handle this excessive load, and cardiac failure will result. The threat of hypovolemia is even more common during hepatic failure. An inadequate circulating blood volume is often associated with decreased renal perfusion and may result in irreversible renal damage. In fact, renal failure is most frequently the terminal event in hepatic disease. Even brief periods of hypovolemia can result in renal destruction, and the prevention of this state is one of the major aims of therapy.

In addition to these derangements in fluid volume, maintenance of electrolyte balance is a further consideration in intelligent treatment. Most patients with hepatic failure tend to become potassium-deficient. Causative factors in this loss of potassium are frequent paracenteses, diarrhea, the use of diuretics, and too frequent use of enemas or laxatives. This potassium loss must be adequately replaced as governed by such factors as the patient's age, renal function, and cardiac status.

## THE NURSING ROLE

### The team approach

Patients with hepatic failure complicated by gastrointestinal hemorrhage are most often critically ill. Their survival is dependent on optimal medical and nursing management. If the outcome of therapy is to be successful, physicians and surgeons must combine their efforts in program planning designed to control hemorrhage, dissipate ascites, and improve nutrition. Treatment methods may vary, depending on the preference and experience of the physicians involved, but the general principles of therapy are fundamentally the same.

Attentive, intelligent nursing care is an integral part of the program for patient survival. Obviously, patients whose central nervous system is grossly impaired (i.e., those with advanced hepatic failure), are incapacitated. Preservation of body function in such patients is dependent on comprehensive nursing care. The customary precautions in treating any comatose patient must be observed, and the nurse should employ those measures required to assure maintenance of an unobstructed airway and to prevent aspiration of vomitus, saliva, and mucus. The nurse must be keenly aware of the clinical status of the patient at all times. Because of her frequent attendance at the bedside she is in the best position to assess any fluctuation in the patient's condition. Her role in this regard is of the utmost importance and is the key to the team approach.

### General considerations

In her assessment of the patient's clinical state, the nurse should consider the following points.

1. Any change in the rate or depth of respiration may indicate a further complication.

2. The development of, or change in cardiac arrhythmias

should be noted. Since it is common practice to monitor patients with hepatic failure continuously (because of the propensity of these patients to develop arrhythmias), the nurse should observe the oscilloscope frequently to ascertain the rhythm of the heart. The fundamentals of cardiac monitoring are discussed on pages 55–56.

3. The nurse should seek evidence of edema when administering nursing care, especially while bathing the patient. Rapid changes in degree of peripheral edema are of vital significance. In addition, the nurse should record measurements of the patient's weight and abdominal girth (using a tape measure) at the same time every day.

4. Careful recording of clinical observations and laboratory data is essential in assessing the patient's course. The form used at the Boston City Hospital for this purpose is found in Fig. 1.

## Control of hemorrhage with esophageal tamponade

1. It is essential that the nurse clearly identify each of the three tube openings and label each correctly before the apparatus is inserted. Serious complications can occur if this is not done. Such labeling is best accomplished with a waterproof marking pencil and small pieces of tape.

2. The nasogastric portion of the tube (lumen #1) should be irrigated every two hours to prevent its occlusion by either clots or food particles.

3. It is extremely important that esophageal balloon pressure be maintained between 35 and 40 mm Hg. The nurse should frequently check the manometer to see whether air leakage is occurring and should adjust the pressure as necessary.

4. The nurse must give continuous attention to ascertain that the balloons are in proper position and have not collapsed. The latter situation can prove fatal for the patient, because if the anchoring gastric balloon ruptures, the entire tube may rise into the nasopharynx and completely obstruct the airway.

*In the event the gastric balloon ruptures, the nurse should immediately deflate the esophageal balloon and withdraw the entire apparatus as a life-saving measure.*

It is a wise prophylactic practice to restrain the arms of disoriented patients in whom these tubes have been placed. If the

| | Day #1 | Day #2 | Day #3 | Day #4 | Day #5 |
|---|---|---|---|---|---|
| Name: | | | | | |
| Date: | | | | | |
| Weight: | | | | | |
| Abdominal Girth: | | | | | |
| Ascites: | | | | | |
| Edema: | | | | | |
| Laboratory Tests | | | | | |
| Bilirubin        Direct: | | | | | |
| Total: | | | | | |
| BSP removal     30 min. retention | | | | | |
| 45 min. retention | | | | | |
| % disappearance rate | | | | | |
| Serum Alkaline Phosphatase: | | | | | |
| Total Serum Cholesterol: | | | | | |
| Proteins:     total serum protein | | | | | |
| albumin | | | | | |
| globulin | | | | | |
| A/G Ratio | | | | | |
| Prothrombin Time: | | | | | |
| Coagulation Time:            11 AM | | | | | |
| 5 PM | | | | | |
| 11 PM | | | | | |
| 5 AM | | | | | |
| Cephalin Flocculation: | | | | | |
| Serum Glutamic Pyruvic Transaminase: | | | | | |
| Serum Glutamic Oxalacetic Transaminase: | | | | | |
| Arterial Blood Ammonia: | | | | | |
| Bleeding Time: | | | | | |
| Icterus Index | | | | | |
| Thymol Turbidity | | | | | |
| Fibrinogen | | | | | |
| Non-Protein Nitrogen | | | | | |
| Urea | | | | | |
| Urea Nitrogen | | | | | |
| Urine Values:    Urobilinogen | | | | | |
| Urobilinogen, feces | | | | | |
| Platelets: | | | | | |

Fig. 1. Daily record form used at Boston City Hospital

patient is in a state of mental confusion, he may attempt to remove the tube himself and obstruct the airway.

5. Antacids are usually ordered as part of the treatment program for hepatic failure as a means of reducing stomach acidity
and to prevent a reflux of acid into the esophagus. The presence
of such acid in the esophagus may precipitate further bleeding by
eroding a varix or the esophageal mucosa.

Usually, antacid drugs are administered through the nasogastric lumen (#1). The lumen is clamped for 30 minutes and is
then irrigated to prevent occlusion from the viscous medication,
and then suction is resumed.

6. Many clinicians use Neomycin to alter the bacterial flora as
a means of reducing ammonia formation in patients with hepatic
failure. This antibiotic is given in the same manner as antacids.

7. Because the esophagus and cardioesophageal junction are
occluded by inflated balloons, secretions frequently accumulate in
the upper esophagus. These accumulations should be suctioned
off by use of a separate small tube inserted into the upper esophagus.

In addition to this esophageal suctioning, it is essential that
the nasopharynx be cleaned as well because of the huge amount
of secretion that develops in this latter site due to irritation from
the tubes.

As a result of this demand for frequent suctioning, crusting
and cracking of the nares is a common problem and requires special nursing care.

Mouth care is also important to prevent parotitis (surgical
mumps), or the formation of ulcerations in the mouth. This
simple nursing measure affords much comfort and relief to the
patient who cannot eat or drink.

8. The patient should be kept as quiet as possible since any
exertion, such as coughing or straining, tends to increase the intra-
abdominal pressure and predisposes the patient to further bleeding. If the patient is conscious and responsive, the presence of this
tube is frightening and a source of great discomfort. Constant
reassurance and explanations are a most important part of his
therapy.

9. When bleeding is controlled and the physician decides to
remove the tube apparatus, the following procedures are followed

by the team: the gastric suction machine is shut off and the gastric tube is irrigated before removal to prevent tearing gastric or esophageal mucosa, and mineral oil is given to the patient to swallow in order to prevent esophageal laceration during removal of the tube. The patient is usually extremely apprehensive, especially at the removal of this appliance. At this time, particularly, he is in need of emotional support from those involved in his management.

### Tracheostomy care

Methods of tracheostomy and the nursing care of a patient with this type of artificial airway are discussed in detail in Chapter I, "Respiratory Insufficiency and Failure."

If the nurse is using tracheostomy tubes with inflated cuffs, it is imperative that this cuff be deflated every two hours for five minutes, to prevent possible development of tracheal erosion. The nurse should realize that a sudden cause of cyanosis due to hypoxia may be rupture of the cuff with resultant obstruction of the airway. At present, we are using rubber tracheostomy tubes with a double inflated cuff; alternating the cuffs reduces the frequency of occurrence of this complication.

### Drug therapy

Because impaired liver function is common in patients with hepatic failure, the nurse must be particularly attentive to the patient's state of responsiveness before and after administering sedatives, analgesics, or narcotics. If there is any suggestion of prolonged drug effect (e.g., periods of long sleep), further doses should be withheld. Dosage and time of administration must be accurately recorded to assess cumulative effects.

### Parenteral therapy

1. It is essential that the nurse repeatedly ascertain patency of the intravenous conduit; it is the patient's lifeline.
2. Because urinary output offers some index to the patient's need for fluid replacement, a Foley catheter must be inserted in

all patients receiving parenteral fluid therapy. The nurse must keep accurate hourly records of urine volumes and specific gravity.

3. Central venous pressure (CVP) monitoring is another important guide to parenteral therapy. The nurse should measure these pressures at hourly intervals and, at the time of each measurement, verify proper function of the system. She should be alert for any variations in central venous pressure which might suggest development of either hypervolemia or hypovolemia.

When measuring central venous pressure it is essential that the bed be kept flat and that a clear reference point be used in positioning the manometer. For this purpose, it is helpful to draw a line with a skin-marking pencil between anterior and posterior axillary lines. In the event that a positive pressure respirator is being used, the machine should be turned off during the period of CVP measurement to avoid false readings due to increased intrathoracic pressure.

4. Since potassium deficiency is a constant threat during the course of hepatic failure, the nurse must be aware of the clinical findings that might suggest this occurrence. The most common manifestations are muscle weakness and cardiac arrhythmias.

5. Pituitrin is administered intravenously to help control esophageal bleeding. The nurse should be aware of possible side effects such as abdominal cramps, evacuation of the bowels, facial pallor, and skin paresthesias.

## Bibliography

ATKINSON, M., and GOLIGHER, J. C.: Recurrent Hepatic Coma Treated by Colectomy and Ileorectal Anastomosis. *Lancet,* I:461–464, 1960.

CHILD, C. G., III: *The Hepatic Circulation and Portal Hypertension.* W. B. Saunders Company, Philadelphia, 1954.

MCDERMOTT, W. V. JR.: Metabolism and Toxicity of Ammonia. *New England Journal of Medicine,* 257:1076–1081, 1957.

MCDERMOTT, W. V. JR., and BROWN, H.: Ascites. *Annual Review of Medicine,* 15:79–92, 1964.

SHERLOCK, S., SUMMERSKILL, W. H. JR., WHITE, L. P., and PHEAR, E. A.: Portal-Systemic Encephalopathy: Neurological Complications of Liver Disease. *Lancet,* 2:453–457, 1954.

STERNBACH, RICHARD A.: *Pain. A Psychophysiological Analysis.* Academic Press, New York, 1968.

# CHAPTER VI

# Metabolic Crises

IRENE L. BELAND, R.N., M.S.
VIRGINIA HILL RICE, R.N., M.S.N.
LAWRENCE POWER, M.D.

This chapter concerns four life-threatening metabolic disturbances, all of which require intensive care:

I. Disturbances of Glucose Metabolism
    A. Diabetic Ketoacidosis
    B. Hypoglycemia
II. Acute Disorders of Calcium Metabolism
    A. Hypocalcemia
    B. Hypercalcemia
III. Acute Adrenal Cortical Insufficiency
IV. Disturbances of Thyroid Function
    A. Hypothyroidism and Myxedema Coma
    B. Acute Hyperthyroidism (Thyroid "Storm")

# I. Disturbances of Glucose Metabolism

## A. DIABETIC KETOACIDOSIS

### THE PROBLEM

Although diabetes mellitus is a common disease, its most severe complication, ketoacidosis, has become infrequent since the advent of insulin. The mortality, previously inevitable from this cause, is now less than five per cent among patients who receive prompt and adequate treatment. When diagnosis is delayed and/or treatment inadequate, the death rate is much higher. Prompt recognition of ketoacidosis and intensive care are essential to survival.

Ketoacidosis, often called diabetic coma, occurs primarily among those patients with the *juvenile* onset form of diabetes, and is seldom seen with the adult (maturity onset) type. When diabetes becomes unregulated in the ketoacidosis-prone patient, the body loses large quantities of glucose, water and electrolytes. Ketone bodies (acids) accumulate and acidosis and dehydration occur; coma and death result unless these disturbances are corrected promptly.

**Glucose metabolism.** To appreciate the pathophysiology of ketosis (and hypoglycemia, to be discussed subsequently) the normal metabolism of glucose, fat, and protein must be briefly reviewed.

A continuous supply of energy is required to support the activities of cells. This energy is obtained from carbohydrates, fats, and proteins by enzymatic action. Tissues differ in their capacity to utilize energy sources. (For example, the nervous system can only use glucose.) The extent to which energy-producing substances can be stored by the body also varies. Thus, glucose can be stored to a limited degree in the liver, as glycogen, but the supply of glycogen is only sufficient to meet the body's demands for a period of about six hours under fasting conditions.

Unlike glucose, fat can be stored in almost unlimited quantities. A well-nourished person has about 10,000 grams of fat that can be utilized for energy. However, this fat is not normally used unless the carbohydrate supply is inadequate. When carbohydrates are not available, the body can synthesize glucose from fat or protein, principally in the liver, by the process of gluconeogenesis.

Despite constant changes in the supply and utilization of glucose, the body is able to maintain a remarkably steady level of blood glucose. By regulating those factors which tend to elevate the level of glucose in the blood and those tending to lower it, blood glucose is maintained at between 80–100 mg% (Folin-Wu method) or 60–90 mg% (Somogyi-Nelson method).

The most significant blood glucose-lowering factor is insulin. Fundamentally there is a negative feedback relationship between the level of glucose in the blood and the secretion of insulin. The exact mechanism by which insulin lowers the level of blood glucose is still uncertain. The two major physiologic actions attributed to insulin are: (a) an increased conversion of blood sugar to liver glucogen; and (b) enhanced utilization of glucose by peripheral tissues. In addition to these effects of carbohydrate metabolism, insulin is also thought to affect fat metabolism by inhibiting the release of fatty acids from fat depots and by stimulating the conversion of glucose into fat (Berson and Yalon.)

Besides a deficiency of insulin, a number of other factors elevate blood glucose. These include: (a) the absorption of glucose from the alimentary canal or parenteral injections of glucose; (b) the conversion of stored glycogen to glucose (glycogenolysis) by the liver, in response to epinephrine and glucagon; (c) the synthesis of glucose from amino acids as mediated through the pituitary-adrenal axis; (d) antagonism of insulin by growth hormone and cortisol; and (e) dehydration.

As long as the regulators of glucose metabolism are in balance and the level of blood glucose is in the homeostatic range, the metabolism of fat is not influenced and proceeds independently at a normal rate. However, when glucose is *not* available in sufficient quantities, fatty acid mobilization and utilization are accelerated. This increased mobilization of fat results in the production of large quantities of the intermediate products of fat metabolism. Normally the liver, and peripheral tissues, can oxidize these intermediate products to a certain degree. However, when this capacity is exceeded, intermediary products called *keto acids* (aceto acetic acid and betahydroxybutyric acid) are retained. These acids, along with acetone, are known as "ketone bodies." When ketone bodies accumulate in the blood, ketonemia results. Although ketones can be excreted in the urine, the capacity of the kidneys is steadily compromised as ketoacidosis progresses. This contributes to a continuous increase of ketones in the blood.

The ketones, being acid in character, cause an increase in the level of hydrogen ions in the blood. This, in turn, causes a decrease in the concentration of bicarbonate ions, which ultimately leads to metabolic acidosis (ketoacidosis). The body attempts to correct this acid-base disturbance by utilizing respiratory and renal mechanisms. The lungs excrete acid, as carbon dioxide and water, by increasing the depth and rate of respiration. This respiratory response of rapid, deep respiration is known as "Kussmaul breathing."

In the presence of acidosis the kidneys increase the excretion of hydrogen ions. In ketoacidosis, from 30–100 grams of ketones may be excreted each day, with lesser amounts as free acids and larger amounts as salts of sodium and potassium. Ammonia, secreted by the tubular cells of the kidney, represents the most effective mechanism for removing excess hydrogen ions (Bradley).

The failure to utilize glucose normally, in addition to producing ketoacidosis, also results in a marked increase in blood glucose. These levels soon exceed the renal threshold and large amounts of glucose are lost in the urine. The loss of both glucose and ketone bodies in the urine causes a profound osmotic diuresis with the loss of large quantities of water, electrolytes and calories from the body. The water loss is further intensified by rapid respirations and by vomiting which accompanies ketoacidosis.

When water loss induced by these causes continues, a decreased blood volume results. As a consequence of this marked hemo-concentration, the capacity of the circulatory system to supply tissues with adequate oxygen fails, and generalized hypoxia develops. In the presence of hypoxia, aerobic metabolism is diminished and there is a shift to anaerobic metabolism with the production of lactic acid. This lactic acidosis places a further strain on those mechanisms that control hydrogen ion concentration.

This combination of dehydration, acidosis, electrolyte imbalance, and caloric waste affect the brain and lead to diabetic coma. Unless these processes are reversed promptly, death can be anticipated.

## ASSESSMENT OF THE PROBLEM

### Clinical picture

*History.* Among ketoacidosis prone individuals, infections of the respiratory and urinary tracts are among the most common precipitating causes. Other causes include omission of insulin, failure to ingest adequate amounts of food and fluid, or some condition increasing insulin requirements. (Excessive food intake, surgery, and trauma are the usual causes of increased insulin requirement.) A point of considerable importance is that a relatively minor threat to the well being of most individuals may be of serious import to the person with the unstable (juvenile) type of diabetes.

*Signs and symptoms.* Depending upon the rapidity with which it develops, ketoacidosis may be preceded by the signs and symptoms commonly associated with uncontrolled diabetes mellitus. They include thirst, polydipsia, polyuria, polyphagia, loss of weight, and malaise. Hours or days after their appearance, these signs and symptoms blend into those of ketoacidosis. Among the signs of ketoacidosis are labored, rapid and increasingly deep respirations, nausea and vomiting, drowsiness, prostration, abdominal or chest pain, oliguria and evidence of shock. (For a more detailed description of the clinical picture see Robert F. Bradley and S. B. Rees, "Water, Electrolyte and Hydrogen Ion Abnormalities in Diabetes Mellitus"—*Clinical Metabolism of Body Water and Electrolytes,* Saunders, 1963.)

*Laboratory findings.* The diagnosis of ketoacidosis can be definitively made only on the basis of laboratory findings.

The major abnormalities include:

a) GLYCOSURIA AND KETONURIA

On admission a urine specimen should be obtained immediately and tested for glucose and aceto acetic acid. In ketoacidosis both of these substances should show 4+ reactions. The information obtained from urinalysis has certain limitations which should be considered in the interpretation of results. For example, in patients with seriously impaired renal function, glucose and ketones in the urine may not markedly increase despite high blood levels of those substances. Conversely, urine that has been present in the bladder over a period of time may contain large quantities of glucose and even ketones in contrast to now normal blood levels.

Measurement of urinary aceto acetic acid is a more reliable index of the degree of ketoacidosis than urinary acetone. The latter, a commonly tested substance, may be formed from sources other than ketoacidosis.

b) MARKEDLY ELEVATED BLOOD GLUCOSE LEVELS (usually 300 to 800 mg% or higher).

c) KETONEMIA as evidenced by the detection of ketones in oxalated blood. The degree of ketonemia can be rapidly assessed by testing for acetone in diluted and undiluted plasma or serum.

d) ACIDOSIS as manifested by decreased blood pH and $CO_2$ levels.

e) HEMOCONCENTRATION as reflected by an increased hematocrit (above 50%) and leucocytosis.

The laboratory findings of ketoacidosis are found in Table 1.

*Table 1*

NORMAL BLOOD VALUES CONTRASTED WITH THOSE FOUND IN KETOACIDOSIS
AND TYPE OF BLOOD SPECIMEN REQUIRED

| *Blood* | *Normal Value* | *Ketoacidosis* | *Type of Specimen Required* |
|---|---|---|---|
| Glucose | 60–90 mg/100 ml | 300–800 mg/100 ml common, may be higher. Lower levels indicative of adequate renal reserve. | Oxalated blood |
| Urea Nitrogen | 10–16 mg/100 ml | 50–200 mg/100 ml | Oxalated blood |
| Ketones | | 50–200 mg/100 ml | Oxalated blood |
| Acetone | | 4+ in undiluted or diluted plasma or serum | |
| Carbon Dioxide | 20–28 mEq/L | 2 to 9 mEq/L | Oxalated blood |
| pH | 7.4 | 6.9–7.3 | |
| Sodium | 132–142 mEq/L | Variable Tend to be normal or low Depends upon degree of hydration | |
| Potassium | 3.5–5 mEq/L | Variable Depends upon degree of hydration | |
| Chloride | 98–106 mEq/L | Variable Depends upon degree of hydration | |
| Leukocyte Count | 7000–9000 cells per cu mm | 15,000–25,000 per cu mm | |
| Hematocrit | 36–47 Vol % | Above 50% with Hemoconcentration | Oxalated blood |

## PRINCIPLES OF TREATMENT

Diabetic ketoacidosis is a true medical emergency and treatment must be initiated as soon as the diagnosis is established if survival is to continue.

The basic aims of treatment are: (1) to initiate insulin treatment immediately; (2) to correct acidosis, dehydration, and electrolyte disturbances; (3) to treat any underlying condition such as infection, which may have precipitated ketoacidosis.

**Insulin Therapy.** Insulin is the cornerstone of therapy in ketoacidosis. It must be administered in quantities large enough to restore normal glucose metabolism and to inhibit further ketone production and prevent additional loss of water, calories and electrolytes.

The dosage of insulin and its method of administration vary primarily with the severity of acidosis, and the age and size of the patient.

The approximate severity of ketoacidosis can be assessed at the bedside by measuring the number of dilutions of the patient's *plasma* that have a 4+ reaction for ketones. The greater the number of dilutions giving this maximal reaction, the more severe the ketoacidosis. Treatment can be initiated on the basis of the degree of ketonemia in accordance with the plan suggested by Duncan (Table 2).

Crystalline insulin is always used as the initial treatment in ketoacidosis because the modified forms are too slow-acting for this critical situation. It may be given intravenously or subcutaneously. Most patients with diabetic coma require an average of 200 units of insulin in the first 3 hours. However, the response to insulin is not predictable and some patients require thousands of units of insulin in the first 24 hours while others, with equally severe ketoacidosis, may respond quickly with lesser amounts. Because of this inability to predict the response to therapy, regular planned observation is essential.

Improvement is usually noted within six hours after the onset of treatment. The most important single index of successful therapy is the degree of lessening of ketonemia. A decreasing concentration of ketones in the blood reflects that glucose and fat metabolism are being restored toward normal levels. Concomitant with

Table 2
CALCULATING INSULIN DOSAGE

| Degree of Ketonemia | Initial Dosage of Insulin | Later Dosages of Insulin |
|---|---|---|
| 4+ ketones of undiluted plasma | 100 units:<br>40 units intravenously<br>60 units subcutaneously | 50 units of insulin at 4–6 hour intervals until the hyperketonemia is corrected |
| 4+ ketones on a 1:1 dilution with physiological saline but not on a 1:3 dilution | 200 units of insulin | |
| 4+ ketones on a 1:3 dilution of plasma with physiological saline— (a profound ketoacidosis) | 300 units of insulin, with 50 units of insulin each ½ hour until a marked improvement in the degree of hyperketonemia occurs | If a marked degree of shock is present, delay in the absorption of insulin can be avoided by administering from one-half to two-thirds of the insulin intravenously |

the reduction in blood ketones there is a decrease in ketonuria. Repeated testing of blood and urine ketones is essential in managing the acute phase of this illness.

During the correction of ketonemia by insulin, it is desirable to accept a moderate degree of hyperglycemia and glycosuria in order to protect the patient from a sudden onset of *hypoglycemia.* As long as ketonemia persists, it is advisable to maintain the blood glucose at levels above 250 mg%. Blood sugar determinations should be made every 2 hours.

**Fluid replacement.** It is necessary that water and electrolyte deficits be corrected simultaneously with the restoration of glucose and fat metabolism. As previously noted, all diabetic patients in ketoacidosis suffer a considerable degree of water and electrolyte depletion. The quantity and type of solution used to replace these water and electrolyte imbalances depend upon the degree of dehydration and the adequacy of renal function. In some patients dehydration may be reasonably well-corrected with as little as 3 or 4 liters of saline. Others may tolerate as many as 8 or 10 liters within the first 12 to 18 hours without showing evidence of overhydration.

At the onset of treatment, at least 1000 cc of normal saline solution (0.9%) should be administered rapidly. This can be followed by a liter of half-strength saline (0.45%), again, given rapidly. These initial fluids help to reduce hemoconcentration and to increase blood volume. Subsequent infusions of saline may follow the second liter, but should be given more slowly. Measurements of hematocrits and urine output must be made frequently to assess additional fluid requirements. As the fluid deficit is corrected, the hematocrit should fall (to 50% or less) and urine volume should increase. Until ketoacidosis is controlled, fluids should not be given by mouth since they remain in the stomach and are of no value in correcting fluid and electrolyte deficits. Further, oral fluids contribute to gastric dilation and may aggravate nausea and vomiting.

**Electrolyte replacement.**

a) *Potassium.*

Potassium replacement is usually not initiated until after the first six hours of treatment. During these early hours when hemoconcentration and ketonemia exist, potassium is usually not required. Once these latter disturbances have been corrected (as evidenced by an increasing urine flow and decreasing hematocrit) potassium chloride, one gram every 4 hours, may be given orally for five doses. The need for potassium therapy may be determined by frequent electrocardiographic tracings. Elevated serum potassium levels (along with electrocardiographic findings of hyperkalemia are commonly found at the time of admission in patients with ketoacidosis. Later, as fluid replacement is achieved, evidence of hypokalemia may appear. The rapid replacement of potassium by intravenous infusion in this situation is dangerous and should not be attempted (Vanderveer and Fisher).

b) *Sodium.*

Although sodium is furnished as sodium chloride in replacing the fluid loss, the sodium ion itself may not necessarily be available to replace the sodium lost in excreting anions of aceto acetic and betahydroxybutyric acids. Therefore, it may be necessary to give additional sodium ions in the form of either sodium bicarbonate or sodium lactate. Although useful in restoring the quantity of sodium in the extracellular fluid, these salts have one disadvantage: they diminish the diagnostic value of the blood $CO_2$ content determination as an index of ketonemia control. This disadvantage is not serious, however, since the degree of ketonemia is a more reliable guide to ketoacidosis than is the $CO_2$ content. A more serious threat from this therapy is that as the ketones are eliminated, large quantities of cations (e.g., sodium) are released into the plasma and alkalosis may result.

**Glucose.** Some clinicians prefer to administer glucose as part of the initial treatment program. It is safe to say that the *early* administration of glucose in the therapy of ketoacidosis does no harm. But it also does no good. As hyperglycemia is controlled, glucose then becomes an essential part of therapy. From 4 to 6 hours after insulin and fluid therapy is initiated, glucose may be given orally as fruit juice. By that time, the patient is usually able to retain and absorb fluids from the intestine. Glucose by intravenous injection is seldom required.

**Gastric lavage.** Gastric distention, due to paralytic ileus and/or potassium depletion, is an indication for gastric lavage. Distention may be indicated by the presence of abdominal pain or vomiting. Following lavage, eight ounces of bicarbonate solution may be left in the stomach.

**Subsequent treatment.** Within 6 hours after therapy is started, the degree of ketonemia, hyperglycemia and hemoconcentration should be appreciably reduced. While urine flow should be obviously increased, vomiting should have ceased. At this time fluids may be given by mouth. Broth, tea and fruit juices may be started cautiously and if tolerated well (that is without causing nausea, vomiting or increasing gastric distention), they may be increased to the point where intravenous fluids can be discontinued.

## THE NURSING ROLE

1. Because the outcome is strongly influenced by prompt and adequate treatment, it is essential that each institution have a treatment plan that is thoroughly understood by the intensive care team. All necessary materials must be available at the bedside and the team members aware of their respective duties. During the first four to six hours, a physician and a nurse should be in continuous attendance at the bedside. Systematic observation, with appropriate actions taken, should be continued for the first 24 hours.

2. The nurse should record the following observations at regular intervals:

    a. state of consciousness

    b. restlessness

    c. type and rate of respiration

    d. color of skin

    e. dryness of skin and mucous membrane

    f. blood pressure and pulse rate

    g. type and volume of fluids administered

    h. urinary output

    i. insulin dosages

3. The nurse should make certain that appropriate laboratory determinations are made promptly at scheduled times and are legibly recorded in an orderly fashion.

4. Because hypoglycemia can develop unexpectedly as a result of excessive insulin (particularly when the blood sugar is approaching normal), the patient should be carefully observed for signs of this emergency (see following section).

5. Prevention. Though not necessarily a part of the emergency care of a patient in diabetic ketoacidosis, the most important form of treatment is prevention. In the patient who is already in ketoacidosis, conditions predisposing to it, such as infection, should be treated. As soon as the patient is able, he and/or his family should learn how to manage his diabetes so that the further threat of ketoacidosis is minimized. He should learn what to do when he develops an infection or other illness. He should be encouraged to seek medical attention early. When a visiting nurse service is available in his community, a few visits from a nurse can be invaluable in helping him to adjust to the management of his disease at home. Emphasis throughout his instruction should be on his controlling the disease rather than the diabetes controlling him.

## B. HYPOGLYCEMIA

### THE PROBLEM

Hypoglycemia may be defined as a blood glucose of 60 mg%, or less, by the method of Folin and Wu, or a level of 45 mg%, or less, when the Somogyi-Nelson technique is used.

Hypoglycemia is not a common cause for admission to an intensive care unit. Patients who present in a comatose state, where the etiology is uncertain, may be admitted to the unit. Hypoglycemia may also be encountered among patients being treated for ketoacidosis.

Hypoglycemia results from excessive amounts of insulin of either exogenous or endogenous origin. Exogenous insulin refers to parenterally administered insulin or the production of insulin by oral hypoglycemic agents; endogenous insulin may be secreted in excessive amounts from adenomas or hyperplasia of the islet cells of the pancreas.

The clinical picture of hypoglycemia varies with the rapidity with which it develops. When blood glucose levels drop *slowly* there may be no clinical manifestations of hypoglycemia despite glucose levels of 30–40 mg%. Conversely, a *rapid* decrease in blood glucose to similar levels is accompanied by obvious symptoms. The latter situation occurs primarily when the hypoglycemia results from overdosages of regular crystalline insulin where the absorption and effect are prompt.

A sudden fall in blood glucose (e.g. from crystalline insulin) stimulates the sympathetic nervous system and some of the *symptoms* are therefore identical to those produced by the injection of epinephrine. These include: (a) nervousness, (b) general weakness and faintness, (c) apprehension, and (d) numbness about the mouth.

The *signs* of acute hypoglycemia are:

a. sweating
b. tachycardia
c. dilated pupils
d. pallor
e. slight increase in systolic blood pressure

The signs and symptoms of hypoglycemia due to overdosages of long-acting insulins are due to the effect of hypoglycemia on the cerebral cortex. With the long-acting preparations, the hypoglycemia may develop slowly but is ultimately of severe degree and of long duration. Once there is evidence of a cerebral effect, the patient may die unless the hypoglycemia is corrected promptly. Among the cerebral manifestations of hypoglycemia are:

a. headache

b. visual disturbances

c. thick speech

d. muscle twitching

e. awkward body movement

f. hemiplegia or paraplegia with tonic or clonic spasms

g. incontinence of urine

h. unconsciousness and convulsion

i. psychiatric reactions including restlessness, personality changes, negativism, catatonia and maniacal behavior.

## ASSESSMENT OF THE PROBLEM

The most likely cause of hypoglycemia is insulin overdosage among patients being treated for diabetes mellitus. Patients with juvenile onset diabetes (the so-called "brittle type") may shift rapidly from hyper to hypoglycemia. If the overdose of insulin is substantial, convulsions and coma may develop. Hypoglycemia and diabetic (ketoacidotic) coma are usually easy to distinguish on a clinical basis. The diagnosis of hypoglycemia can only be proven by the demonstration of markedly decreased blood glucose levels. Urine analysis is undependable in this regard since urine specimens obtained at the onset of a hypoglycemic episode may or may not contain glucose. Urine that has been in the bladder over a period of several hours may contain considerable amounts of glucose despite the presence of hypoglycemia.

## PRINCIPLES OF TREATMENT

1. The diagnosis must be established promptly. A blood glucose determination will reveal levels of 60 mg% or less.

2. When the clinical picture suggests hypoglycemia, it is wise to institute treatment immediately and prior to the report of the blood glucose determination. If the patient is unconscious, 100 grams of glucose is given by intravenous infusion after a blood sample has been drawn. If the patient is able to swallow, orange juice or some other readily available source of glucose is given orally.

3. Once the hypoglycemia has been corrected and signs and symptoms controlled, it is important to repeat the blood sugar

levels at periodic intervals thereafter because of the tendency of hypoglycemia to recur in certain circumstances (particularly when the hypoglycemia has resulted from absorption of oral hypoglycemic agents).

4. A program for the prevention of further episodes of hypoglycemia should be instituted. This would include restandardization of insulin requirements and dietary adjustment or, where appropriate, further diagnostic studies.


**THE NURSING ROLE**

1. Since death or cerebral damage can result from prolonged hypoglycemia, it is important that this state be controlled as promptly as possible. The nurse should be aware of the possibilty of hypoglycemia in diabetic patients under her care and should seek those symptoms which would reflect hypoglycemia.

2. When the condition is suspected (particularly in a high-risk candidate for hypoglycemia), blood should be drawn for a blood sugar determination, then orange juice given the patient.

3. Patients admitted in an unconscious state without a diagnosis should be managed in accordance with principles of prevention of aspiration, adequate airway assurance, etc. (see Chapter I, "Respiratory Insufficiency and Failure").


# II. *Acute Disorders of Calcium Metabolism*

Calcium, the most abundant cation in the body, is vital to many physiologic mechanisms. Normally, the concentration of calcium in the blood is maintained at a remarkably constant level. This homeostasis is achieved by the balance of several interrelated factors including gastrointestinal absorption of calcium, parathyroid hormone (parathormone), and vitamin D. Because of disturbances within this metabolic system, the concentration of blood calcium may exceed or fall below physiologic levels. This variation results in either hypercalcemia or hypocalcemia, both of which can be life-threatening emergencies.

To appreciate the clinical picture of disturbed calcium metabolism, some functions of this cation should be considered:

**Neuromuscular system.** Calcium plays an important role in regulating the excitability of nerve and muscle tissue. A *decrease* in serum calcium results in an *increase* in neuromuscular activity even to the point of spontaneous discharge of nerve and muscle fibers. (This observable phenomenon is known as *tetany*.) In contrast, elevation of serum calcium levels causes a decrease in the excitability of these tissues. These effects appear related to alterations of cell membrane permeability induced by calcium ions. An excess of calcium decreases permeability of the cell membrane to sodium and potassium while a reduction in calcium enhances this permeability.

**Circulatory system.** The action of calcium on cardiac muscle is probably similar to its action on skeletal muscle and nerve tissue. Calcium exerts its effect by altering cell membrane permeability and by indirectly antagonizing the action of potassium. An increase in calcium concentration tends to slow cardiac impulses and their transmission; prolonged systole develops and contractility of the myocardium is increased. In this sense calcium and cardiac glycosides (digitalis) have similar influence on myocardial function. Digitalis administered during periods of hypercalcemia may lead to serious cardiac arrhythmias, while the glycoside may have decreased effectiveness if hypocalcemia exists.

**Blood coagulation.** Calcium is necessary to activate the enzyme, thromboplastin, which is required for the conversion of prothrombin to thrombin. In the absence of adequate calcium ions blood will not clot.

**Bone.** Calcium and phosphates are the two principal mineral constituents of bone. Throughout life these substances are continuously deposited in, and removed from, bone. When there is a reduction in blood calcium levels (for one of several reasons to be described), calcium stored in bones is released in an attempt to preserve homeostasis. If this demand is chronic, the bones become depleted of calcium (osteomalacia) and fractures or deformities may develop.

**The regulation of plasma calcium levels.** Under normal physiological conditions, plasma calcium is maintained within a narrow range of 9–11 mg per 100 ml. This constant level is achieved by adjustments made by the body, in the amount of calcium absorbed by the gastrointestinal tract, the amount excreted by the kidneys, and the amount of calcium deposited or resorbed from bone.

Calcium ions exist in a state of equilibrium with phosphate ions and the product of calcium ions (e.g. 10 mg%) and phosphate ions (normal: 3–5 mg%) is constant (i.e. 30–40). Thus if calcium ions are *increased,* phosphate ions *decrease,* and vice versa. The preservation of this relationship between calcium and phosphate and the maintenance of constant plasma calcium levels is largely dependent on parathormone, the hormone secreted by the parathyroid glands. (The parathyroid glands are situated in the neck closely related to the upper and lower poles of the thyroid gland.) There are normally four glands but occasionally five or six may be found. Parathormone enhances the intestinal absorption of calcium (in the presence of Vitamin D) and also increases renal tubular reabsorption of calcium. Both of these effects tend to raise plasma calcium. At the same time, parathormone promotes excretion of phosphate by the kidneys thus maintaining a constant product of these ions.

The secretion of parathormone is controlled mainly by the level of ionized calcium in the blood plasma through a negative feedback mechanism. If the plasma calcium level rises (e.g. from the continuous dissolution of bone) the activity of the parathyroids is decreased and, if the calcium level falls, parathyroid activity increases.

In addition to parathormone, vitamin D plays a role in maintaining calcium equilibrium. The vitamin influences the absorption of calcium from the gastrointestinal tract.

## A. HYPOCALCEMIA

### THE PROBLEM

Hypocalcemia may be defined as a plasma calcium level of less than 9 mg%. This decrease in ionized calcium results in increased neuromuscular excitability which presents as tetany in most patients. Other serious manifestations of hypocalcemia include convulsions and epileptic seizures. In addition, muscle cramps, paresthesias, numbness, palpitations and cardiac arrhythmias commonly occur with this disturbance in calcium metabolism.

Low plasma calcium levels may develop acutely or gradually. The most common cause of *acute* hypocalcemia is parathyroid deficiency (hypoparathyroidism) secondary to the inadvertent removal of the parathyroid glands during thyroidectomy. (*Transient* parathyroid deficiency is not unusual after thyroid surgery and is the result of temporary edema or ischemia of the parathyroids.) Acute hypocalcemia may also develop after the transfusion of large volumes of citrated blood (citrate binds calcium producing hypocalcemia). In addition to these acute forms, hypocalcemia may be noted with rickets and osteomalacia (due to a deficiency of vitamin D); steatorrhea (where large quantities of calcium are lost with fatty stools), and renal insufficiency (where calcium and phosphate excretion is disturbed). In these latter chronic states, decalcification of bone usually accompanies hypocalcemic symptoms.

## ASSESSMENT OF THE PROBLEM

**Clinical manifestations of hypocalcemia.** The most striking sign of hypocalcemia is *tetany*. This reflection of increased neuromuscular irritability may be manifested in a variety of ways:

1. *Carpopedal spasm*—the hand is held in a hollowed position with rigid fingers flexed at the metacarpo-phalangeal joints. The wrists, elbows, legs and feet are kept in an extended position.

2. *Trousseau's sign*—when the circulation to the arm is occluded by a blood pressure cuff just above systolic levels, the hand develops carpopedal spasm within 2–3 minutes.

3. *Chvostek's sign*—light finger tapping over the area of the facial nerve (in front of the ear) results in contraction of the facial muscles. This sign is almost always positive with hypocalcemia.

4. *Erb's sign*—on mild electrical stimulation, muscular hyperexcitability is noted.

5. *Convulsions*

6. *Laryngeal stridor* with or without cyanosis.

In chronic hypocalcemia there may be extensive ectodermal changes including rough, dry skin, sparse hair and deformed nails. Cataracts are frequently observed, as are dental abnormalities. Papilledema and signs of increased intracranial pressure may be detected.

A summary of the physiologic manifestations of hypocalcemia is found in Table 3.

**Laboratory manifestations of hypocalcemia.** In acute hypocalcemia the following abnormalities are found:

    1. Plasma calcium—lower than 9 mg%.

    2. Plasma phosphate—more than 7 mg%.

    3. Urinary calcium—usually absent. (The presence of calcium in the urine can be estimated roughly at the bedside by Sulkowitch's test. 5 cc of urine are added to 5 cc of Sulkowitch solution and the appearance of a milky cloud is noted and graded from 0 to 4+, depending on the amount of calcium present.)

    4. Electroencephalogram—characteristic findings of a convulsive disorder may be found.

    5. Electrocardiogram—prolongation of the QT interval is a generally reliable index of low plasma calcium.

## PRINCIPLES OF TREATMENT

    1. Immediate correction of hypocalcemia is essential. An intravenous injection of 10 cc of a 10% calcium gluconate will usually control the acute episode. *Calcium replacement must be given carefully and slowly in patients receiving digitalis because of the danger of provoking cardiac arrest.*

    2. Parathyroid extract (100–200 units) may be administered intravenously or intramuscularly but is rarely used.

    3. Maintenance dosages of vitamin D (50,000–100,000 units daily) are given orally thereafter to maintain calcium in the urine (at a 2+ Sulkowitch test level).

    4. In chronic hypoparathyroidism serum calcium levels are maintained by a combination of vitamin D and diet.

## THE NURSING ROLE

    1. The nurse should think of the possibility of hypoparathyroidism and hypocalcemia among patients who have had any thyroid surgery.

    2. Because the immediate correction of serum calcium with

intravenous calcium is transient (lasting only a few hours), the nurse should watch for recurring signs of hypocalcemia during the early stages of the treatment period.

3. Blood samples should be drawn frequently for calcium determinations and urines saved for 24-hour calcium determinations or Sulkowitch testing.

4. Continuous electrocardiographic monitoring may be utilized during this phase along with frequent serum calcium determinations.

5. Patients presenting with laryngeal stridor must have adequate airway maintenance. A tracheostomy set should be available at the bedside.

6. The convulsive tendency associated with hypocalcemia necessitates adequate padding of the rails and head of the bed to protect the patient from injury.

7. Hypocalcemia may also precipitate congestive heart failure, and careful observation for this complication is required. The pulse rate and blood pressure should be monitored.

8. During the correction of hypocalcemia with intravenous calcium gluconate, there is a slight risk of cardiac arrest and resuscitative equipment should be available.

9. The following data should be available for repeated evaluation of the patient:

    a. Plasma calcium
    b. Plasma phosphate
    c. Urinary calcium
    d. ECG interpretation
    e. EEG interpretation
    f. Dosage of cardiac glycosides
    g. Dosage of calcium given
    h. Number, type, and nature of convulsions
    i. Fluid intake and urinary output

## B. HYPERCALCEMIA

### THE PROBLEM

When the level of plasma calcium exceeds 11.5 mg% (hypercalcemia) serious consequences may be expected in cardiac, renal, and neuromuscular function (see Table 3). Unless the elevated blood calcium level is corrected, the central nervous system becomes markedly depressed and coma may develop (hypercalcemic crisis). Ventricular fibrillation is often the terminal event.

Hypercalcemia may result from the following causes:

*Hyperparathyroidism.* An overproduction of parathormone by a parathyroid adenoma is a reasonably common cause of hypercalcemia.

*Metastatic malignancy.* Elevated plasma calcium levels are frequently observed in patients with metastatic disease. A rise in plasma calcium can be associated with tumors found in almost any part of the body, but it is more commonly seen with malignancies of the breast and lungs (Fraser). At one time it was thought that the hypercalcemia was the result of metastasis to bone, but it became apparent that tumors not associated with overt radiographic evidence of bone involvement could also be accompanied by hypercalcemia. The exact mechanism to explain this latter circumstance is still lacking but many believe that certain tumors release a humoral factor which promotes hypercalcemia.

*Sarcoidosis.* This systemic granulomatous disease of unknown etiology is associated with a high incidence (5% to 30% of cases) of hypercalcemia. The etiology of this hypercalcemia is, again, uncertain but appears to result from unusual sensitivity to vitamin D, or a similar substance in increasing gastrointestinal absorption of calcium.

*Other causes of hypercalcemia* include multiple myeloma, excessive milk and alkali ingestion (the milk-alkali syndrome) and excess vitamin D intake.

## ASSESSMENT OF THE PROBLEM

**Clinical manifestations.** The clinical picture of hypercalcemia varies with the etiology of the underlying pathologic process producing the elevated calcium levels. Early in the course of the illness the symptoms are vague and seldom lead to diagnosis. Often the first specific suggestion of hypercalcemia is a renal stone or a spontaneous fracture. The most common symptoms of hypercalcemia are:

*musculoskeletal:* weakness, fatigue, localized or generalized bone pain, or a spontaneous fracture. With hypercalcemic crisis there is marked muscle weakness, headache, stupor and coma.

*genitourinary:* polyuria frequently accompanies hypercalcemia and results from the excretion of large amounts of calcium by the kidneys as well as from renal damage. Renal stones and their sequelae are common. In hypercalcemic crisis, anuria may supervene.

*gastrointestinal:* anorexia, nausea, weight loss, constipation, and polydipsia all usually occur. Vomiting can be conspicuous.

In hypercalcemic crisis, hypotonicity of the muscles, lethargy, confusion and coma are the dominant features.

## Laboratory findings

### Biochemical:

1. The plasma calcium and phosphorus levels are diagnostic. Plasma calcium is increased well above 11.5 mg% while plasma phosphate is usually below 3 mg%.

2. Urine calcium and phosphate are increased. Despite a low calcium diet, excretion of calcium still exceeds 200 mg per day.

3. When hypercalcemia is due to increased bone destruction, the alkaline phosphatase is generally elevated.

### X-ray studies:

1. Skeletal—generalized demineralization and subperiosteal resorption of bone is noted; bone cysts may occur.

2. Intravenous pyelography may reveal calcium stones in the kidneys or bladder.

*Electrocardiogram:*—shortening of QT interval is expected.

## PRINCIPLES OF TREATMENT

The basic plan of treatment is:

a. to reduce the serum calcium levels as rapidly as possible.

b. to correct associated electrolyte imbalances.

c. to prevent further dehydration.

d. to control cardiac arrhythmias and avoid renal complications.

e. to prepare the patient for surgery in the event the hypercalcemia is due to a parathyroid adenoma.

## Table 3

### PHYSIOLOGICAL MANIFESTATIONS OF HYPERCALCEMIA AND HYPOCALCEMIA

| | Hypercalcemia | Hypocalcemia |
|---|---|---|
| HEART | decreased heart rate—vagal stimulation<br>increased contractility and excitability<br>prolonged systole<br>shortened Q-T interval<br>depressed S-T segment<br>bradycardia<br>premature ventricular contractions<br>ventricular fibrillation in severe hypercalcemia<br>increased systemic pressure | impaired contractility and prolonged diastole<br>prolonged diastole<br>lengthening of the Q-T interval<br>elongation of the S-T interval<br>decreased cardiac output<br>hypotension |
| BONE | increased bone resorption—many osteoclasts<br>generalized decalcification<br>increased bone formation—many osteoblasts | inadequate resorption of bone<br>decreased density of bone on x-ray<br>excessive formation of bone |
| RENAL | decreased tubular reabsorption of phosphate<br>(hypophosphatemia)<br>increased phosphate clearance (hyperphosphaturia)<br>increased tubular reabsorption of calcium<br>(hypercalcemia)<br>increased clearance of calcium (hypercalcuria)<br>impaired acidification<br>impaired concentrating ability | increased tubular resorption of phosphate<br>(hyperphosphatemia)<br>decreased phosphate clearance (hypophosphaturia)<br>decreased tubular resorption of calcium (hypocalcemia)<br>low or normal clearance of calcium (hypocalcuria) |
| NEUROMUSCULAR | decreased irritability<br>increased pressure<br>stabilized transmissions | increased irritability (tetany)<br>labilized transmissions<br>increased CSF pressure (common)<br>EEG changes, possibility of convulsions<br>papilledema (in some cases) |

The methods of treatment are as follows:

a. When hypercalcemic crisis is suspected, blood determinations of calcium and phosphorus should be made at once.

b. Continuous ECG monitoring should be initiated.

c. An intravenous infusion of a chelating agent, EDTA, (Versonate, or Endrate sodium), should be initiated: usually 5 grams of EDTA in 500 cc of 5% glucose or normal saline are given over a period of two hours. This chelating agent binds the calcium ions and the bound product is excreted in the urine. This reduces the blood calcium level promptly. If EDTA is infused too rapidly or the total amount is excessive, the fall in serum calcium may be precipitous and induce *hypocalcemia* (tetany).

d. Hypercalcemia can also be controlled with oral prednisone (except when due to hyperparathyroidism). Prednisone is started at a dose of 10 mg q.i.d. for the first two days. Reduction of hypercalcemia takes several days to accomplish.

e. Intravenous fluids should be given to replace fluids and electrolytes lost by vomiting and polyuria.

f. Urinary volume should be measured.

## THE NURSING ROLE

a. As soon as the diagnosis of hypercalcemia (or hypercalcemic crisis) is made or suspected, the nurse should be sure an intravenous infusion is started (normal saline or 5% glucose in water). She should have a supply of disodium EDTA (Endrate) on hand to be added to the I.V. fluid as soon as it is ordered.

b. ECG leads should be attached to the patient and monitoring started. If premature ventricular contractions or ventricular tachycardia develop, the physician should be notified promptly. In the event of ventricular fibrillation, immediate electrical defibrillation should be performed (see page 91).

c. Once the EDTA is started, the nurse should observe the patient carefully for signs or symptoms of tetany. Burning sensations at the site of the infusion or along the course of the vein are common and the nurse should slow the infusion rate at this point but not discontinue it solely for this reason.

d. Careful intake and output records should be kept because of the disturbed fluid and electrolyte balances which exist in hypercalcemic states.

e. Great care must be taken in moving the patient because of the danger of fracture of demineralized bone.

f. Patients with hypercalcemic crisis are often stuporous or comatose and care must be directed at the prevention of respiratory complications from this condition (see Chapter 1, "Respiratory Insufficiency and Failure").

# III. Acute Adrenal Cortical Insufficiency

## THE PROBLEM

When the adrenal cortex fails to secrete its characteristic hormones (collectively called steroids), a marked disturbance occurs in sodium metabolism which, if uncorrected, leads to death in a few days. Although more than 30 different hormones have been isolated from the adrenal cortex, only three are of proven importance to body function. These are: (a) the glucocorticoids (cortisol), (b) the sex steroids (ketosteroids), and (c) aldosterone. Although these hormones have certain activities in common, each has a dominant function. Thus cortisol exerts at least 95% of the glucocorticoid activity influencing carbohydrate metabolism, while the mineralocorticoid, aldosterone, is concerned primarily with the regulation of electrolytes, sodium and potassium.

If adrenal cortical hormone production becomes insufficient, there is a marked loss of sodium in the urine.

The loss of sodium results in a state of hypovolemic shock, and death follows unless replacement therapy with sodium chloride and adrenal cortical hormones is immediately instituted. This situation may occur abruptly and is known as *adrenal crisis*. Other factors which contribute to death in this circumstance are hypoglycemia and hyperkalemia, both of which are related to steroid insufficiency.

Adrenal insufficiency, leading to adrenal crisis, is of three types:

**Chronic adrenal insufficiency (Addison's disease).** Either because of atrophy, or destruction from some other cause, a loss of function of the adrenal cortex occurs usually taking place slowly over a period of years.

Generalized infection, exposure to extreme weather changes, strenuous exertion, surgical procedures or trauma may precipitate adrenal crisis in patients with chronic adrenal insufficiency. In fact, any condition making increased demands on this individual may lead to adrenal crisis.

**Secondary adrenal insufficiency.** Patients who receive cortisone compounds for prolonged periods of time (e.g., those with rheumatoid arthritis or blood dyscrasias) may develop secondary adrenal insufficiency. These exogenous steroids, when administered in large amounts on a chronic basis, inhibit the negative feedback response for adrenal function. Specifically the pituitary hormone, ACTH, is depressed with a resulting loss of stimulation of the adrenals. While the body can tolerate reduced amounts of *endogenous* steroids as long as adequate *exogenous* therapy is given, adrenal crisis may occur if the drug is withdrawn abruptly, or if there is an increased demand for adrenal hormones. This latter circumstance may arise as a result of infection, surgery, or other stress.

**Acute adrenal destruction.** Occasionally adrenal failure may develop abruptly in the absence of pre-existing adrenal disease. In these instances, the adrenal glands are destroyed rapidly as a result of overwhelming septicemia, usually meningococcic in origin. Hemorrhage and necrosis of the adrenal tissue (Waterhouse-Friderichsen syndrome) results.

## ASSESSMENT OF THE PROBLEM

### Clinical manifestations of acute adrenal crisis

a. There is severe prostration. When the crisis has followed chronic adrenal insufficiency there is usually a history of marked weakness and asthenia preceding this extreme prostration. Lethargy progresses to somnolescence.

b. The patient is likely to be in shock. The blood pressure is very low (usually below 70 mm Hg systolic), and the heart sounds and peripheral pulses are very weak.

c. Abdominal pain may be present and can resemble an acute abdominal process. Uncontrolled diarrhea is usually seen during the period of crisis. Earlier gastrointestinal symptoms are anorexia, nausea, and vomiting.

d. Patients with chronic adrenal insufficiency will exhibit typical pigmentation of the skin. This appears as a general darkening of the skin of the exposed areas of the body (hands, arms, neck, face), as well as deepening of the color of the nipples and genitalia.

e. Fever may occur during crisis or the body temperature may be subnormal even in the presence of severe infection.

**Laboratory studies**

a. Serum sodium and chloride levels are distinctly decreased while serum potassium is elevated.

b. Hypoglycemia is common.

c. Blood and urine cortisol levels are depressed (17-hydroxy steroids).

d. Plasma volume is low reflecting dehydration.

## PRINCIPLES OF TREATMENT

Adrenal crisis is a medical emergency and survival depends on prompt and adequate therapy. The aims of treatment are:

a. To provide adequate circulating adrenal cortical hormone. The usual program involves either the administration of 100 mg of hydrocortisone intravenously over several hours, or the infusion of 1000 cc 5% glucose in NSS to which 100 mg of hydrocortisone has been added.

b. To support the cardiovascular system and restore blood volume. This is accomplished in many instances by the infusion of normal saline. If the hypotension is severe, plasma expanders or vasopressors may be used.

c. Correction of sodium and chloride deficits. Depending on the degree of hyponatremia, 3–5 liters of normal saline may be required to restore normal levels of sodium and chloride.

d. Control of infection. Since many episodes of adrenal

insufficiency are precipitated by systemic infections, it is essential to obtain appropriate specimens for culture and sensitivity determinations, after which intensive and definitive antibiotic therapy is begun.

e. To protect the patient from further stress until the crisis is controlled.

## THE NURSING ROLE

On admission to the intensive care unit, the nurse member of the team should assist in the immediate treatment program in the following ways:

1. Blood should be drawn promptly for determinations of CBC, Na, K, Cl, BUN, glucose, and plasma cortisol levels.

2. An intravenous infusion of 1000 cc of 5% glucose in normal saline solution should be started.

3. Hydrocortisone hemisuccinate should be available at the bedside.

4. Blood and urine cultures should be obtained.

Informed observation of the clinical condition by the nurse is essential to therapy. Blood pressure should be recorded at regular intervals. Decreasing blood pressure levels or failure of pressure to rise after therapy should be reported to the physician promptly.

Because of the severity of dehydration and its threat to life, it is important that the type and volume of fluid given intravenously, as well as the volume of urine excreted be recorded accurately and currently.

Since the patient in acute adrenal crisis is unable to adapt to any increase in stress and strain, the importance of reducing all unnecessary demands made upon him cannot be overemphasized. Talking should be limited to giving necessary directions or brief explanations of what to expect. Tone and volume of the voice should be quiet. Care should be taken to avoid giving the impression of hurry, though therapy should be initiated with all due haste. Relatives should be asked to be quiet and to avoid spirited conversations. When a relative has an obviously quieting effect on the patient and is able to do so, he may be encouraged to sit at the bedside of the patient. The positive support that some family members give is all too often overlooked and patients are thereby deprived of an important source of security. (If the relative's presence interferes with necessary treatment of the patient, he should be directed to the waiting area.) The environment should be carefully controlled: room temperature should be regulated to approximately 70 degrees Fahrenheit. Drafts should be prevented by screening the patient or by other suitable measures. Bright lights should be dimmed or the patient's eyes protected from them. Loud and/or sudden noises should be prevented. Attention should be given to body positioning so that comfort is maintained. Insofar as possible, removing sources of interpersonal or environmental stress is essential.

# IV. Disturbances of Thyroid Function

## THE PROBLEM

Marked oversecretion of thyroid hormone (thyroxin) may result in a lethal syndrome known as *"thyroid crisis or storm."* Conversely, patients with severe hypothyroidism may also become dangerously ill with *myxedema coma.* Both of these situations demand intensive care.

Disturbances in the production of thyroid hormone have far-reaching metabolic consequences. Perhaps the most important function of this hormone is the control of oxidation at the cellular level. In its presence, oxygen consumption by the tissues is stimulated and in its absence, oxygen consumption is decreased. In addition, thyroid hormone has the following major effects:

a. It influences the rate of growth. Hypothyroidism in childhood leads to dwarfism and mental retardation (cretinism).

b. It affects the metabolism of protein, carbohydrates and lipids. Specifically, it promotes protein synthesis and increases nitrogen retention. It enhances the rate of intestinal absorption of glucose as well as its peripheral utilization. A deficiency of thyroid hormone results in an elevation of serum cholesterol.

    c. Thyroid hormone has a stimulating effect on the myocardium and increases the rate and force of contraction. It also accentuates the vascular effects of epinephrine and norephinephrine and patients with hyperthyroidism should not receive these agents.

The production and secretion of thyroxin are controlled by the pituitary through its thyroid-stimulating hormone (TSH). When the thyroid gland produces adequate amounts of thyroid hormone, there is a concomitant decrease in TSH and conversely, when thyroxin levels are inadequate, TSH levels increase to stimulate the thyroid to produce additional hormone.

## A. HYPOTHYROIDISM AND MYXEDEMA COMA

### THE PROBLEM

    Hypothyroidism refers to the deficiency state which results from an insufficient supply of thyroid hormone. Thyroid deficiency, resulting from disease or deficiency of the thyroid gland itself, is known as "primary" hypothyroidism. Insufficiency that develops as a result of anterior pituitary gland failure is described as "secondary" or "pituitary" hypothyroidism.

    Regardless of the etiology, the major physiological and biochemical alterations of hypothyroidism include: decreased cellular metabolism, decreased energy production, decreased mental and physical abilities, and a peculiar collection of proteins, water, and electrolytes in the extracellular spaces. The last condition is described as myxedema.

    The patients who have severe hypothyroidism associated with myxedema may develop acute respiratory distress and become comatose. This crisis is precipitated by infection, trauma, convulsion, a surgical procedure, or barbiturate administration. During the period of myxedema crisis, carbon dioxide retention develops but the respiratory center appears insensitive and carbon dioxide narcosis ensues. The patient is usually hypothermic and a shock state exists. Unless the problem is recognized and treated promptly, death follows.

## ASSESSMENT OF THE PROBLEM

**Clinical manifestations of myxedema crisis.** The typical presenting picture is that of a patient with known hypothyroidism who is admitted in a deep stupor, with or without evidences of shock. The respirations are shallow and breathing is obviously labored. The body temperature is also obviously reduced. The physical finding of long-standing hypothyroidism are apparent (see pages 222–225).

*Laboratory manifestations.* There is biochemical evidence of severe hypothyroidism (see Table 4).

The $pCO_2$ is distinctly elevated, reflecting depression of the respiratory center.

Hypoglycemia is common.

*Table 4*
LABORATORY FINDINGS IN HYPOTHYROIDISM

| Test | Normal Range | Anticipated result |
|---|---|---|
| PBI | 4–8 mcg % | Less than 3.5 mcg % |
| I[131] UPTAKE | 20–50% | Less than 15% |
| $T_3$ | 0.9–1.1 | Less than .80 |
| FREE THYROXIN INDEX (FTI) | 2.2–7.0 | Less than 2.0 |
| BASAL METABOLIC RATE | −15%–+15% | Less than −20 |

## PRINCIPLES OF TREATMENT

The basic program for combating myxedema crisis includes the following objectives:

1. to establish and maintain an adequate airway
2. to treat shock if present
3. to initiate replacement therapy with thyroid hormone
4. to correct hypoglycemia if present
5. to restore body temperature to normal
6. to control infection if present

These objectives are accomplished in the following ways:

     a. The patient usually requires tracheostomy to assist

respiration. Intermittent positive pressure breathing can be used. Repeated determinations of $pCO_2$ are valuable.

b. The shock state accompanying myxedema coma is usually treated with hydrocortisone therapy. Hydrocortisone (100 mg) may be given intravenously during the first 12 hours of treatment. Vasopressor drugs must be used with caution, as they have a synergistic action with thyroid hormone which may provoke serious ventricular arrhythmias.

c. Replacement therapy with thyroid hormone is instituted very cautiously. Most programs use *small* dosages of triiodothyronine (2.5 to 5.0 micrograms), administered either intramuscularly or by nasogastric tube twice daily.

d. Control of hypoglycemia can be achieved by intravenous infusion of 5% glucose in distilled water.

e. The use of external heat for the hypothermia is contraindicated as it may exaggerate or precipitate circulatory collapse. One or two blankets are all that should be used. Body temperature generally begins to return to normal within 24–48 hours after triiodothyronine has been started.

f. Care should be taken not to stress the patient with examinations, exposure, etc., during this period.

g. Appropriate antibiotic therapy may be used to combat existing infection.

## THE NURSING ROLE

1. Tracheostomy care and maintenance of airway. The details of this care are described in Chapter I, "Respiratory Insufficiency and Failure."

2. The nurse should carefully observe the patient for evidence of $CO_2$ narcosis. Dangerously high levels of $CO_2$ in the blood can be suspected from changes ranging from confusion to deep coma.

3. Because of the tendency to ventricular arrhythmias and sudden death, patients should have constant ECG monitoring. The nurse should be aware of the possibility of ventricular tachycardia and ventricular fibrillation (see pages 59–60). Necessary resuscitative equipment including defibrillators and pacemakers should be available.

*Table 5*

## HYPOTHYROIDISM

| | |
|---|---|
| Associated conditions | Cretinism (infants, small children) |
| | Hypopituitarism (secondary hypothyroidism) |
| | Autoimmune thyroiditis (Hashimoto's disease, primary adult hypothyroidism, or myxedema.) |
| | Riedel's thyroiditis |
| | Surgical removal (excessive) |
| | Atrophy |
| | Hyperplasia |
| Physiological alteration | Decreased production of thyroid hormones |
| Effects of alteration | Decreased energy production (heat) |
| | Decreased metabolic activity with carbohydrate protein, lipid, water and mineral disturbances. |
| | Abnormal collection of protein, electrolytes, and water in the extracellular spaces. |
| | Failure of normal mental and physical development in infants and children. (Slowing of mental and physical activities in adults.) |

Circulatory System:

| | |
|---|---|
| Cardiovascular | Pseudohypertrophy of chamber walls, dyspnea, peripheral edema may be present, hypertension, pulse rate and pulse pressure decreased. Decrease in stroke volume, minute volume, and circulation rate. |
| Blood constituents | Decreased plasma volume |
| | Increased protein concentration |
| | Decreased PBI |
| | Increased cholesterol level |
| | Increased phospholipids |
| | Increased carotene |
| | Decreased Vitamin A |
| | Albuminuria |
| Blood cells | Anemias (a) hypochromic |
| | (b) macrocytic |
| | (c) pernicious (secondary) |
| | Increased capillary fragility |
| Ectodermal structures | *Skin*—pale, cool, dry, scaly, puffy, and inelastic. Pitting edema in prolonged disease. Wounds heal slowly. Jaundice coloring due to carotemia. |
| | *Hair*—Decreased in scalp, pubis, axillae, eyebrows and most everywhere. Tends to regrow very slowly. Dry, brittle, and without gloss. |
| | *Fingernails*—Brittle and break easily. |

* Adapted from Irene L. Beland, *Clinical Nursing*, New York, Macmillan

## HYPERTHYROIDISM

Exophthalmic goiter or Graves' disease
Plummer's disease (toxic modular goiter)
Toxic adenoma
Ectopic thyroid tissue
Thyrotoxic factitia

Increased production of thyroid hormones

Increased combustion of food with increased absorption rate of glucose, and glycogenolysis. May lead to glycosuria
May have increased use of fat and proteins for fuel, leading to depletion of body stores
Increased liberation of energy (heat)

Tachycardia, palpitations and exertional dyspnea. Auricular fibrillation may be evident. Forceful contractions, increased cardiac output. Increased stroke volume, rate, pulse volume, systolic pressure. Peripheral pulsations. Decreased circulation time. Congestive heart failure not uncommon in older age group.

Plasma volume increase
Decreased protein concentration
Elevated PBI
Increased concentration of creatine
Decreased concentration of creatinine
Increased ratio of blood cell phospholipids to serum phospholipids
Hyperglycemia

Low white cell count
Agranulocytopenia
Lymphocytosis
Monocytosis

*Skin*—warm, moist or cold and moist depending on external temperature and vasomotor function. Pink and smooth.

*Nails and scalp hair*—friable

*Sweat glands*—overactive

Company, New York, 1965, pp. 1045–1047.

*223*

*Table 5 (continued)*

HYPOTHYROIDISM

| | |
|---|---|
| Central nervous system | Slow mentation, poor memory, decreased sensory perception. Emotional reactions slow. Deep tendon reflexes slow to respond. Patient usually lethargic, good-natured, and pleasant. May develop psychosis of paranoid type ("myxedema madness"). Infants and young children, mental retardation. |
| Gastrointestinal system | Anorexia, constipation and achlorhydria. Increased weight gain due to fluid retention. Decreased absorption of glucose. Dysphagia. |
| Muscles | Weakness, fatigue and crampy. Muscle striations indistinct due to fluid accumulation. Hypotonia. |
| Skeletal system | Excess loss of calcium and phosphorus in urine and stools. If severe enough, renal calculi and pathological fractures may develop. |
| Temperature sensitivity | Increased sensitivity to cold. |
| Eyes | |
| Gonads | Decreased libido and fertility. Abnormal menstruation—prolonged to absent Impotence common in males. |
| Speech | Edema of tongue and larynx. Hesitating, slurred, and hoarse speech. |
| Immune reaction | Increased susceptibility to infections. |

4. There is often a marked sensitivity to thyroid hormone, even very small doses, among patients with severe hypothyroidism. For this reason the nurse should record the vital signs at frequent intervals during the early period of thyroid replacement. Increases in the pulse rate or pressure, or variation in the rate and depth of respiration should be reported to the physician.

5. If hypoglycemia is a conspicuous feature, blood for sugar determinations should be drawn at regular intervals by the intensive care team to estimate the response to therapy.

6. Recognizing the potential danger of the application of external heat, the nurse should refrain from adding extra blankets to the customary bed covering. It is wise to place the patient in a warm, draft-free area of the intensive care facility.

## HYPERTHYROIDISM

Hyperactive and nervous (mental and physical jitteriness).
Flight of ideas, tremors, hyperactive reflexes, lability of emotions, hypersensitive, and agitated.
May have bouts of depression. Older patients may be diagnosed as having senile dementia.


Hyperphagia, diarrhea, nausea, vomiting, and anorexia in older patients.
Weight loss dependent on ratio of food intake to metabolic activity.


Weakness and fatigue.
Twitching and tremors.


Increased density of bone.


Increased sensitivity to heat.

Exophthalmia, lid-lag, infrequent blinking, and poor convergence.

Menses may be scanty and irregular
Oligomenorrhea, amenorrhea


Rapid and excited.
Local pressure on recurrent laryngeal nerves may cause hoarseness.

Infection susceptible.

7. Care should be taken to avoid cross-contamination in the unit. To this end the nurse should see that the patient is placed in an area remote from patients with infections. Be certain that all personnel in contact with the patient wash their hands carefully and wear masks. Relatives and friends should be screened for infections before visiting the patient.

8. Protect the patient from further stress or injury. Padded bed rails are helpful in this regard.

9. The unconscious patient is predisposed to the development of decubiti and the usual precautions regarding turning, etc., should be observed.

10. As the patient recovers from myxedema coma, psychotic manifestations may emerge. Slow mentalization is to be expected.

The nurse-physician team should understand this aspect of the illness and must not become impatient or exasperated with the patient's behavior.

11. Constipation is a constant problem in hypothyroidism and fecal impactions occur.

# B. ACUTE HYPERTHYROIDISM ("THYROID STORM")

## THE PROBLEM

It is unlikely that patients with hyperthyroidism would be admitted to an intensive care unit unless the problem was that of severe thyrotoxicosis or *"thyroid storm."* With earlier recognition of hyperthyroidism and improved medical arrangement the occurrence of this acute problem is now rare.

Hyperthyroidism is characterized by an overproduction of thyroid hormone which results in major physiological and biological disturbances. (See Table 5.) Thyroid storm represents one of the severest complications of hyperthyroidism. It is thought to be precipitated by trauma to the thyroid region, infections, emotional upsets, and especially thyroid surgery undertaken on poorly prepared patients with hyperthyroidism.

The characteristic findings of acute hyperthyroidism include:

    a. fever (up to 106° F.)
    b. tachycardia (up to 200/min.)
    c. A marked nervousness with extreme irritability or, conversely, apathy.
    d. delirium or coma.
    e. diarrhea, and later, vomiting.

## PRINCIPLES OF TREATMENT

Thyroid storm is seldom seen today because of careful preparation preoperatively. The single most important factor for successful surgery is that the patient be in a euthyroid state at the time of operation. This usually takes 6–12 weeks of treatment with antithyroid drugs. Two weeks prior to surgery, Lugol's solution or saturated solution of potassium iodide is added to the treatment program.

In the unlikely event that thyroid crisis develops post-operatively, the following program is carried out:

1. Iodine is administered intravenously and antithyroid drugs are initiated.

2. Glucose and water are given intravenously in large amounts.

3. Hydrocortisone (100 mg.) is used intravenously at the start of treatment and repeated as indicated every 12 hours.

4. Hyperpyrexia may require hypothermic blankets and oxygen.

5. Agitation is usually controlled with barbiturates, including sodium pentothal.

6. Since heart failure may accompany the tachycardia, digitalis is commonly used, along with the oxygen therapy.

## THE NURSING ROLE

Confusion and agitation may be present. It is important that the patient's behavior be closely observed. It is a wise practice to seclude the patient as much as possible (a private room is desirable) during this disturbed period, and care must be taken to protect him from injury. Sedatives should be given.

Body temperature should be carefully monitored by rectal probe. Hypothermic blankets should be used but wet packs or ice can be substituted. Try to maintain a body temperature under 100° F.

### Bibliography

ARKY, RONALD A. and HURWITZ, DAVID: Management of Emergencies. VII. The Therapy of Diabetic Ketoacidosis. *New England Journal of Medicine,* 274:1135–1137, May 19, 1966.

DAVIES, D. R. and FRIEDMAN, M.: Complications After Parathyroidectomy. *Journal of Bone and Joint Surgery,* 48B:117–126, February 1966.

Emergency Treatment of Hypercalcemia, *Lancet,* 2:501–502, September 2, 1967.

JOHNSON, ROBERT D.: Management of Diabetic Ketoacidosis. *Postgraduate Medicine,* 39:246–255, March 1966.

LIBERMAN, BERNARDO, WAJCHENBERG, BERNARDO L. and PIERONI, ROMULO R.: Water and Electrolyte Metabolism in Adrenal and Pituitary Insufficiency. *Metabolism,* 15:992–1001, November 1966.

MAYNARD, DONALD E., FOLK, ROBERT A., RILEY, THOMAS R., et al.: A Rapid Test for Adrenacortical Insufficiency, *Annals of Internal Medicine,* 64:552–556, March 1966.

NUTTALL, FRANK Q.: Metabolic Acidosis-Diabetic. *Archives of Internal Medicine,* 116:709–716, November 1965.

RANDALL, RAYMOND V.: Hypoglycemia. *Mayo Clinic Proceedings,* 41: 390–398, June 1966.

SEFTEL, H. C. and KEW, M. C.: Early and Intensive Potassium Replacement in Diabetic Acidosis. *Diabetes,* 15:694–696, September 1966.

# Chapter VII

# Water and Electrolyte Imbalances

ISABEL E. DUTCHER, R.N., M.A.
HAROLD C. HARDENBURG, JR., M.D.

## THE PROBLEM

Water and electrolyte disturbances occur in nearly every patient whose medical or surgical problem demands intensive care. Obviously, an understanding of the etiology of these disturbances is essential for successful therapy. The physiology of water and electrolytes is a massive subject, about which volumes have been written. It is not our purpose here to consider this topic in a truly comprehensive manner; instead, this chapter is presented as an introduction to the fundamental concepts, and as a practical guide to rational therapy of fluid and electrolyte imbalances.

**Basic principles of fluid and electrolyte balance.** To comprehend the clinical aspects of maintaining water and electrolyte balance, it is important to consider the following subjects initially:

1. The total volume of body fluids.
2. The composition of body fluids.
3. The sources of water and electrolyte intake to the body.
4. The routes by which water and electrolytes are lost from the body.
5. The body's mechanisms for preserving water and electrolyte balance.

**1. The Total Volume of Body Fluids.** Water is the largest single constituent of all living organisms. In man it constitutes about 55% of the total body weight and varies with age, sex, and, most significantly, with the amount of body fat. Fat is relatively free of water as compared to other tissues, and therefore women and obese persons have a lower proportion of water to their total body weight. An average 150 pound (70 kg) male has total body fluids approximating 42 liters of water.

Although all body water can be considered to be in a continuous phase, since it is freely diffusable and reaches all tissues, it is nevertheless customary (and practical) to divide the total body water into *functional* compartments. This division is based on differences in the chemical composition of the fluids in various parts of the body.

The two major fluid compartments are classified as *intracellular* and *extracellular*. The intracellular compartment represents the fluid found within cells and accounts for about 30 liters of the total 42 liters of body water (of a 150 pound male). All of the fluid located outside the cells is described as *extracellular*. The extracellular compartment is further subdivided into two classes, *intravascular* water, the fluid within the blood vessels (i.e., plasma), and *interstitial* water, the water in the tissues surrounding the cells. Thus, in a 150 pound male, the *intravascular* water volume is about 3.5 liters. (This volume, along with 3 liters of red blood cells, constitutes the total *blood* volume of 6.5 liters.) The *interstitial* water volume is about 7.7 liters.

Fluids within the gastrointestinal tract, as well as fluid located within the ducts of glands and in the urinary collecting system, are categorized as *transcellular* fluids. These fluids may be considered as a specialized portion of the *extracellular* compartment. When they are lost in large quantities, a serious imbalance of extracellular fluid can occur.

The volume of water in the various compartments expressed as a percentage of *total body weight* is shown in the following table.

*Table 1*
BODY WATER EXPRESSED AS A PERCENTAGE OF BODY WEIGHT

| | |
|---|---|
| Total Weight of the Body | 100% |
| *Weight of Body Solids* | 45% |
| *Weight of Water* | 55% |
| Intracellular water | 40.3% |
| Extracellular water | 14.7% |

**The Internal Transfer of Fluids.** Theoretically, water can move freely from one compartment to another because the separating membranes are freely permeable to water. This movement, however, is regulated by the composition of dissolved materials (solutes) contained within the water (solvent). This control is mediated in two ways:

DIFFUSION

This is the simplest type of fluid transfer and represents spontaneous movement of the solutes and solvent from areas of high concentration to areas of low concentration until a state of equilibrium is established. For example, a dye added to a container of water will diffuse until a uniform color of the solution results. Diffusion occurs even though the watery medium is separated by membranes, provided the membranes are permeable (i.e., permit passage) to the diffusing molecules of solute and solvent.

OSMOSIS

In a true solution, molecules of the solvent water are in constant random motion. As a result, these molecules continuously collide against each other or against any surface in their way; this motion creates a form of pressure called *osmotic pressure*. Such pressure is proportional to the number of dispersed solute molecules in the solvent; the higher the concentration of these particles the greater the number of impacts between solute and solvent molecules and the greater the osmotic pressure of the solution.

An important physiologic phenomenon resulting from osmotic pressure is osmosis, which can be defined as the passage of water (solvent), or of water and solutes, through a semipermeable membrane separating two solutions of unlike composition or concentration. A semipermeable membrane is one which is freely permeable to water but relatively impermeable to solute particles. Water moves across the membrane from a solution with a lesser concentration of particles (a hypotonic solution) into one with a higher concentration of particles (hypertonic), i.e., "water goes where the salt is."

The most important forces which tend to pull water into, or prevent the escape of water from, the intracellular and extracellular compartments are the osmotic pressures exerted by the solutes in these compartments. In extracellular fluid the major osmotic effect is exerted by sodium and chloride ions. In the intracellular compartment potassium, magnesium, phosphates, and proteinates are the underlying controlling forces. When the concentration of ions on either side of a membrane is altered, water moves quickly to re-establish osmotic equilibrium.

The laws of osmosis and diffusion cannot, however, fully explain the movement of ions in solution. Despite a concentration gradient created by forces of diffusion and osmosis, solutes can penetrate cell membranes. This opposed movement requires the expenditure of energy that is derived from metabolic activity. The term *active transport* is applied to any movement of solutes where energy is expended.

**2. The Composition of Body Fluids.** Essentially, body fluids are solutions in which water is the solvent and various organic and inorganic chemical substances are dissolved as solutes. Solutes are conveniently divided into two classes: *electrolytes,* substances capable of dissociating into ions which in solution will conduct an electric current, and *non-electrolytes,* substances such as sugar or urea, which in solution do not dissociate into ions, and are thus electrically neutral. Ions are defined as atoms, or groups of atoms, which have either a positive charge (cations), or have a negative charge (anions). The electrical activity of ions in solution results from a net loss, or gain, of negatively charged particles (electrons), which are a basic component of every elemental atomic structure. When electrons are lost, the ion then has a net positive charge and is attracted to the negative pole of a battery. This pole is known as a cathode, hence the term "cation" for a positively charged ion. Conversely, when electrons are gained, the net charge of the ion is negative and it is attracted to the positive pole of a battery, the anode, and is called an anion.

In solution, ions of like charge (e.g., anions) cannot exist alone and must be balanced by an equivalent number of oppositely charged ions (cations). For this reason, the solution as a whole is electrically neutral.

The following list indicates the electrolytes of biological significance:

| Cations | Anions |
|---|---|
| Sodium (Na+) | Chloride (Cl−) |
| Potassium (K+) | Bicarbonate ($HCO_3$−) |
| Calcium (Ca++) | Phosphate ($HPO_4$)= |
|  | and ($H_2PO_4$)− |
| Magnesium (Mg++) | Proteinate |

The electrolyte composition of body fluids is as follows:

A. EXTRACELLULAR FLUID

The principal cation of extracellular fluid is sodium. The main anions are chloride, bicarbonate, and proteinate. The sum of all the cations expressed in *milliequivalents* per liter exactly equals the sum of all the anions. (See appendix at end of chapter.)

B. INTRACELLULAR FLUID

Intracellular cations are potassium and magnesium, the former being the more abundant ion. There is relatively little sodium in the intracellular fluid. The anions are organic phosphates and proteins.

It is essential that differences in the composition of intracellular and extracellular fluids be maintained. For example, sodium plays a dominant role in maintaining extracellular water osmotic pressure and hence the volume of extracellular fluids. Potassium has a somewhat similar role in intracellular water. However, these cations are decidedly *not* interchangeable in their function. Potassium, when in its intracellular location, is nontoxic over a wide concentration range, but in the extracellular fluid this cation is highly toxic when the concentration is above normal.

**3. The Sources of Fluid and Electrolyte Intake to the Body.** There are three normal sources of body water: oral fluids, water found within foods (e.g., cooked lean meat is from 65% to 70% water), and water formed by oxidation of foods or by oxidation of body fat and protein. If food and fluid intake are inadequate or lacking, this latter source may become a major factor.

The average daily water intake in an adult male, performing moderate activity, is as follows:

| | |
|---|---|
| Beverages | 1350 ml |
| Water content of food | 1000 ml |
| Water of oxidation | 350 ml |
| Total | 2700 ml |

The sources of electrolytes are also food and drink. Normally, a person ingests larger amounts of sodium chloride, calcium, potassium, protein, and other salts than are required. The body maintains a balance for each substance by excreting the excess.

**4. The Routes by Which Fluids and Electrolytes Are Lost from the Body.** The channels of exit for both water and electrolytes are skin, lungs, gastrointestinal tract, and kidneys. The daily water output through these various channels in an average size adult male, performing moderate activity at room temperature and humidity, is as follows:

| | |
|---|---|
| Skin and lung (insensible loss) | 600–1200 ml |
| Gastrointestinal (feces) | 150 ml |
| Kidneys (urine) | 1500 ml |

A. THE SKIN

Water loss through the skin occurs in two ways: as sensible sweat and as insensible sweat. The sensible loss is that which is produced by the sweat glands and of which the person is aware. Its volume varies with the atmospheric conditions and with body temperature. Such sweat contains electrolytes and can be considered a hypotonic solution, since it has less concentration of solutes than internal fluids. Because of its hypotonicity, profuse sweating tends to deplete the body of water more than sodium and chloride. In patients who are losing large volumes of water in other ways (e.g., diarrhea), sweating can be dangerous.

Insensible sweat refers to the water lost as vapor on the surface of the skin, by evaporation. This loss is not visible and is obligatory (i.e., it is continuous without regard to intake of fluid or the body's needs). It amounts to 300 to 600 ml daily. It is essentially electrolyte-free, unlike sensible sweat, which contains salts.

B. THE LUNGS

The expired air is saturated with water vapor. The magnitude of water loss from this source varies with the rate and depth of respiration and the volume of exchange. An average adult loses 300 to 500 ml of water daily in this manner.

This water vapor loss from the lungs and insensible sweat are jointly classified as *the insensible water* loss of the body (600 to 1200 ml per day).

### C. THE GASTROINTESTINAL TRACT

Enormous quantities of water and electrolytes are secreted into the stomach and intestines daily as part of the digestive process. Of the estimated 8000 ml secreted into the gastrointestinal tract, almost all is subsequently reabsorbed so that the material (feces) reaching the sigmoid contains only 100 to 150 ml of water, with little electrolyte content. Sodium is the chief cation of these secretions, and chloride and bicarbonate are the main anions. The relative concentration of anions varies at different sites in the gastrointestinal tract; thus, chloride predominates in the acid medium of the stomach, while bicarbonate is the major anion in the intestines where the secretions are alkaline. The concentration of potassium in the stomach is 2 to 5 times that of the serum.

The enormousness of the volume of electrolyte-containing liquids which pass from the extracellular fluid to the gastrointestinal tract and then return to this compartment must be appreciated. The volume (8000 ml) represents 2 to 3 times the *total* plasma volume of the body and is many times in excess of the total water intake. For this reason, loss of gastrointestinal secretions from the body is one of the most serious causes of water and electrolyte depletion.

Although the concentration of solutes in the gastrointestinal secretions differs from that of the other body fluids (e.g., the concentration of potassium), osmotic equilibrium nevertheless exists. This is achieved by the transfer of water and electrolytes to and from the extracellular compartment until equilibrium is reached (*isotonic* state).

Ingested liquids or other materials, passing through the gastrointestinal tract, assume the same electrolyte pattern as the fluid present in the particular site. For this reason there is danger in irrigating a gastrointestinal tube with water. In this situation, water, which is hypotonic, draws sodium chloride and potassium from the extracellular compartment into the stomach or bowel while establishing equilibrium of the solutes so that isotonicity is achieved. This creates a depletion of extracellular electrolytes. The lower the tube is positioned in the gastrointestinal tract, the more marked the electrolyte disturbance will be. Thus, patients on gastrointestinal suction should not be allowed water and ice, because these liquids will promote excessive intestinal secretion and loss of electrolytes. Irrigation should be carried out with isotonic sodium chloride solution.

### D. THE KIDNEYS

The kidneys assume a major role in the regulation of fluid, electrolyte, and acid-base balance. The fluid passing through from the glomerulus to the proximal tubule is a protein-free filtrate of plasma. Within the proximal tubule about 80 per cent of the water and all of the glucose of this filtrate are reabsorbed, along with small amounts of sodium and a large fraction of urea. During the passage through the loop of Henle and the distal tubules, further reabsorption occurs. The reabsorption of sodium, chloride, water, bicarbonate, and phosphate are individually regulated by specific control mechanisms in the kidney to maintain normal electrolyte and osmotic concentration of the extracellular fluid. In addition to the process of reabsorption, the kidney has the ability to secrete potassium and hydrogen ions in accordance with the needs of the extracellular fluid.

The average excretion of urine is about 1500 ml per day.

## 5. The Body's Mechanisms for Preserving Fluid and Electrolyte Balance.

### A. THIRST

Thirst is one of the major factors in determining fluid intake and maintaining the balance between intake and output. The chief stimuli to this subjective sensation are cellular hypohydration and an increase in the hypertonicity of the body fluids due to an increased solute concentration and a resultant increase in osmotic pressure. This latter effect is illustrated by the increased desire for water after eating salted nuts, potato chips, etc., all of which increase hypertonicity. Additional stimuli to thirst include a decreased circulating blood volume (e.g., shock), drying of the mucous membranes, and emotional factors such as anxiety. In the sick individual the usual stimuli may be inadequate or absent, and cannot serve to indicate the need for fluids.

### B. ANTIDIURETIC HORMONE (ADH)

ADH regulates osmotic pressure of the extracellular water by controlling the reabsorption of water in the distal tubules of the kidney. Specifically, the antidiuretic hormone increases reabsorption of water and therefore decreases the urine volume. The usual stimulus for the secretion of the antidiuretic hormone is water loss, so that when there is need for the conservation of water by the body as in states of dehydration, ADH is elaborated.

Additionally, pain, fear, acute stress, or the administration of analgesics such as morphine and Demerol, barbiturates, or most anesthetics, may stimulate excessive ADH production. On this basis postoperative oliguria may often be the result of ADH secretion, and in this circumstance, forcing fluids will not appreciably increase the urine output, but may instead lead to water intoxication.

### C. ALDOSTERONE

Aldosterone, a hormone secreted by the adrenal cortex, regulates the extracellular volume by affecting the renal control of sodium and potassium. Specifically, aldosterone promotes *retention* of sodium and water by the kidney, while causing increased urinary *excretion* of potassium.

Aldosterone secretion is stimulated by low blood sodium levels, high blood potassium level, and dehydration. The hormone causes an increase in sodium reabsorption by the renal tubules. The sodium retained for this reason holds tenaciously to water (because of osmolarity) and the urinary excretion of water decreases. In addition to its role in balancing the water volume, aldosterone also promotes a reduction of excessive amounts of potentially toxic potassium found in the extracellular fluid, a circumstance partially responsible for aldosterone secretion in the first place.

**The balance of fluid intake and output.** Because many of the systems of calculation used to establish fluid and electrolyte balance rely primarily on accurate intake/output records, it is essential that the nurse appreciate the need for precision in making these measurements and recording the data. Many nurses apparently feel that intake/output assessment is a menial task which can be ignored or merely approximated. The difficulty in getting the nursing staff to perform this simple, but nevertheless vital, task and record the results on proper forms is perplexing to many physicians. Nursing educators cannot stress too heavily the significance of this nursing duty.

A. *The measurement of fluid intake.* The intake of fluids can be calculated with reasonable certainty. The volume includes liquids given orally, fluids administered intravenously (or by clysis) and the amount of water in ingested foods (determined from standard tables). Water formed from oxidation of food is normally disregarded in calculations of total fluid intake.

B. *The measurement of fluid output.* Fluid output is more difficult to measure accurately than fluid intake. In uncomplicated situations the output volume includes urine, vomitus, tube or fistulous drainage, and an estimate of insensible water losses from the lungs and skin.

In critical situations (e.g., patients with metabolic crises or severe burns) greater accuracy is demanded.

Periodic measurement of the body weight affords a measure for estimation of fluid loss (or gain). Patients should be weighed on the same scale every 12 hours. The patient should void prior to the weighing procedure and the amount of bed clothing should be constant. Metabolic bed balances offer even further accuracy.

**Acid-Base Balance.** Hydrogen ions (H+) are present in the extracellular fluid in minute amounts, approximately 0.0000001 gm/L. This very low concentration of hydrogen ions in the extracellular fluids is conveniently expressed as a logarithm to the base 10 and represented by the term pH. The concentration of hydrogen ions determines the acidity or alkalinity of the solution; the more hydrogen ions present, the more acid the solution. The normal pH of the extracellular fluid (and blood) is between 7.35 and 7.45. A pH above 7.45 indicates alkalosis, and a pH less than

7.35 indicates acidosis. A pH of 7.0 or lower (marked acidosis) or a pH greater than 7.8 (marked alkalosis) usually results in death.

The body's ability to maintain pH within this very narrow range (7.35 to 7.45) is a remarkable achievement, because cellular metabolism is a hydrogen-ion-producing process and thus there is a continuous tendency toward acidosis. Acid-base balance is achieved through a number of regulating systems within the body. These control mechanisms include:

**A.** *An acid-base buffer system within the body fluids.* This mechanism behaves, in a sense, as a sponge and either absorbs H+ ions or frees them, depending on the need.

**B.** *The lungs.* When the H+ ion concentration increases beyond the normal limits (acidosis), the respiratory center in the brain is stimulated and the rate of respiration is increased. In this way large amounts of carbon dioxide are blown off and the amount of carbonic acid in the extracellular fluid is decreased; this combats acidosis. The normal respiratory system responds within minutes to change in the pH and is a continuous guard against incipient acidosis.

**C.** *The kidneys.* The buffer systems within the kidneys represent the most powerful homeostatic mechanism to control acid-base balance. The acidity or alkalinity of the urine reflects the activities of this regulatory mechanism. Unlike the pulmonary control system (which works in minutes), the renal mechanism takes several hours to readjust the hydrogen ion concentration. Normally, these systems can handle moderate disturbances in the acid-base balance resulting from some kinds of disease processes; but with overwhelming loads of acids, as occurs in diabetic acidosis, these mechanisms become insufficient, and intravenous infusions are necessary to combat developing acidosis. Diseases of the kidneys or lungs can upset acid-base balance, for obvious reasons.

## ASSESSMENT OF THE PROBLEM

A general estimate of fluid and electrolyte deficiency can be obtained from the medical history and physical examination. Some pertinent factors in this regard are:

1. The specific diagnosis and the duration of the disease.

Obviously, patients with abnormal losses of fluids or blood are high risks for fluid and electrolyte disturbances.

2. The patient's general condition and mental state. The presence of confusion or a lack of alertness may reflect an underlying fluid and electrolyte disturbance.

3. The turgor of the skin, the intraocular pressure, and dryness of the tongue are classical physical signs of adequate or inadequate hydration. Similarly, the presence of congestive heart failure or the presence of pitting presacral or dependent edema are obviously significant signs of imbalance.

4. The deep tendon reflexes, muscle tone, or Chvostek's sign may reflect serious electrolyte changes.

5. A history of both the patient's former weight and his weight on admission are of special importance. (If the patient is a child, the height must also be recorded.) Because calculations to determine fluid and electrolyte replacement are based on body weight (or corrected to reflect total body surface area), the nurse must recognize the importance of this simple determination. Weighing the patient on a bed scale should not be considered a "nuisance chore," but rather the collection of fundamental data required for therapy.

Laboratory studies are essential in assessing fluid and electrolyte problems. The standard basic studies include CBC, urinalysis, blood sugar, blood urea nitrogen, serum Na, K, and Cl, blood $CO_2$ and pH, a chest film, and an electrocardiogram. The serum electrolyte determinations and the electrocardiograms must be made serially to assess the effectiveness of therapy.

## PRINCIPLES OF TREATMENT

Intravenous therapy is required for two fundamental purposes: to maintain adequate fluid and electrolyte balance (i.e., to prevent *deficits*) particularly in the postoperative state when the patient cannot take fluids orally, and *to replace* existing deficits that have occurred because of the disease state.

### Maintenance therapy

Maintenance therapy includes the administration of water, dextrose, and electrolytes.

**A. *Water*.** The maintenance requirement of water is best calculated on the basis of body surface area, rather than on the patient's weight. Children and small adults require more water per pound than do large adults, so that weight alone may be a misleading index.

A useful formula to calculate the maintenance water is that maintenance water = 1600 ml water per square meter of body surface per day. The body surface area can be derived from height and weight measurement and can be simply calculated from prepared tables. With obese or edematous patients, the "ideal" weight, rather than the actual weight, should be used in the calculation.

**B. *Dextrose*.** All maintenance solutions should contain at least 5% dextrose for purposes of caloric balance. The use of dextrose minimizes ketosis (which accompanies "starvation" and reduces the accumulation of "starvation solutes," urea, phosphates, and other protein breakdown products).

**C. *Electrolytes*.** Maintenance requirements of electrolytes are more difficult to estimate than water requirements, because the renal excretion of sodium, potassium, bicarbonate, and chloride varies markedly in response to factors such as diet, fluid intake, acid-base balance, and endocrine function.

The components of several commercially available premixed electrolyte solutions used for maintenance purposes are given in Table 2.

*Table 2*

PREMIXED ELECTROLYTE SOLUTIONS FOR MAINTENANCE

| Solution | Supplier | Na | K | Cl | $HCO_3$ | Mg | P |
|----------|----------|----|----|----|---------|----|----|
| Ionosol MB | Abbott | 25 | 20 | 22 | 23 | 3 | 3 |
| Electrolyte 4 | Baxter | 35 | 15 | 22 | 20 | – | 3 |
| Electrolyte 48 | Cutter | 25 | 20 | 22 | 23 | 3 | 3 |
| Electrolyte 4 | McGaw | 30 | 15 | 22 | 20 | – | 3 |
| Isolyte P | McGaw | 25 | 20 | 22 | 23 | 3 | 3 |

**Infusion Rate.** It is important that the physician indicate precisely how rapidly an intravenous infusion should be given. The rate of administration of intravenous fluids can be calculated from the following equation:

Drops per minute × drop factor = ml per hour.

To utilize this formula it is first necessary to know how many drops are required to deliver 1 ml of fluid with the equipment being used. (Infusion sets from various manufacturers deliver different size drops.)

The drop factor is obtained by dividing the number of drops required to deliver 1 ml into 60. For example, if 15 drops = 1 ml, the drop factor is $\frac{60}{15} = 4$. Thus if the infusion is running at a rate of 25 drops per minute, the volume per hour would be 25 × 4 = 100 ml fluid per hour. The hourly infusion rates for various solutions are shown in Table 3.

## Replacement therapy

### Basic principles

It is considered more physiologic to replace salts in a dilute solution distributed equally over a 24-hour period than to use a more concentrated solution for a few hours and then maintain a 5% glucose in water infusion for the remaining 24-hour period. For example, if a patient needs 4000 cc of fluid of which half should be 0.9% NaCl, it is wiser to administer all 4000 cc as 0.45% NaCl in 5% glucose, rather than to use 2000 cc of 0.9% NaCl in 5% glucose/water followed by 2000 cc of 5% glucose/water. It is believed that the "pouring" of a heavy salt load on the kidneys for a few hours is disadvantageous.

The replacement of potassium, calcium, and sodium bicarbonate should be individualized for each patient. The use of prepared multielectrolyte solutions for replacement is a popular practice, but one that cannot be wholly recommended. These standardized solutions are prepared to resemble extracellular fluid and, while useful in many instances, may create electrolyte imbalances in certain situations. For example, patients with renal disease, particularly those with uremia or acute tubular necrosis, poorly tolerate potassium, magnesium, and phosphates, which are included in most premixed solutions. In these circumstances, it is safer to add specific electrolytes to a dilute sodium chloride solution. When these particular problems do not exist, standard solutions can be used for the rapid replacement of water and electro-

*Table 3*

INTRAVENOUS FLUIDS—USUAL HOURLY INFUSION RATES

| Solution | Usual Hourly Rate* | Comments |
|---|---|---|
| **Dextrose solutions:** | | |
| 5% Dextrose | 400–500 cc/hour | Up to 2000 cc 5% dextrose or 1000 cc 10% dextrose solution per hour can be given for rapid replacement therapy |
| 10% Dextrose | 200–250 cc/hour | |
| **Saline solutions:** | | |
| Isotonic (0.85%) saline | 300–400 cc/hour | If rapid replacement therapy needed (e.g., shock) 1000–2000 cc isotonic NaCl can be administered per hour |
| 3%–5% saline (hypertonic) | 100 cc/hour | No more than 400 cc of 5% NaCl should be given in 24 hours |
| **Alkalizing solutions:** | | |
| Sodium bicarbonate (isotonic) | 200–400 cc/hour | Sodium bicarbonate can be administered very rapidly when used to combat lactic acidosis |
| Sodium lactate (⅙ molar solution isotonic) | 200–400 cc/hour | If *hypertonic* alkalizing solutions are used, the hourly rate is same as for hypertonic saline |
| **Multi-electrolyte solutions:** | | |
| Homeolyte (Mead-Johnson) Inosal (Abbott) Trovert (Baxter) Polysol (Cutter) | Adults: 400 cc/hour Children: 100–200 cc/hour Infants: 150 cc/kg body weight per day | |
| **Potassium-containing solutions:** | | |
| (When potassium is added to infusion bottle) | As ordered by physician | Urine output must be measured hourly when potassium is being administered |

* The rate of administration of fluids must be adjusted to each patient's needs. The values shown here are those generally employed for maintenance purposes.

lyte deficits. Some typical solutions available for this purpose are listed in Table 4.

Table 4

SOLUTIONS RESEMBLING EXTRACELLULAR FLUID FOR *Rapid* REPLACEMENT OF WATER AND ELECTROLYTE DEFICITS

| Solution | Supplier | Milliequivalents per Liter | | | | | |
|---|---|---|---|---|---|---|---|
| | | Na | K | Cl | HCO₃ | Ca | Mg |
| Hartmann's | Abbott; Cutter; McGaw | 131 | 4 | 110 | 28 | 3 | – |
| Ionosol D-CM | Abbott | 138 | 12 | 108 | 50 | 5 | 3 |
| Normosol R | Abbott | 140 | 5 | 98 | 27 | – | 3 |
| Plasmalyte | Baxter | 140 | 10 | 103 | 55 | 5 | 3 |
| Polysal | Cutter | 140 | 10 | 103 | 55 | 5 | 3 |
| Equivisol | McGaw | 140 | 10 | 103 | 55 | 5 | 3 |
| | | 150 | — | 100 | 50 | – | – |

After initial replacement is accomplished, additional fluid and electrolyte therapy is necessary to satisfy maintenance requirements as well as to continue replacement of ongoing losses. Solutions useful for these purposes are listed in Table 5.

Table 5

SOLUTIONS FOR MAINTENANCE AND ADDITIONAL REPLACEMENT OF FLUIDS AND ELECTROLYTES

| Solution | Supplier | Milliequivalents per Liter | | | | | | |
|---|---|---|---|---|---|---|---|---|
| | | Na | K | Cl | HCO₃ | Ca | Mg | P |
| Darrow's | Abbott; Baxter | 121 | 35 | 103 | 53 | – | – | — |
| | Cutter; McGaw | Dilute with equal parts of 10% dextrose | | | | | | |
| Ionosol B | Abbott | 57 | 25 | 49 | 25 | – | 5 | 13 |
| Normosol | Abbott | 40 | 13 | 40 | 16 | – | 3 | — |
| Electrolyte 2 | Baxter | 61 | 25 | 50 | 25 | – | 6 | 13 |
| Polysal M | Cutter | 40 | 16 | 40 | 24 | 5 | 3 | — |
| Electrolyte 2 | McGaw | 58 | 25 | 51 | 25 | – | 6 | 13 |

## Water imbalance

### Dehydration

Although a deficit of water by itself is not a common cause of dehydration among hospitalized patients, there are certain situations that can create this particular state: when swallowing is difficult or impossible; with impairment of the sense of thirst (e.g., cerebral injury); because of inability of the kidneys to concentrate urine (e.g., diabetes insipidus, alcoholism, or water-losing nephrites); or, with hyperventilation causing excessive loss of water from the lungs.

The clinical picture of water deficit from the above causes is quite distinctive, and includes symptoms of thirst and dryness of the mouth, oliguria, weight loss, fever, and flushed, dry skin having a thick, "doughy" feeling. In severe water loss, other findings may involve the central nervous system with the development of hallucinations, delirium, or coma. If the vascular volume deficit is great, hypovolemic shock may develop.

A second basic cause of water deficit relates to water loss due to solute excess. For example, when the unconscious patient is given nasogastric feedings which supply a large solute load *without* an adequate volume water intake, a solute excess is created. A similar situation can develop in patients with bleeding gastric ulcer disease where frequent feedings of milk and cream are given *without* water. In these situations there is an oligatory loss of water by the kidney which is demanded to secrete the excessive amounts of solute.

The signs and symptoms in these latter conditions are similar to those of dehydration mentioned previously, except that the patient may gain rather than lose weight and polyuria may exist rather than oliguria.

Dehydration can be considered significant when there is a deficit of 6% or more in the total body weight of an adult or 10% of the body weight of infants. Deficits of 3% in adults or 5% in infants can be classified as mild dehydration. The actual total loss of body weight is particularly important in this regard. As a general practice, this weight should be replaced in fluid, with one-half the volume being given over the first 24 hours and the remainder over the next day or so.

### Water excess

When the vascular system receives more water than a patient's kidneys can excrete, a state of overhydration develops. This can occur from two major sources: when antidiuretic hormone (ADH) secretion is excessive as with pain, fear, or the acute stress of trauma, and when renal blood flow is decreased as the result of adrenal cortical insufficiency or low cardiac output syndrome.

The clinical picture of overhydration is usually sudden and dramatic. It is characterized by the following findings:

1. behavioral changes: inattention, staring, confusion, shouting, and violence are common characteristics;
2. convulsive seizures;
3. anorexia, nausea, and vomiting;
4. hyperventilation;
5. abrupt weight gain;
6. edema of the skin.

In most instances, restricting fluids and sodium chloride will correct the problem. Occasionally, dialysis is necessary to remove the excessive fluid load.

## Specific Fluid and Electrolyte Problems
### Sodium imbalance

A normal 70 Kg male has a total body sodium of about 3000 meq. Most of this (about 2000 meq) is in the extracellular fluid, only a small amount being in the cells. Thus, the normal concentration of sodium in the extracellular fluid is about 140 meq/L (normal range 136 to 143). This concentration can be easily determined by measuring the amount of sodium in serum (which is, of course, part of the extracellular fluid).

In the healthy individual the excretion of sodium each day is about equal to the intake of sodium in the diet. The average diet contains about 100 meq of sodium (1 milliequivalent of sodium weighs 23 mgm; thus, in milligrams the diet contains about 2300 mgm of sodium). In patients with congestive heart failure or other forms of edema, the dietary intake of sodium is usually restricted to 1000 mgm or less per day.

About 1200 meq of sodium is secreted into the gastrointestinal tract each day. Under *normal* circumstances almost all of this is reabsorbed and the stool contains only trivial amounts. Thus, vomiting and diarrhea can obviously create marked depletion of sodium. Under these circumstances replacement can be made only by intravenous infusions. Solutions of choice are normal isotonic sodium chloride solution containing 154 meq/L of sodium or whole blood containing about 145 meq/L of sodium.

There are two major derangements of sodium imbalance,

namely a loss of sodium and sodium excess; the former is far more common than the latter.

**1. *The sodium loss syndrome* (*deficit*).** A loss or depletion of sodium from the extracellular fluid is one of the most common electrolyte imbalances.

*Etiology*
    a. *Loss of sodium through gastrointestinal secretions.*
        1. Vomiting;
        2. diarrhea, ulcerative colitis;
        3. continuous nasogastric or intestinal suction;
        4. fistulous drainage.
    b. *Loss of sodium through skin.*
        1. Excessive sweating;
        2. burns;
        3. cystic fibrosis.
    c. *When sodium is isolated or loculated within the body and is not physiologically available.*
        1. Within the large fluid volume sequestered in the small bowel in obstruction.
        2. In the edema fluid beneath burns.
        3. In the abdominal fluid in peritonitis.

*Signs and Symptoms.*
The clinical picture of sodium depletion is the result of actual loss of sodium as well as the accompanying loss of body fluids. The symptom complex varies with the degree of depletion of salt and water.

Typical symptoms include:
    a. weakness, apathy, and lassitude;
    b. fatigue;
    c. muscle weakness;
    d. muscle cramps;
    e. headache;
    f. vertigo.

Accompanying physical signs are:
    a. skin shows a loss of turgor;
    b. eyeballs may be soft;

c. cardiovascular;
    1. tachycardia;
    2. loss of peripheral pulse;
    3. slow filling of peripheral veins;
    4. shock may occur with severe sodium loss.

*Treatment*

The aim of treatment is to restore balance by replacing the sodium and water deficits. A method of calculating the replacement requirement of sodium is demonstrated in the following example: A 40-year-old male weighing 70 Kg (150) pounds) is admitted with a history of frequent vomiting for 48 hours. He complains of weakness and fatigue. The serum sodium is 128 meq/L. Replacement of sodium to achieve a normal serum level of 140 meq/L is desired. Thus, there is a deficiency of 12 meq per liter (140 meq − 128 meq = 12 meq).

Because sodium is mainly an extracellular ion, the patient's extracellular volume must be determined in order to calculate the amount of sodium required for replacement. This is done as follows: Knowing that 20% of the total body weight represents extracellular fluid, the weight of extracellular fluid can be calculated by merely multiplying the body weight by 20%.

$$\begin{array}{r} 70 \text{ Kg} \\ \times\ .20 \\ \hline 14 \text{ Kg} \end{array}$$

This weight, 14 Kg, is the equivalent of 14 liters of extracellular fluid. On this basis, we must replace 12 meq Na/liter for each of 14 liters, i.e.,

$$\begin{array}{r} 12 \text{ meq Na/L} \\ \times\ 14 \text{ L} \\ \hline 168 \text{ meq of sodium} \end{array}$$

This means that to achieve a normal sodium level, the patient must receive 168 meq of sodium (in addition to the amount needed to maintain a daily balance). A liter of 0.9% saline solution contains 154 meq of sodium. When the amount of sodium required is of this great a magnitude, the correction of imbalance must not be rapid, but should be accomplished over a 2- to 3-day period (unless a marked continuing depletion is occurring). Such balance can be achieved only by measuring the total number of meq of sodium in a 24-hour urine specimen. Replacement must include the daily loss in addition to the actual amount of sodium needed for correction of the existing deficit.

**2. *The sodium excess syndrome.*** Under normal temperature conditions, practically all of the loss of sodium from the body each day occurs through the kidneys. (The loss of sodium through the skin is negligible unless the environmental or body temperature is high.) The kidneys regulate the excretion of sodium in the healthy person in accordance with dietary intake. Thus, if there is a large intake, the kidneys do not reabsorb sodium in the tubules and allow it to be excreted in the urine. On the other hand, when there are modest losses of sodium, the kidneys can conserve the body stores by excreting urine that is practically free of sodium.

If the kidneys fail in this regulatory capacity, because of hormonal or hemodynamic effects, an excess of total body sodium can develop. This type of sodium excess is associated with the retention of fluid (edema) and is seen in the following circumstances:

    a. *Circulatory.*
        1. congestive heart failure;
        2. cirrhosis;
        3. ascites;
        4. nephrosis.
    b. *Hormonal.*

        1. The adrenal cortical hormones (corticosteroids) tend to increase the reabsorption of sodium by the renal tubules and promote sodium excess and edema. Thus, edema is characteristic of Cushing's syndrome and is seen in patients receiving long-term steroid therapy.

        2. Excessive secretion of the antidiuretic hormone (ADH). As previously noted, ADH secretion is increased in postoperative states, acute infections, stress, and with certain kinds of drug therapy (particularly morphine or meperidine).

The excess of sodium in these instances may not be found primarily in the vascular portion of the extracellular compartment, but in the tissue fluid itself. For this reason the serum level may be near normal despite an excess of total body sodium. The clinical picture of sodium excess relates to the source of the edema. The treatment is directed at the underlying cause, and includes the use of agents to promote excretion of sodium by preventing renal tubular reabsorption (diuretics).

**B.** *Potassium imbalance*

The total body potassium is about 3200 meq in an average male and about 2000 meq in the female. Most of the potassium is intracellular. The extracellular level (i.e., serum potassium) is between 4.5 and 5.0 meq/L. (Note the marked differences in the serum levels of sodium and potassium, reflecting their intracellular and extracellular concentrations.)

Potassium is ingested with the diet and the intake and output are essentially balanced, as is the situation with sodium, by renal excretion. The excretion of potassium in the stool is negligible.

**1.** *Potassium deficit (hypopotassemia)*. There are several causes for potassium depletion:

a. Vomiting, diarrhea, gastrointestinal suction.

b. Excessive or prolonged parenteral administrations of solutions not supplemented with potassium.

c. Adrenal cortical steroid increases the urinary excretion of potassium. Thus, Cushing's disease and prolonged steroid therapy are associated with hypopotassemia.

d. Diuretics of the thiazide class inhibit reabsorption of both sodium and potassium. Although they serve a useful purpose in states of sodium excess, they frequently cause potassium depletion.

e. In diabetic acidosis, potassium escapes from the cells into the extracellular fluid, resulting in an intracellular depletion of potassium, but an extracellular excess.

f. Inadequate diet or semistarvation with low intake of potassium ultimately produces a depletion state because the daily turnover (and excretion) of potassium continues without adequate replacement.

A potassium deficit affects cellular metabolism. This is manifest particularly in muscle tissue where there is loss of tone. This is shown in the following ways:

a. The skeletal muscles are soft and flabby, while the patient complains of marked weakness.

b. The smooth muscles of the gastrointestinal tract relax to produce a paralytic ileus and abdominal distention.

c. When potassium deficit is marked, the heart muscles can be injured and congestive failure may develop. In this circumstance the electrocardiogram shows flattened or inverted T waves with a prolonged QT interval. These changes are often the best index of a decrease in cellular potassium, because the serum potassium level does not necessarily reflect the concentration in the cells.

Potassium depletion is treated by the addition of potassium to intravenous fluids. The amount of potassium needed for replacement cannot be calculated in the same way as the amount of sodium needed because of the intracellular location of most of the body's potassium. Prompt improvement of the findings described above is the most useful guide.

**2. *Potassium excess (hyperpotassemia)*.** The varied etiologies of potassium excess (hyperpotassemia) include:

a. Renal failure where excretion of potassium decreases or fails.

b. Adrenal cortical insufficiency. In untreated Addison's disease the concentration of potassium is markedly increased because of decreased potassium excretion.

c. Excessive parenteral administration of potassium, or the *overly rapid* administration of solutions containing potassium.

d. Trauma of tissues (e.g., crush injuries), where potassium escapes from the cells.

The major danger of increased serum potassium is its effect on the myocardium. When the extracellular potassium reaches levels of 7 meq/L or more, heart block and ventricular standstill may occur. The presence of hyperpotassemia can usually be demonstrated by the appearance of tall peaked T waves on the electrocardiogram in the absence of cardiac failure before the onset of lethal arrhythmias. The shortening of the QT interval and the alterations of the T wave are important signs of hyperpotassemia to be recognized.

Other symptoms and signs of hyperpotassemia are vague muscle weakness, paresthesias of face, tongue, hands, and feet, and flaccid paralysis (first noted in legs).

The treatment of potassium excess depends on the etiology. Renal failure, probably the most common source of this problem, is the most difficult problem to treat. Ion exchange resins (e.g., Kayexalate, etc.) which bind potassium in the gastrointestinal tract, are sometimes helpful. Dialysis, either peritoneal or hemodialysis, is usually effective. (This problem is discussed in detail in Chapter XIII, "Renal Dialysis.")

## APPENDIX

### Units of Measurement

Since the solutes of extracellular water interact with one another as molecules and ions, it is best to express the concentration of the components in divisions that permit comparison of the interrelationship of ions. Units of measurement for this purpose are mol (M), millimol (mM), milliequivalent (mEq), and milliosmol (mOsm).

**Mol and Millimol:** A mol of a substance is the molecular weight of that substance in grams. For example, the chemical formula for potassium hydroxide is KOH. The molecular weight is (K) 39 + (O) 16 + (H) 1 = 56 gm. Thus, one mol of potassium hydroxide equals 56 gm. One *millimol* of potassium hydroxide is 1/1000 of 56 gm, or 56 mgm. Mol or millimol is applicable to any ion and represents its atomic weight in grams. For example:

|  | Atomic Weight |  |  |
|---|---|---|---|
| Sodium | 23.0 | 1 mol $Na^+$ | 23.0 gm |
| Potassium | 39.1 | 1 mol $K^+$ | 39.1 gm |
| Calcium | 40.0 | 1 mol $Ca^{++}$ | 40.0 gm |
| Chloride | 35.5 | 1 mol $Cl^-$ | 35.5 gm |
| Sulfate | 96.0 | 1 mol $SO_4^{--}$ | 96.0 gm |
|  | (Sum of atomic weights) |  |  |

One millimol of any of these ions is 1/1000 of a mol.

**Milliosmol:** The unit of measurement of osmotic pressure is the *osmol*. If one molecular weight of a *un-ionized* substance is dissolved in a liter of water, it exerts one osmol or 1000 milliosmols of pressure. However, if the substance is completely *ionized* (e.g., $K^+OH^-$), then the solution which contains one molecular weight of substance actually contains *twice* as many osmotically active particles (because of the ionization there is one force from K and another from OH) and this solution is said to exert 2 osmols or 2000 milliosmols of osmotic pressure.

**The milliequivalent:** The term "milliequivalent" is employed more extensively than "milliosmol" in clinical practice. Provided one has a clear idea of the mol, the milliequivalent falls neatly into place. As we have seen, the osmol (and milliosmol) is the unit of choice to describe concentration relative to osmotic pressure. However, this latter unit of measurement does not account for electrical forces of electrolytes. Whereas in osmosis one ion exerts the same influence as any other ion, such is not the case in electrolytic reactions.

If we divide the atomic weight of $Na^+$ (23) by its valence (1), we obtain 23. (See Table 6.) If we divide the atomic weight of $Ca^{++}$ (40) by its valence (2), we obtain 20. Therefore, 23 gm $Na^+$ and 20 gm $Ca^{++}$ are equivalent, or (stated in terms of electrical charges) both quantities possess the same number of positive charges. This means that one equivalent of sodium is equal, chemically, to one equivalent of calcium. Further, as cations of equal value they can react with equivalent anions. For example, one equivalent of $Cl^-$ (an anion) will exactly react with either one equivalent of $Na^+$ or one equivalent of $Ca^{++}$. Because a solution of an electrolyte is neutral, it will always contain the same number of equivalents of anions as cations. Normal saline, for instance, contains 0.2 equivalents (Eq) $Na^+$ and 0.2 Eq $Cl^-$ per liter.

*Table 6*

ATOMIC (OR IONIC) WEIGHTS AND
VALENCES OF THE BODY'S CHIEF IONS

| Ion | Symbol | Weight | Valence | mEq |
|---|---|---|---|---|
| Sodium | $Na^+$ | 23 | 1 | 0.023 |
| Potassium | $K^+$ | 39 | 1 | 0.039 |
| Calcium | $Ca^{++}$ | 40 | 2 | 0.020 |
| Magnesium | $Mg^{++}$ | 24 | 2 | 0.012 |
| Chloride | $Cl^-$ | 35.5 | 1 | 0.035 |
| Bicarbonate | $HCO_3^-$ | 61 | 1 | 0.061 |
| Phosphate | $HPO_4^{--}$ | 96 | 2 | 0.048 |
| Sulfate | $SO_4^{--}$ | 96 | 2 | 0.048 |

Like the osmol, the equivalent is much too large a unit to express physiologic concentration, and for this reason the milliequivalent (mEq) is employed. Unfortunately, many common solutions are described in milligrams percent rather than in milliequivalents. In this case it is necessary to convert mg% to mEq. This is accomplished as follows:

$$\frac{mg\%}{atomic\,weight} \times 10 \times valence = mEq/Liter$$

Example:
The normal value for serum calcium ($Ca^{++}$) is 10 mg%. What is this value in terms of milliequivalents?

$$\frac{10}{40} \times 10 \times 2 = 5\,mEq/Liter$$

**Bibliography**

BLAND, JOHN H.: *Clinical Metabolism of Body Water and Electrolytes.* W. B. Saunders, Phila., 1963.

DUTCHER, ISABEL and FIELO, SANDRA: *Water and Electrolyte Balance: Implications for Nursing.* Macmillan Company, New York, 1967.

GAYTON, ARTHUR: *Textbook of Medical Physiology,* third edition. W. B. Saunders Co., Philadelphia, 1966.

GOLDBERGER, E.: *A Primer of Water, Electrolyte and Acid-Base Syndromes.* 3rd Ed. Lea & Febiger, Philadelphia. 1965.

GOLDSMITH, R. and INGBOR, S.: Inorganic Phosphate Treatment of Hypercalcemia of Diverse Etiologies. *New Eng. J. of Med.* 274:1–7, Jan. 6, 1966.

# Chapter VIII

# Burns

TRUMAN G. BLOCKER, JR., M.D.
DELILAH BULLACHER BREEN, R.N., B.S.
RITA GASTON LUNG, R.N., B.S., M.S.

## THE PROBLEM

During the last twenty-five years, more than 30 million persons have received burns serious enough to require medical treatment and in many instances sufficient to keep them away from work. Of these, more than 70,000 persons have required prolonged hospitalization. At least half of all burn injuries occur in the home, and more than 8,000 persons die every year in house fires and other conflagrations. Half of all hospitalized burn patients are under 20 years of age; in these patients, therefore, the burn injury affects subsequent physical and emotional development in both early and later life.

The physiological and biochemical changes that occur following severe thermal trauma distinguish the burn patient as a special medical and nursing problem. The early alterations following burn injury occur in two stages: the acute, or shock-edema phase, and the sub-acute phase. In the acute phase, which lasts for 48 hours as a rule, clinical shock, external loss of plasma, loss of circulating red cells, and burn edema usually occur simultaneously. The sub-acute phase is associated with diuresis, clinical anemia, accelerated metabolic rate, nitrogen disequilibrium, disordered fat metabolism, abnormal vitamin metabolism, endocrine disturbances, bone and joint changes, impairment of hepatic function, and electrolytic and chemical imbalance. Circulatory derangements usually occur, and loss of function of the skin as the organ of integument further complicates the clinical picture.

In the acute phase, the medical procedures and the nursing care methods should be geared toward meeting the immediate urgent needs of the patient. During the sub-acute phase, the physician should anticipate the various metabolic complications and be prepared to treat changes as they occur. Emergency therapy may be needed at any time. Recovery depends primarily on the competence of the physician-nurse team in recognizing and treating physiological and biochemical changes that occur with burns. Both the burn syndrome as such and the processes of repair are continuing events which require intensive care.

## ASSESSMENT OF THE PROBLEM

The magnitude of injury is determined by the percentage of total body surface involved and the depth of the burn wound. A simple but practical method of estimating the amount of body surface involved in adults can be derived from the use of the Rule of Nine, designed by Tennison, Pulaski, and Wallace (Fig. 1). The head-neck area is considered to be 9% of the total body surface, as is each upper extremity. The anterior trunk, posterior trunk, and each lower extremity are each considered as 18% of the total body surface. The perineal region is designated as the remaining 1%.

The Rule of Fives, advocated by Lynch and Blocker, utilizes multiples of 5% in assessing the extent of burn damage. This method is particularly applicable in estimating the involvement in infants and small children. In infants, the head-neck area is considered 20% of the total body surface; each extremity, whether upper or lower, 10%; and the anterior and posterior trunk, each 20%. For a child aged 5, the head and neck represent 15% of the total body surface; each upper extremity, 10%, and each lower extremity, 15%; and 20% is allotted for the anterior and posterior trunk surfaces, respectively. In adults, the head-neck area is considered 5%; each upper extremity, 10%; each lower extremity, 20%; and the anterior and posterior trunk surfaces, 15% each. (Figs. 2, 3)

It is difficult to determine the depth of the burn wound with any accuracy immediately after the occurrence because of various combinations of injury in and around an extensive burn. The

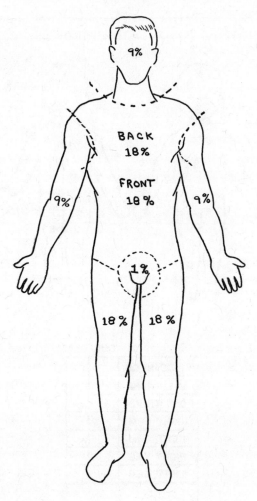

*Fig. 1. Percent of Body Burn, Rule of Nine*

depth of injury in one area often fades into other areas in such a manner that definite demarcation cannot be recognized. It is nevertheless important to make as accurate an approximation as possible because the systemic derangements and prognosis are directly related to the amount of tissue destroyed. The depth of injury also determines the necessity for subsequent skin grafting. First-degree and superficial second-degree burns will heal spontaneously. Third-degree (or full-thickness) burns will eventually

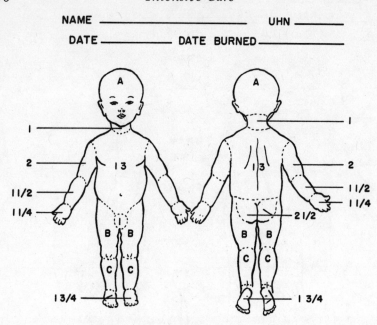

NAME _____ UHN _____

DATE _____ DATE BURNED _____

| | Total | 3° |
|---|---|---|
| HEAD-NECK | | |
| ANT. TRUNK | | |
| POST. TRUNK | | |
| RIGHT ARM | | |
| LEFT ARM | | |
| RIGHT LEG | | |
| LEFT LEG | | |
| TOTAL | | |

| | | |
|---|---|---|
| | 1° | RED |
| | 2° | BLUE |
| | 3° | BLACK |

| AREA | Age 0 | 1 | 5 |
|---|---|---|---|
| A = 1/2 of HEAD | 9 1/2 | 8 1/2 | 6 1/2 |
| B = 1/2 of ONE THIGH | 2 3/4 | 3 1/4 | 4 |
| C = 1/2 of ONE LEG | 2 1/2 | 2 1/2 | 2 3/4 |

*Fig. 2. Percent of Body Burn, Rule of Five (Children)*

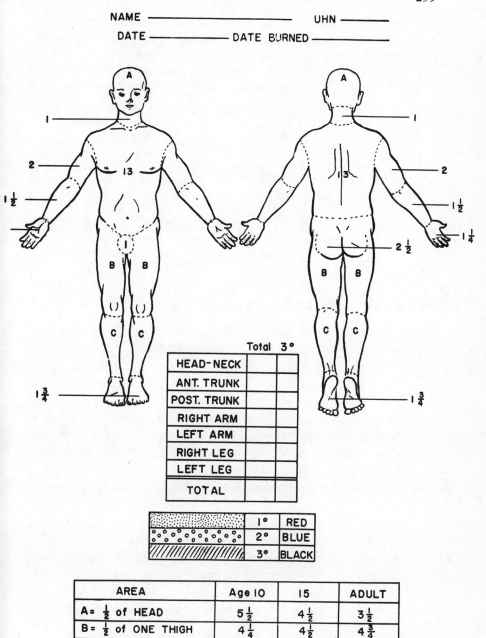

| Total 3° | | |
|---|---|---|
| **HEAD-NECK** | | |
| **ANT. TRUNK** | | |
| **POST. TRUNK** | | |
| **RIGHT ARM** | | |
| **LEFT ARM** | | |
| **RIGHT LEG** | | |
| **LEFT LEG** | | |
| **TOTAL** | | |

| | | |
|---|---|---|
| 1° | RED |
| 2° | BLUE |
| 3° | BLACK |

| AREA | Age 10 | 15 | ADULT |
|---|---|---|---|
| A = ½ of HEAD | $5\frac{1}{2}$ | $4\frac{1}{2}$ | $3\frac{1}{2}$ |
| B = ½ of ONE THIGH | $4\frac{1}{4}$ | $4\frac{1}{2}$ | $4\frac{3}{4}$ |
| C = ½ of ONE LEG | 3 | $3\frac{1}{4}$ | $3\frac{1}{2}$ |

*Fig. 3. Percent of Body Burn, Rule of Five (Adults)*

require grafting for coverage. Sometimes deep second-degree burns may be converted to third degree by maceration and infection. Guides for estimating the depth of injury are as follows:

|  | Second-Degree Burn | Third-Degree Burn |
|---|---|---|
| Cause | Hot liquids splashed on skin Flash fires | Flame, electricity, chemicals, immersion in hot liquids |
| Color | Pink or mottled red | White or charred |
| Surface Appearance | Blisters and weeping | Dry, as a rule |
| Pin-Prick Test | Painful | Anesthetic (although maximum nerve destruction may be delayed) |
| Microscopic Pathology | Involvement of the dermis | Involvement of the entire thickness of the skin |

## PRINCIPLES OF BURN THERAPY

**On admission.** When the burn team has been notified of the expected arrival of a patient with severe burns, plans for his care should be initiated immediately.

We believe that the patient should be initially placed in the area where he will remain throughout his hospital stay and that the Emergency Room should be bypassed unless there is an urgent need to establish a patent airway. Optimal care can be best offered in the prepared setting of an intensive care unit. The need for prior preparation cannot be overemphasized.

The following equipment should be available in the patient's room:

1. Tracheostomy tray with tubes #6 and #7.
2. Cut-down tray with #16 catheter, suture.
3. An adequate supply of intravenous fluids and medications (tetanus toxoid, antitoxin, antibiotics).
4. A tray containing the following:
   a. blood tube for electrolytes, complete blood studies, type and cross match.
   b. syringes—30 and 50 cc, needles #19, #20.
   c. tourniquet, alcohol sponges.
   d. instrument set.

  e. sterile bandages—small and large gauze flats, kerlix rolls, Ace bandages, adhesive tape, towels, gloves.
  f. intravenous and blood administration sets.
5. Catheterization tray and #18 Foley catheter.
6. Records for charting: burn diagrams, hourly output sheet, vital signs sheet.
7. Stryker frame or Circ-O-Lectric bed if requested.
8. Oxygen and suction equipment.
9. Bed cradles and a footboard.
10. I.V. standards.

As soon as the patient is brought into the area designated for care of patients with burn injury, all personnel in contact with the patient should wear masks and gowns to protect the patient from organisms carried by hospital personnel. This precaution must extend to the family, who should be instructed accordingly. The patient, as a rule, has intense anxiety and the nurse should give simple, direct information with regard to all that is happening to him. Careful explanation should be offered to the patient and his family about various treatments and inconveniences (e.g., why the hands may have to be restrained and elevated), if cooperation is to be achieved.

The attending physician and his assistants should remove the patient's clothing, as well as any constricting jewelry on the hands or wrists, and completely expose all burn areas for evaluation. Careful observation of vital signs should be recorded. Intravenous fluid therapy is indicated in all burns involving 20% or more (15% in children) of the body and in any patient in whom shock is evident. Such therapy is best administered by way of a large-bore polyethylene catheter which should be inserted into the most available peripheral vein. If the burns are extensive or the patient is in shock, plasma should be started initially; otherwise Ringer's lactate should be used. If the burn covers considerable body surface area, survival in the early post-burn phase will depend fundamentally on whether or not adequate fluid balance can be maintained. For this reason, the intravenous pathway is the patient's lifeline.

At the time of insertion of the catheter, blood should be drawn to obtain baseline values for hemoglobin, hematocrit, sodium, potassium, chloride, carbon dioxide combining power, blood urea nitrogen, blood sugar, as well as for purposes of typing and cross matching. Initially, in adult patients, 600 cc of plasma and 1000 cc lactated Ringer's solution are administered intravenously. Children are given smaller volumes according to weight and age.

The majority of burn patients do not require narcotics for control of pain and can be kept relatively comfortable with oral or parenteral analgesics. This is particularly true with full-thickness burns which are anesthetic because of pain receptor destruction. Patients in shock frequently require narcotics, and the choice of therapy is morphine sulfate administered intravenously. Morphine is usually diluted in 3 to 5 cc of saline and injected intravenously over a period of one to two minutes. It is not advisable to use the intramuscular route in this situation, because absorption may be delayed until the blood volume is restored. Where circulatory efficiency is impaired, there is a threat of sudden absorption of the narcotic with toxic effects if multiple injections have been given.

Following the establishment of a venous pathway, a Foley catheter should be inserted into the bladder for subsequent determination of urinary output.

**Initial Care.** The following program is that employed at the University of Texas Medical Branch at Galveston. Physician's orders are written for the following procedures, which are initiated as soon as possible after admission:

1. Insert a large-bore polyethylene catheter (#16) into a vein.
2. For an adult, administer plasma (600 cc) and lactated Ringer's solution (1000 cc) intravenously to keep the urine output between 25 and 50 cc per hour, while fluid requirements are being calculated. In a child, give proportionately smaller amounts.
3. Insert a Foley catheter.
4. Give morphine intravenously, if necessary (1/10 mgm per kilogram). (No narcotics are ordinarily given after 24 hours except in relation to surgery or for pain associated with infectious complications.)

5. Administer oxygen if indicated.
6. Give aqueous penicillin, 250,000 units in each liter of intravenous fluid administered during the first 24 hours. Procaine penicillin, 600,000 units, should be given intramuscularly twice per day thereafter.
7. Obtain a brief history (from the family if necessary).
8. Examine the patient for concomitant injuries.
9. Chart estimation of percentage of depth of burn.
10. Send urine specimen to laboratory for urinalysis.
11. Obtain blood for laboratory studies and cross matching.
12. Determine fluid requirements for first 24 hours and number all bottles.
13. Give a booster injection of tetanus toxoid or prophylactic tetanus immunization after appropriate skin testing.
14. Weigh the patient.
15. Place patient on critical list if indicated.
16. Give nothing by mouth except occasional ice chips if burn injury exceeds 20% of body area in adults or 15% in children. In deep burns of limited extent and extensive *second-degree* burns, oral hypotonic saline solution may be given unless the patient is nauseated or vomiting.
17. Record hourly intake and output, blood pressure and pulse.
18. Place cradle over bed to keep bedclothes off patient.
19. Give Vitamin B Complex (2–4 capsules or tablets), and 150 mgm Vitamin C daily.
20. Give barbiturates or tranquilizers as necessary in appropriate doses.
21. Insert nasogastric tube, if vomiting or gastric distention occurs.
22. Order photographs of burned areas.
23. Elevate burned extremities and place footboard at the end of the bed.

For circular burns of the trunk, place the patient on a Stryker frame or Circ-O-Lectric bed. Turn every 3 hours.

## Specific Considerations

**Fluid Therapy.** The burn patient requires large amounts of fluids, because of obligatory accumulation of edema in the burn wound and adjacent areas. This edema is secondary to an increase in capillary permeability to proteins as well as to vasodilation, both being a direct result of capillary injury caused by heat. Because of stress elaboration of mineral corticoids, retention of sodium chloride and water occurs and also contributes to edema. In addition to edematous fluid loss, there is loss of fluid at the burn surface itself. This volume may average 100 to 300 cc per hour in a large burn and may be doubled in a setting of increased heat and decreased humidity. (For this reason, the patient should be placed in an area where the temperature and humidity can be controlled.)

During the first forty-eight hours, the use of a fluid formula guide can be helpful in estimating fluid replacement in the burn patient. It is impossible to determine in advance the fluid requirements in simple arithmetical terms, and therapy must be adjusted in accordance with the clinical response of the patient. The Brooke Formula, a modification of the Evans Formula, is most commonly used in this country:

DURING FIRST 24 HOURS

1. *Colloids*

　　*Formula:* 1 cc × body weight in *kilograms* × percentage of body surface burn (or 0.5 cc × weight in *pounds* × percentage of burn area).

　　*Example:* A 70 Kg man with a 40% burn area would require the following amount of colloids:

$$1 \text{ cc} \times 70 \times 40 = 2800 \text{ cc}$$

　　*Method:* This volume may be given as blood plasma or dextran according to the depth of burn and the preference of the surgeon.

2. *Electrolytes*

　　*Formula:* 3.0 cc × body weight in *kilograms* × the per cent of body surface burn (or 1.5 cc × weight in pounds × per cent).

　　*Example:* A 70 Kg man with a 20% surface area burn would require the following volume:

$$3 \text{ cc} \times 70 \times 20 = 4200 \text{ cc}$$

*Method:* Lactated Ringer's solution is generally preferred to normal saline for electrolyte replacement.

3. *Water*

*Formula:* Adults 1500–2000 cc

Children: 6 months: 100 cc per kilogram (200 cc per pound)

1 year: 80 cc per kilogram (160 cc per pound)

5 years: 60 cc per kilogram (120 cc per pound)

8 years: 40 cc per kilogram (30 cc per pound)

*Method:* 5% dextrose in water.

*Plan for administration of initial fluids.* The aim of therapy during the first 24 hours should be to administer colloids and electrolytes at a rate that approximates that of the obligatory edema formation in the wound and at the same time provides water for urinary and insensible losses. (See Chapter VII, "Water and Electrolyte Imbalances".)

One-half of the estimated daily amount of each of the replacement solutions should be administered during the first eight hours after injury, if possible, because the physiological disturbances and rate of edema formation are maximal during this initial period. The remaining half of the estimated fluid requirement should be divided equally and given during the second and third eight-hour intervals of the first day.

DURING SECOND 24 HOURS

During the second day, the same amount of 5% dextrose in water and $\frac{1}{2}$ to $\frac{2}{3}$ of colloids and electrolytes given during the first 24 hours should be given.

A basic rule in the care of the burn patient during the first 48 hours is to administer sufficient fluids to *maintain the urinary output between 25 cc and 50 cc per hour in an adult.* A urinary output over this amount may indicate overhydration, in which case the amount or the rate of fluid administration should be decreased. Decreasing blood pressure and decreasing urinary output may indicate the need for more colloids.

Solutions containing potassium (for example, milk and citrus fruit juices), should be avoided during the first 48 hours post burn except for lactated Ringer's solution, which contains minimal amounts. Early in the postburn course there is a tendency toward hyperkalemia secondary to the release of potassium from the red cell and tissue cell destruction. Tap water should be avoided for 48 hours, and all oral solutions such as water, tea, and soft drinks should contain salt (½ tsp. per 8 ounces) and sodium bicarbonate (⅛ tsp. per 8 ounces of fluid).

In mild burns and in severe burns, after 24 hours a cold oral hypotonic saline-sodium bicarbonate solution may be made up by the liter (3.5 grams of sodium chloride, 1.5 grams sodium bicarbonate in 1000 cc distilled water), and given *ad lib* provided that it is well tolerated and the patient is not vomiting. The amount of oral solution given is then subtracted from intravenous electrolyte and water requirements estimated according to the Brooke formula.

**Transfusion Therapy.** Blood transfusions are required in deep, extensive burns throughout the entire period of treatment, although opinion differs as to whether or not blood should be administered during the immediate shock period. The anemia seen in the burn patient is due to several factors and must be corrected:

1. A number of cells are destroyed by heat at the time of the burn.
2. Red cells are trapped in dilated capillaries and sludging occurs.
3. The life of the red blood cell is shortened in burn patients because of abnormal fragility.
4. Infection depresses the function of the hematopoietic tissues.
5. Blood is lost at each dressing change.

**Tracheostomy.** Steam burns of the head and neck, burns occurring in an enclosed space, and explosions may result in airway obstruction that may require tracheostomy. The tendency in burn centers recently has been to perform a tracheostomy only when respiratory distress is anticipated or when it develops in severe facial burns, rather than as a routine procedure. Respiratory distress is usually characterized by restlessness, hoarseness, coughing, rapid respirations, cyanosis, or crowing noises as local edema develops. The nurse should be on the alert for these symptoms of respiratory embarrassment and report them immediately.

**Local Therapy.** Between 1950 and 1960 there was considerable controversy concerning whether exposed or closed treatment (occlusive dressings technique), was preferable in the case of acute burns. The problem has been resolved, in a sense, in that most centers now employ both techniques, often concurrently in the same patient for different body areas. Each method has its advantages and disadvantages, but the two types of therapy can be complementary rather than antagonistic. Most clinicians employ exposure treatment initially for the face, perineum, and genitalia. Closed methods of treatment have gained acceptance for third-degree burns of the hands. A third method of treatment, silver nirate therapy, has fallen into disfavor recently in many centers.

*The exposure treatment* (**Fig.** 4) consists of careful positioning of the patient so that no bed clothing touches the areas involved (except in a circumferential burn of the trunk where a pad is placed underneath the back). The patient is then turned frequently to permit drying. This is accomplished in an ordinary or special type of bed, using a pad under the chest to prevent contact.

With this technique, the patient is placed on sterile or laundry-clean sheets, using wire cradles to suspend bed clothing and to prevent it from touching exposed surfaces. Vigorous washing is not carried out; only gross debris is removed. Blisters are left intact, since epithelization is known to be improved under the covering of a blister. Drafts should be avoided, since they are a source of patient discomfort.

Within 48 hours of adequate exposure technique, the burn will form a dry coagulum or eschar. As a rule, superficial second-degree burns will heal within two weeks without incident and will not require grafting if the process is not impeded by infection or added trauma.

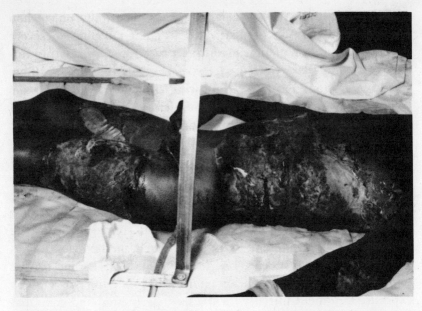

*Fig. 4. Exposure Treatment of Burns*

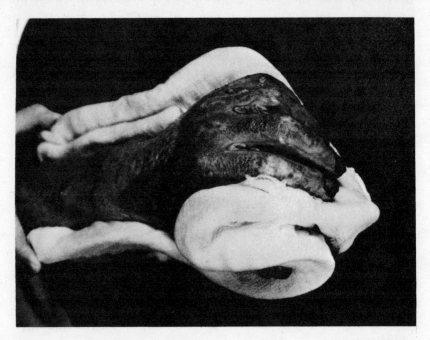

*Fig. 5. Properly positioned burned hand*

**The closed method** of therapy is used primarily for severely burned hands. Some believe it is also the treatment of choice for circumferential burns of the lower extremities. The occlusion dressing (boxer type), is offered with the hands in a position of function. The dressing should consist of only one layer of grease gauze placed between the fingers and over the burned surface. A large amount of fluff gauze is then placed so that the wrist is maintained cocked up (in extension), with the thumb and forefinger in opposition and the fingers moderately flexed (Fig. 5). A hand splint may be used instead of the gauze (Fig. 6). Unless the hand

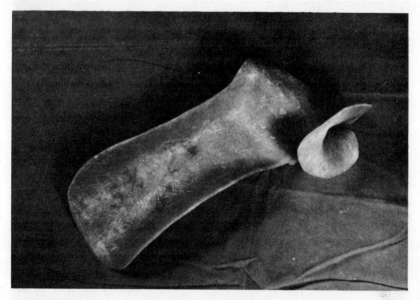

*Fig. 6. Modified Brooke Splint of fiberglass used by The University of Texas Medical Branch.*

is maintained in this way severe deformities may result (Fig. 7). A bulky dressing is then applied and held in place with an elastic bandage. The hand should then be elevated either with pillows or a suspension device (metal standard). Sulfamylon, gentamycin, and furain dressings can also be used with the occlusive technique.

The *silver nitrate method* is also a closed technique. It consists of the use of pads or dressings which are kept constantly saturated with 0.5% silver nitrate solution. These dressings are

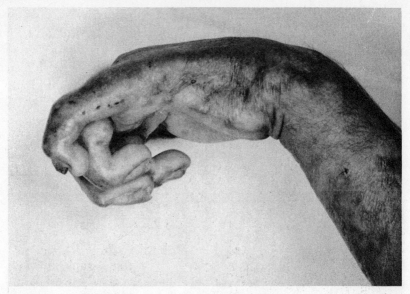

*Fig. 7. Deformity resulting from improper positioning*

applied over plain mesh gauze strips and are changed every 12
hours or less by the nurse. Saturation is accomplished by applying
the silver nitrate solution every two hours with an asepto syringe
or by continuous drip. We have discarded the silver nitrate method
on our service because it prolongs the period of hospitalization
and requires more blood for transfusion therapy.

**Physical therapy.** After the technique of local therapy has been
adopted and the schedule of turning the patient established, the
nurse should receive specific instructions regarding the proper
positioning of the patient. It will be her responsibility to maintain
proper alignment of the patient, including the normal positions
of function of the head, spine, hands, and feet. The amount of
joint motion to be allowed should be discussed by the nurse-
physician team and plans made for preventing osteoporosis and
contracture deformities.

**Nutrition.** A severe burn is accompanied by gastrointestinal
edema and hypomotility; therefore, oral intake of foods or fluids
may result in gastric distention, vomiting, and possibly even
aspiration (especially in infants).

After the first forty-eight hours, the patient should gradually be allowed a liquid diet, followed by a soft diet. Usually by the end of the first week, intensive feedings may be initiated to meet the needs for increased protein, calorie, and vitamin requirements. This high-protein, high-calorie need is demanded by the systemic response to trauma as well as the need for tissue repair and for red cell regeneration.

The recommended total intake is two to four grams of protein per kilogram daily, 50 to 70 calories per kilogram daily, and a routine daily vitamin supplement of ascorbic acid 150 mgm, thiamine 50 mgm, riboflavin 50 mgm, and nicotinamide 500 mgm, plus the fat-soluble vitamins in approximately twice the normal dosage employed by proprietary preparations.

**Tetanus prophylaxis.** Anaerobic microbes frequently colonize the surface of deep burns, and tetanus has been reported as a cause of death following acute burns. For this reason, routine tetanus prophylaxis should be given initially and should be repeated during the course of therapy. Patients who have been previously immunized with tetanus toxoid should be given a booster injection of 1 cc of toxoid. Tetanus antitoxin 5000 units (or more), is recommended for patients who have not been previously immunized. Human gamma globulin preparation may eventually replace the present tetanus antitoxin.

**Antibiotic therapy.** The employment of routine systemic antibiotics during the first five to seven days post burn is believed to be of value in the prevention of invasive infection from hemolytic streptococcus. If the patient has a history of hypersensitivity to penicillin, erythromycin ethyl carbonate (Ilotycin) or erythromycin lactobromate (Erythrocin) may be given. Penicillin has been shown to reach a high concentration in the burn wound in a very short time. An injection site for the administration of drugs may be a problem in the patient with extensive burns, but any muscle may be used.

## THE NURSING ROLE

**The team approach.** The nursing care required for the burned patient is continuous, concentrated, comprehensive, and prolonged. The nurse with her intimate knowledge of the patient's clinical course and her active participation in therapy is the person through whom many aspects of the care are coordinated, both officially and unofficially. It is the nurse who implements the directives of the attending and consulting physicians and organizes the immediate environmental regimen of the ward.

A well-informed staff of nurses is an essential part of the burn team. The team effort should have as its goals first, the preservation of life, second, the restoration of the patient to his maximum functional capacity, and, third, a decrease in the over-all morbidity.

Since the patient must receive intensive treatment from the moment the burn occurs until grafting has been accomplished, *the key* to successful care is the *establishment of a team* who understand the physiologic alterations produced by thermal trauma and are trained in concerted efforts to expedite details of therapy. All nursing personnel must be aware of the problems of care of severely burned individuals. Close and continued attention is required during the early phases of burn therapy, far in excess of those required by the majority of other patients. The attending nursing personnel cannot leave the bedside for long periods, and thus must continually rely on the floor nurse for assistance.

A "nursing methods coordinator," a nurse who keeps abreast of new procedures and available materials, is invaluable in the over-all care of patients with burn injuries since the clinical nurse specialist in burn therapy is a rarity. Also, because of the depressing influence of high mortality and prolonged morbidity associated with burns, few choose to work with these patients on a permanent basis unless they have unusual motivation.

In order for the physician-nurse team to function effectively, the hospital administration should realize the special needs of the burned patient. Burn patients require more hospital days, more nurse hours, and more supplies than the average surgical patient. The demands of caring for the patient with burn injuries with regard to the supportive services of a hospital are of great significance. Because of the contaminated environment of the burn and the necessity for infection control, the facilities of the hospital are taxed. Linens should be separated from those of the regular hospital laundry. The hospital central supply unit should exclude items used for burned patients from the supply chain so they will not re-enter and be distributed to other areas of the hospital. This requires close supervision and often necessitates procurement of additional items. Frequent changes of burn dressings and grafting procedures require large amounts of materials. Bulk items must be purchased in large quantities, and many special items must be made by hand. Heavy demands are made on the autoclaving facilities for sterile supplies. Intelligent management of supplies and careful projection of future needs are essential if burn patients are to receive optimum care.

Other hospital personnel are involved in burn care. For instance, the operating room supervisor must cooperate with the burn team by arranging facilities and personnel effectively to accommodate these patients during multiple trips to the operating room. This need is particularly apparent in those hospitals with large burn services.

Also essential to the care of the burned patient is the anesthesiologist. Pulmonary complications of thermal injury as well as copious secretions in the tracheobronchial tree make aeration difficult in many patients. The maintenance of a patent airway requires the patience and skill of an anesthesiologist; his role is of singular importance in this respect.

Laboratory facilities of the hospital are similarly strained by the care of burned patients. Large quantities of blood may be required to treat the secondary anemia of burns and to meet the patient's needs at the time of surgery. This burden on the blood bank facilities continues throughout the patient's therapy. Multiple laboratory determinations, including surface and blood cultures (and antibiotic sensitivity tests), are usually necessary in large numbers.

**Fluid therapy.** Because the intravenous pathway is essential to life in most burn patients, it is extremely important that the nurse verify the patency of this conduit at frequent intervals. Any sign of leakage about the catheter site or evidence to suggest local infection or phlebitis should be reported immediately.

There is a mandatory need for adequate hydration to combat the enormous loss of fluid associated with burns. The best gauge to fluid replacement is urinary output, particularly in the absence of detailed laboratory studies along with the inability to weigh the patient frequently.

The nurse must impress on all personnel the absolute importance of the hourly recording of urine output. In the event that the output decreases to levels of less than 25 cc per hour, the physician should be notified promptly. A calibrated urine collector is best used for this purpose, and should be securely attached to the bed to prevent accidental spillage. The patency of the Foley catheter should be specifically ascertained during each nursing shift.

Oral fluid intake should be guided by the principles (chapter VII) regarding the prevention of hyperkalemia and hypernatremia. Both the type of fluid and its volume must be carefully recorded. The intake and output sheet should be left in a conspicuous place near the patient's bed.

The rate of intravenous fluid administration must be regulated according to the output. In elderly patients the nurse should be cognizant of the signs of overloading the cardiovascular system. Careful assessment of central venous pressure, when possible, is helpful.

**Transfusion Therapy.** Since most patients develop either a primary or secondary anemia after extensive burns, transfusions are used frequently. The nurse should be totally familiar with signs of transfusion reactions.

**Tracheostomy Care.** The nursing care of the patient with a tracheostomy is described in Chapter I, "Respiratory Insufficiency and Failure."

**Local Burn Therapy.** As soon as possible a schedule should be established for turning the patient. When such turning is done on a regular bed, it is advisable to have at least three persons available to assist. If a Stryker frame or Circ-O-Lectric bed is employed, the patient should be strapped in securely and turned rapidly by at least two persons. During the turning process every effort should be made to avoid touch-contamination of the burn wound and the dislodging of catheters and intravenous tubing.

The nurse should examine the burn wound frequently to determine whether any purulence has developed beneath the eschar or whether any cracks have occurred in the eschar. In the event of cracking, wet gauze should be applied at the site. If the eschar is lost, the denuded areas should never remain exposed. When the eschar becomes loose with normal healing, the area is cleansed every three to four days with soap and water in the operating room. At the time, loose shreds of tissue are clipped away and a single layer of fine-mesh gauze is applied to all raw areas in a pattern that covers the defect. Dressings are continued in this way until the patient is ready for grafting.

**Burns of head and face.** These are especially difficult to treat because bandages may shut off sight and speech, making the patient very apprehensive and often psychotic. In nursing the patient with burns of the head and face, it may be necessary for the nurse to reassure the patient with regard to fear of blindness, which may result from edema around the eyes.

When the patient is unable to see, the nurse should speak to the patient before touching him, put facial tissues and urinal within easy reach, and assist the patient in eating his meals. Irrigation of the eyes with saline or boric acid solution or application of ophthalmic ointments may be ordered to keep the cornea moist. Burns of the ears should be observed closely for signs of chondritis, which is a common complication.

Oral hygiene is important in burns of the lower part of the face. There may be excessive mucus secretions, and the nurse should employ frequent oral suctioning to avoid aspiration and prevent hypostatic pneumonia. A toothbrush and mouthwash should be employed unless contraindicated. The use of glycerin and lemon juice is often soothing and is recommended for the prevention of mouth sores.

**Physical therapy.** The nurse should work closely with a physical therapist or orthopedic consultant to encourage active patient participation in physical therapy as soon as feasible. Until this is possible, preventive use of footboards and pillows should be utilized to maintain proper positioning of the patient. The size of the pillow should be selected according to the body area to be supported. In children, only a small pillow should be placed beneath the head, to obviate the possibility of a "batwing" deformity.

**Maintenance of adequate nutritional status.** A knowledge of the patient's cultural background, dietary habits, and food idiosyncracies will help the nurse and dietary consultants to prepare appetizing trays. Initially, small frequent servings are preferable to larger meals. It is often necessary to administer supplementary nourishment prepared with high protein concentrates such as Provimalt, Geveral, and Sustagen. The addition of certain flavoring syrups (cherry, chocolate) may increase the palatability of the preparations, especially for children. High-protein formulas may first be offered to the patient orally between meals and at bedtime. If the required intake is not achieved voluntarily, a high-protein formula should be given through a nasogastric polyethylene tube. Such feedings should be administered hourly, or every other hour, rather than as a constant drip.

If tube feedings are indicated, the nurse should irrigate the tubing with water following each use. Extreme care must be exercised in giving tube feedings to burned children and to older critically injured patients who may vomit and aspirate or who may develop acute gastric dilation with resulting respiratory embarrassment. Diarrhea, a frequent complication of tube feedings, may be caused by giving too large a volume of mixture or a formula too high in concentration of carbohydrate or fat.

**Other Considerations.** Psychiatric consultation is often valuable in the management of the burn patient. Having sustained a severe burn, a previously active, independent person becomes totally dependent upon others for even the most elemental functions. In addition, large bulky dressings covering extremities exclude tactile sensations, while head dressings shut out sight and hearing. Under such circumstances the individual may become irrational and psychotic, belligerent, infantile, or completely withdrawn. In these situations psychiatrists are of great aid, not only to the patient, but to the family as well.

Visits from a clergyman may be of great practical and spiritual comfort. At times the busy physician does not think of enlisting the help of a clergyman, and the thoughtful nurse should take the initiative in consulting the patient or the family in this matter. The clergy are often of assistance by helping to secure blood for transfusions, in finding donors for homograft skin, and, especially, in contacting home, church and friends when necessary.

As the patient progresses, the assistance of a social worker, and of vocational rehabilitation consultants is frequently necessary to help the patient plan his future. Again, communication between members of the nurse-physician team is necessary to ascertain the expected capabilities of the individual patient.

A hospital in-service program, which educates not only those in nursing service but the allied disciplines involved in burn-patient care, is important. Monthly programs in which each section demonstrates its unique contribution to total care provide members of the paramedical team with a greater insight into the problems and contributions of each.

The intensive care of the burn patient is a serious financial burden to the patient, his family, the community, and the hospital. For this and other reasons, burn centers have been initiated in this country and abroad through the combined efforts of health professionals as well as concerned business and industrial leaders. A great variety of clinical and fundamental research is being sponsored at these burn centers. Grants for research are available from the Federal Government to institutions concerned with problems of burn injury and treatment.

The Federal Government also finances a variety of state assistance programs which make funds available for the care of such patients. Among these is the Crippled Children's program to provide aid to the medically indigent. Private groups, such as the Shriners of North America, have also become interested and are giving their financial support to studies of problems relating to the prolonged care of the burned patient, as well as the many factors which contribute to the rehabilitation of such patients.

**Bibliography**

ALLEN, CHARLES R., VIRGINIA BLOCKER and T. G. BLOCKER, JR.: The Medical Aftermath of the Texas City Disaster. 15th National Con-

Intensive Care

ference on Disaster Medical Care, *American Medical Association Publications,* Chicago, 1965.

ARONS, MARVIN S., S. R. LEWIS, J. B. LYNCH, and T. G. BLOCKER, JR.: The Use of Unburned Skin from Burned Animals as Homografts with the Adjunctive Use of Convalescent Burn Serum. *The Journal of Surgical Research,* 4:6:253–256, 1964.

ARONS, MARVIN S., J. B. LYNCH, S. R. LEWIS, and T. G. BLOCKER, Jr.: Scar Tissue Carcinoma—Part I. A Clinical Study with Special Reference to Burn Scar Carcinoma. *Annals of Surgery,* 161:2:170–188, 1965.

ARTZ, CURTIS and REISS, ERIC: *The Treatment of Burns.* W. B. Saunders Company, Philadelphia, 1957.

BLOCKER, T. G., JR.: Burns, in *Reconstructive Plastic Surgery,* John M. Converse, ed., W. B. Saunders Company, Philadelphia, 208–265, 1964.

BLOCKER, T. G., JR.: The Acute Burn As a Catastrophic Illness. *Bulletin, American College of Surgeons,* 2–5, 1965.

BLOCKER, T. G., JR., LEWIS, S. R. and LYNCH, J. B.: Trends Away from Blood and Plasma in the Early Treatment of Severe Burns. *Annals New York Acad. Science,* 150:912–920, 1968.

BRANTL, V. M., BROWN, B. J. and MORELAND, M.: The Care of Patients With Burns: Comprehensive Nursing Care. *Nursing Outlook,* 6:383–385, July 1958.

COATS, ALMA W., BLOCKER, T. G., JR., and ESTES, FRANCES L.: Effect of Thermal Burn on the Total Sulfur Content in Liver and Kidney of Rats. *Texas Reports on Biology and Medicine,* 22:3:440–443, 1964.

DECKER, R. and NEMEC, B. M.: The Care of Patients With Burns, Convalescent and Rehabilitative Care. *Nursing Outlook,* 6:386–387, July 1958.

DERRICK, JOHN R., REA, VAN and BLOCKER, T. G., JR.: Constriction of the Renal Vein—A New Concept in Renal Hypertension. *Annals of Surgery,* 160:4:589–595, 1964.

DUNTON, E. FRANK, BLOCKER, T. G., JR., LEWIS, S. R. and PADEREWSKI, JOSEPH: A Compromise Approach to Total Ear Reconstruction. *Plastic and Reconstructive Surgery,* 34:3:247–251, 1964.

LARSON, D. L., LEWIS, S. R., RAPPERPORT, A. S., COERS, C. R., III, and BLOCKER, T. G., JR.: Lymphatics of the Mouth and Neck. *The American Journal of Surgery,* 110:4:625–630, 1965.

LYNCH, J. B., LEWIS, S. R. and BLOCKER, T. G., JR.: Chronic Cystic Parotitis. *Annals of Surgery,* 161:5:693–700, 1965.

LYNCH, J. B., LEWIS, S. R., BLOCKER, T. G., JR.: Chronic Cystic Parotitis. (Abstract) *Modern Medicine,* 33:16:150–152, 1965.

LYNCH, J. B., LEWIS, S. R., BLOCKER, T. G., JR., and BRELSFORD, H. G.: Maxillary Bone Grafts in Cleft Lip-Cleft Palate Reconstruction, *Texas State Journal of Medicine,* 61:172–180, 1965.

MAXWELL, PATRICIA, et al.: Routines on the Burn Ward. *American Journal of Nursing,* 66:522–525.

MOYER, C. A., et al.: The Treatment of Large Human Burns with 0.5% Silver Nitrate. *Archives of Surgery,* 90:812–867, June 1965.

NOWINSKI, W. W., BLOCKER, T. G., JR., and OHKUBO, TATSUYA: Tricarboxylic Acid Cycle in Wound Healing by Granulation. *Proceedings of the Society for Experimental Biology and Medicine,* 119:1011–1014, 1965.

SAKO, Y.: The Emergency Care of Burns. *Medical Clinics of North America.* 46:383, March 1962.

WOOD, MACDONALD; KENNY, HELEN; and PRICE, WILLIAM: Silver Nitrate Treatment of Burns: Technique and Controlling Principles. *Amer. J. of Nursing,* 66:3:518–521, March 1966.

*Film:* "Basic Principles in the Management of the Local Burn Wound." Davis and Geck Pharmaceuticals, Division of American Cyanamid, Danbury, Connecticut.

# CHAPTER IX

# The Complications of General Surgery

MARIE KURIHARA, R.N., M.A.*
FRANK G. MOODY, M.D.

The magnitude of operative surgical therapy has progressed to the point where complications, when they occur, often demand the full resources of a highly skilled physician-nurse team. Although most of these complications can be well managed within the traditional hospital environment, there are several which are life-threatening and which may place excessive demands on available personnel and resources. These complications can best be managed in an intensive care unit. The advantages of this specialized type of care will be discussed as they may relate to the general surgical patient.

It should be emphasized that the responsibility for postoperative care of the surgical patient continues to rest with the surgeon, even though the environment in which this care is rendered may change. The availability of highly skilled personnel within a special unit can lead to a false sense of security concerning the patient's welfare. Since admission to an intensive care unit implies the presence of a serious complication, the physician's responsibility increases proportionately. Fulfillment of this responsibility involves frequent and sometimes continuous medical attention by the surgical team familiar with the patient's illness and operative procedure.

## GASTROINTESTINAL SURGERY

Complications following operations on the gastrointestinal tract are usually manifested by: (1) disturbances in gastrointestinal motility, (2) intraluminal or intra-abdominal hemorrhage, and/or (3) leakage of intestinal contents into the peritoneal cavity.

* Contributed while an Instructor in Medical-Surgical Nursing and post-master's student at the University of California School of Nursing in San Francisco.

# 1. Disturbances of Gastrointestinal Motility

## THE PROBLEM

Acute gastric dilatation is a life-threatening and dramatic disturbance of gastrointestinal motility. This problem may occur after surgery involving vagal denervation of the stomach, but in most instances the cause cannot be identified. Massive distention of the stomach with fluid and air leads to abdominal discomfort, respiratory distress, and, ultimately, vasomotor collapse.

Paralytic ileus, a disorder of decreased small and large bowel motility, is a common sequela of intra-abdominal surgical procedures. Distention of the gastrointestinal tract leads to a rise in intra-abdominal pressure. This increased pressure not only jeopardizes the union of a recent abdominal incision, but also contributes to the severity of incisional pain. Furthermore, the pressure rise within the peritoneal cavity causes elevation of the diaphragm, which markedly impairs ventilation. The resulting hypoxia, along with depression of normal cardio-respiratory reflex patterns, leads to vasomotor collapse in the form of shock; unless the process is interrupted, death may result.

## ASSESSMENT OF THE PROBLEM

Early findings of this complication, as well as of the others to be discussed, may be obscured by the effects of anesthesia and the metabolic consequences of surgical stress on the patient. Careful examination is necessary to detect the complication near its onset, particularly when the incisional site is heavily covered with dressings.

**Signs and symptoms of disturbances in gastrointestinal motility.**

1) Gastrointestinal distention can be recognized by finger percussion over the upper abdomen. A tympanitic sound can usually be elicited.

2) With more advanced degrees of distention (including acute gastric dilatation) the patient may complain of chest pain and appear acutely ill. The skin is frequently moist, cool, and

ashen grey in color. The respirations are rapid and ventilation is shallow. There is often a sharp drop in blood pressure and the pulse rate may be very slow.

## PRINCIPLES OF TREATMENT

1) In anticipation of the decreased intestinal motility which may follow intra-abdominal procedures, a nasogastric tube is often positioned in the stomach prior to operation to reduce passage of air and secretions into the lower gastrointestinal tract. The continuous functioning of this tube in the postoperative period is sometimes critical to the patient's recovery. The loss of gastrointestinal secretions through nasogastric and intestinal tubes represents one of the most common causes of water and electrolyte imbalance following surgery. These problems have been considered in specific detail in Chapter VII, "Water and Electrolyte Imbalances," and are not discussed here.

When continuous gastric aspiration is essential, it is wise to use a double lumen tube that provides a "sump" effect. By way of a vent situated close to the end of the tube positioned in the stomach, continuous passage of air is assured. This vent prevents trapping of mucosa against the lumen of the tube after the stomach has been emptied of its contents. The cessation of the low-pitched hissing sound from the vent suggests obstruction of the tube orifice. In this situation, suction may be re-established by instilling saline or water into the aspirating lumen.

2) Acute gastric dilatation may be dramatically relieved by nasogastric intubation. The tube should be left in place for 24 hours after the stomach has been fully emptied.

3) If gastrointestinal distention develops (despite nasogastric suction), decompression should be attempted by means of a longer tube (Miller-Abbott or Cantor tube). Segmental areas of active peristalsis may exist (in the presence of paralytic ileus), which permit the passage of such mercury-weighted tubes into the lower intestinal tract. The combined efforts of the patient and nurse are needed to successfully pass the tube from the stomach into the small bowel. (See nursing role.) The presence of the tube in the duodenum should be confirmed by x-ray of the abdomen. In fact,

the simplest way to intubate the duodenum is to utilize fluoroscopic control. If the tube is to be passed further, it is necessary to allow for slack so that the tube may be moved forward by peristaltic action. This slackening of the tube is accomplished by inserting an additional 10 cm of the tube into the stomach every hour. We do not recommend instilling fluid into the intestinal lumen to promote local peristalsis, nor do we use cholinergic drugs to stimulate motility. There is, however, some value in evacuating the colon by enema while the tube is being passed. Patients with tight anal sphincters may be benefited by insertion of a rectal tube.

The best method of managing paralytic ileus is to control the contents of the intestinal tract from above.

## 2. *Intra-abdominal and Intraluminal Hemorrhage*

### THE PROBLEM

Although postoperative hemorrhage may occur following any procedure within the peritoneal cavity, it is most common when vessels within the mesentery or retroperitoneum are divided and ligated, as during radical pancreatoduodenectomy. In this procedure the pancreas is transected and several major vessels are divided. Proteolytic enzymes from the remaining pancreatic tissue may cause digestion of tissue at the point of vessel ligature, resulting in massive intraperitoneal hemorrhage.

Intraluminal hemorrhage occurs most frequently following operations upon the stomach (peptic ulcer disease or neoplasm) and is related to the extensive distribution of vessels within the submucosa of the gastric wall. If the surgeon fails to identify and secure these vessels when the stomach is transected, massive intragastric hemorrhage may develop in the immediate postoperative period.

### ASSESSMENT OF THE PROBLEM

It is a common practice to place multiple drains within the peritoneal cavity when extensive surgical procedures are performed. The leakage of bright red blood from these drainage sites may be the first sign of intra-abdominal hemorrhage. Similarly, an inordinate amount of blood on the dressings should arouse suspicion that a serious hemorrhage has developed within the peritoneal cavity. The absence of visible bleeding or dry dressings, however, does not negate the possibility of intraperitoneal hemorrhage.

Progressive distention and generalized abdominal tenderness are often noted during periods of bleeding. Unfortunately, these findings may be obscured or suppressed by the lingering effects of anesthesia or by sedatives and analgesics used to control postoperative pain.

When intraperitoneal hemorrhage is suspected, confirmation can be obtained by aspiration (or tap) of the peritoneal cavity.

Intraluminal bleeding can be recognized simply and promptly by the presence of fresh blood in the nasogastric drainage.

The degree of hemorrhage (intra-abdominal or intraluminal) can generally be gauged by the relative decrease in successive hematocrit values, as well as by an increased pulse rate and a fall in blood pressure.

## PRINCIPLES OF TREATMENT

The treatment of intra-abdominal hemorrhage consists of blood volume replacement followed by re-exploration and ligature of the bleeding sites.

Intragastric bleeding involves blood replacement and decompression of the stomach initially. This decompression not only determines the rate of blood loss, but allows compression of bleeding vessels passing through the muscular layer of the stomach as the lumen is reduced in size.

Distention of the stomach may result in secretion of large amounts of hydrochloric acid, which tends to inhibit clot formation at the ends of open vessels. Gastric lavage should be used as necessary to keep the nasogastric tube open and the stomach decompressed. Lavage with cold saline, while a common procedure, is probably of little value; as with intra-abdominal hemorrhage, early re-exploration is usually the safest course of action.

## 3. Leakage of Intestinal Contents into the Peritoneal Cavity

Inflammation within the peritoneal cavity, whether from a perforated viscus or anastomotic leak, is a life-threatening complication which frequently requires the facilities of an intensive care unit because of the severe metabolic disturbances that accompany peritonitis. Regardless of whether the origin of peritonitis is chemical or bacterial, there is an immediate and voluminous outpouring of fluid into the peritoneal cavity. This may soon lead to a decrease in circulating blood volume, resulting in peripheral vascular collapse. This sequence of events is often accompanied by a decreased urinary output, excessive thirst, dry mucous membranes, warm dry skin, increased pulse rate, and loss of skin turgor. A sharp rise in venous hematocrit is an early sign of fluid loss into a hidden space, such as the peritoneal cavity. These changes in fluid distribution and their sequelae must be anticipated in a patient with peritoneal inflammation. Early fluid replacement is mandatory, and should include colloid, usually in the form of plasma, as well as saline solutions, since not only sodium chloride and water but also protein are lost within the peritoneal cavity. Antibiotics are of value in the treatment of peritonitis, regardless of its origin, since these agents are readily secreted into the peritoneal contents and help to control bacterial growth within this protein-rich fluid.

## SURGERY OF THE GALL BLADDER AND COMMON DUCT

Operations on the gall bladder and biliary tree are among the most common surgical procedures in daily hospital practice. The incidence of complications is normally very low.

For chronic gall bladder disease without a history of jaundice the usual procedure is a cholecystectomy. In the event of an acute gall bladder attack when cholecystectomy may be contraindicated, a cholecystostomy may be performed. This interior procedure, which consists of the removal of calculi from the gall bladder and the insertion of a self-retaining drainage catheter (e.g., a Malecott catheter) into the fundus of the gall bladder, may be performed under local anesthesia. The wall of the catheter is sutured to the peritoneum and to the posterior rectus fascia. The distal portion of the catheter is brought through the abdominal wall and attached to a drainage bottle. This technique provides for decompression of the biliary tract and averts the danger of peritonitis.

If there is a history of jaundice or if calculi are found within the ductal system by exploration, the common duct must be opened to ascertain and establish its full patency (choledochostomy). Following this procedure a T tube is usually inserted into the common duct through the choledochostomy incision. This tube consists of a short proximal arm which extends from the site of the ductal incision half the distance to the bifurcation of the bile ducts. The distal arm of the tube extends one-half the distance to the opening of the common bile duct into the duodenum (the ampulla of Vater). Bile drains from the long arm of the T tube, which is brought out through a small incision through the abdominal wound. Some surgeons prefer direct catheter drainage by way of remnant of the cystic duct. The appearance of more than 500 cc of bile within 24 hours may indicate a distal obstruction of the common duct resulting from mechanical obstruction or kinking of the drainage system.

Two serious complications may follow surgery of the gall bladder and biliary tree:

1. *Acute obstructive suppurative cholangitis.* This acute illness results from obstruction of bile flow from the biliary tree (usually by a stone). This occlusion creates increased pressure within the bile ducts and allows bacteria to multiply rapidly. The infection ultimately finds its way into the blood stream and is characterized by shaking, chills, fever, progressive jaundice, lethargy, and severe right upper quadrant pain. Recommended treatment is massive antibiotic therapy and operative drainage of the bile duct.

2. *Gas-gangrene wound infection.* This rare, but extremely grave, complication occurs early in the postoperative course and is marked by severe toxemia and disorientation. Although the

surface of the wound may appear grossly normal, subcutaneous crepitus is usually elicited by careful palpation.

Treatment consists of opening the wound and incising the underlying fascia for the full extent of the involvement. Massive doses of penicillin (up to 20 million units or more), and clostridia antitoxin must be promptly administered. Even with such vigorous therapy, the chances for survival are extremely poor.

## FISTULOUS DRAINAGE

While gastric or enterocutaneous fistulas are usually chronic conditions, occasionally patients with such a problem demand intensive care because of other complications. Accurate replacement of fistulous losses is essential to the body's economy, and successful treatment depends in large part on the ability to measure these losses. If the drainage is from a small wound, e.g., a drain site, then fluid loss can easily be collected in a small, disposable plastic bag (see nursing role). Samples of the drained material should be analyzed at intervals for electrolyte composition. If the fistula arises deep within an infected wound, sump drainage must be instituted.

Skin care is particularly important to patients with fistulas. The wound edges can be protected from maceration and digestion in several ways, but the prime need is to keep the skin free from contact with draining fluid. After gentle skin cleansing with soap and water, and drying, an ointment with an aluminum base may be applied. If the fistula drains pancreatic juice in high concentration, the proteolytic activity of this secretion can be counteracted by yeast paste or a thick protein emulsion made from chunks of beef.

## THE NURSING ROLE: GASTROINTESTINAL SURGERY

**General considerations.** Discussion between nurse and operating surgeon regarding patient management is essential in planning nursing care following general surgery. Identifying and comprehending the objectives of the surgeon is beneficial to both nursing and surgical members of the team. When nurses recognize and appreciate the treatment plan, they are better prepared to anticipate and watch for early signs of complications, particularly those which may indicate the need for further surgical intervention.

Nurses must be alert to patient attitudes, including response to the intensive care unit. Every nurse in the unit should be alert to adverse patient response to therapy, and, in some instances, should even terminate treatment to prevent further complications until the physician arrives. In order to assume this responsibility and provide a high quality of patient care, nurses must continually update their knowledge and understanding of the problems involved.

**Preoperative preparation of patients.** It is vitally important that patients be prepared for *postoperative* care prior to surgery.

Deep breathing and coughing exercises to reduce the threat of postoperative atelectasis are essential. Since most patients are distressed by endotracheal suction, it is of value to forewarn the patient of its possible necessity in the event of inadequate coughing following surgery.

**Deep-breathing exercises**
   a. *Position of the patient.*
   Assist the patient to relax in either the supine or sitting position, with the head and neck in a neutral position; a position of comfort will facilitate maximum expansion of the thorax. If the patient lies flat on his back, with his knees flexed, the abdominal muscles relax and permit maximal excursion of the diaphragm.
   b. *Diaphragmatic-abdominal breathing.*
   Instruct the patient to inhale quietly through the nose, using the diaphragm to balloon the upper abdomen, and then to exhale through the mouth by contracting the abdominal muscles. In learning this maneuver, patients often find it helpful to place one hand on the midabdomen. After learning this exercise in the supine-knees-flexed position, the patient should practice diaphragmatic breathing in the sitting and standing positions.

Because of incisional pain, patients who have had abdominal surgery tend to splint their chests, producing a shallow type of breathing which predisposes to alveolar hypoventilation. To ventilate the alveoli, particularly in the periphery and the lower lobes of the lung, and to prevent atelectasis, deep-breathing 5 to

10 times hourly is helpful. Most patients in bed maintain a lower than adequate tidal volume at rest, unless they have been instructed and assisted with deep-breathing exercises every hour to increase the tidal volume.

**Coughing exercises.** Instruct the patient to inspire and expire several times. On expiration, the patient should be instructed to force the air by making an explosive sound. Emphasize the importance of making a deep, forceful expiration, rather than short coughs which are unproductive and ineffective. These exercises are explained in detail in the appendix of this chapter.

Exercises should be demonstrated and repeated by the patient until he is proficient. Teach these maneuvers preoperatively, rather than in the postoperative period when the patient is usually quite uncomfortable.

**Lower extremity exercises.** Preoperatively, the patient can also be taught lower extremity exercises involving flexion and extension of hip, knee, and ankle joints to help prevent thrombophlebitis. During the postoperative period the nurse can assist with these as well as resistive exercises of the joints to facilitate venous return.

**Psychologic preparation for surgery.** In most situations surgical patients are not sent to intensive care units unless a complication develops after surgery; however, on some occasions where the complication risk is known to be high (either because of age, obesity, the procedure itself, etc.), it is beneficial to advise the patient of the plan to transfer him to the ICU following surgery.

As part of preoperative preparation, the nurse should determine the extent of the patient's knowledge of his disease and of the surgical procedure planned. In the event of misunderstanding, it is appropriate to clarify these points with the surgeon before surgery. It is necessary to provide time and opportunity for the patient to ask questions about his illness and care. By listening and answering these questions, the skillful nurse establishes a valuable rapport with the patient as a person.

**Postoperative care of patients.** The nurse should carefully observe the postoperative patient for signs indicative of disturbed gastrointestinal motility, hemorrhage, or peritonitis. These observations should be performed in a planned manner, with the results recorded for comparative purposes.

**Detection of abdominal distention.** The girth of the abdomen should be measured hourly when there is suspicion of abdominal distention. Although such measurement can be accomplished with a tape measure, a simple method involves the use of ties taped to the abdominal wall in the following manner:

a. a string is taped to each side of the abdomen;

b. the point at which the two strings overlap at mid-abdomen is marked as the starting point in succeeding measurements;

c. if the end points overlap, the abdominal size has decreased;

d. and, if the midpoints cease to meet, the abdominal size has increased.

**Care of Patients with Nasogastric and Intestinal Tubes**

a. It is essential to maintain patency of these drainage tubes. Mucus and blood clots can obstruct the lumen of gastric and intestinal tubes and defeat their purpose to encourage decompression. To prevent such blockage, gentle irrigation of nasogastric tubes with 10 to 15 cc of saline or air every hour is imperative. The amount of saline or air used for this purpose should be limited in order to minimize the amount of pressure exerted on the stomach. In the event that the tube is lying near the site of surgical anastomosis, unduly high pressures can disrupt the suture line.

Irrigation of intestinal tubes requires large amounts of fluid, usually 30 cc to 60 cc of normal saline every hour.

b. The drainage tube should be connected to a low-pressure suction apparatus. It is important to record the type and volume of drainage at least every 8 hours, so that the amount of fluids, electrolytes, and blood required for replacement can be accurately determined. Normal drainage from the lower intestinal tract is brown or bile-colored, but active bleeding may change the fluid color to "coffeeground" color or to a dark red hue.

c. Patients with these drainage tubes require more than usual care of the mouth. Poor oral hygiene in this setting may lead to parotitis (surgical mumps), a condition recognizable by the presence of a swollen, tender area just above the angle of the jaw.

**Care of patients with intra-abdominal bleeding.** When there is intraluminal bleeding, patients have frequent, tarry stools, often liquid, reddish to dark black-red in color, which may occur as often as 10 times in an 8-hour period. These stool specimens should measured, and a simple guaiac test should be performed by the nurse to ascertain the presence of blood. Patients frequently develop perianal excoriation from repeated liquid bloody stools; this can be prevented by meticulous skin care and cleanliness. A heat lamp applied to the irritated skin is sometimes effective.

Bleeding from drain sites after a radical procedure (such as pancreatoduodenectomy) can be measured by weighing the blood-soaked dressings on a small scale. The amount of blood lost can be estimated by subtracting the weight of an equal number of dry dressings from the weight of the saturated dressings. In general, one gram weight of blood is equivalent to one cc of blood in volume.

Because changes in the pulse rate, blood pressure, and urinary volume may reflect active hemorrhage, it is essential that the nurse measure these parameters at frequent intervals and record them in sequence. A sudden increase in pulse rate, a fall in blood pressure, or a decrease in urinary output may indicate serious bleeding which the nurse should report promptly to the physician. When such sudden changes in the patient's status occur, blood should be drawn for hematocrit, type, and cross-match at once.

**Care of patients with fistulous drainage.** In conditions of fistulous loss of intestinal fluids (e.g., with an ileostomy) the fluid drainage is usually voluminous and rapid. Because the skin is vulnerable to the high concentration of proteolytic enzymes found in this fluid, every effort must be made to protect the skin by channeling the flow into a system of suction drainage. This may be accomplished by the use of a commercially available disposable plastic bag in which an opening is cut to fit the stoma of the fistulous tract. Care must be taken that the opening of the bag does not fit too tightly about the stoma and constrict the blood supply, or too loosely, permitting drainage fluid to seep underneath the bag and spill onto the skin. A plastic catheter can then be placed in one of the upper corners of the bag to permit constant suction drainage. (See Fig. 1).

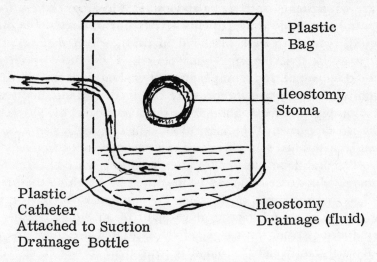

Fig. 1. *Suction drainage used for fistulous tracts*

This type of suction drainage is suitable for ileal and pancreatic fistulas.

In some instances the fistula involves the colon and the drainage contains fecal matter. This overflow may be a source of contamination to the abdominal incision, and particular care must be given to contain these bowel contents. In addition to the risk of infection, fecal spillage is obviously disturbing to the patient because of the constant soiling of his clothing and bed linens.

All fistulous drainage should be carefully measured to allow for accurate fluid and electrolyte replacement.

**Measurement of central venous pressure**

In instances of hemorrhage or when there is massive outpouring of fluid into the peritoneal cavity (peritonitis), the circulating blood volume can be markedly decreased, resulting in peripheral vascular collapse (shock). The hemodynamic changes associated with circulatory volume depletion can be assessed by measuring the central venous pressure and used as an index for volume replacement.

Central venous pressure (CVP) is a measurement of the pressure within the superior vena cava which reflects the pressure of the right atrium. When the blood volume is reduced (e.g., following hemorrhage or other fluid loss), the CVP will be lower than normal, and conversely, when the circulatory system is overloaded (e.g., as may occur with congestive heart failure or overadministration of fluids), the CVP is elevated.

Central venous pressure is measured directly by using a polyethylene catheter placed in the superior vena cava; the pressure is expressed in centimeters of water pressure. The normal CVP is usually between 5 and 10 cm of water. Values below 5 cm may reflect a decreased circulating volume, and those above 10 cm may indicate overloading of the right heart, as seen in congestive heart failure.

**Method of CVP measurement**

**1. *Insertion of Catheter*.** A disposable venous polyethylene catheter is inserted through an appropriate-sized needle in either the jugular, subclavian, or an arm vein; the arm vein is the most convenient site for the patient. Sometimes a venous section is performed when the arm veins are used. The manufacturers are designing teflon catheters with plastic styluses which make insertion simple and easy.

Once the physician has placed the catheter at the desired site in the vena cava, and has removed the plastic stylus, the nurse has available a 500 cc bottle of 5% dextrose in water to which sometimes 10 mg of heparin has been added (as preferred by many physicians). The infusion is started promptly to prevent clotting in the lumen of the catheter as with any intravenous fluids. This bottle is referred to as the "flush bottle"; it is regulated to drip slowly thereafter, through use of the microdrip technique to maintain patency. This venous line can serve as a source for intravenous fluids also. There is a tendency to over-hydrate the patient by forgetting that the flush bottle can account for significant fluid load unless it is carefully watched and regulated to drip slowly.

**2. *Establishing a Baseline for Manometer Position*.** The manometer is so positioned that the zero mark is at the level of the right atrium, using the left or right midchest. (See Fig. 2.) The right atrium is located inferiorly to midsternum and half-way between the front to the back of the chest laterally. A carpenter's

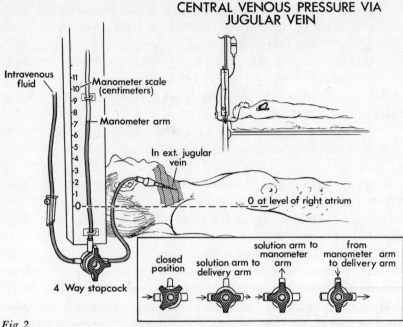

CENTRAL VENOUS PRESSURE VIA
JUGULAR VEIN

*Fig. 2.*

level is very useful in establishing the parallel line between the zero mark and the right atrium. If the patient has pulmonary emphysema or lung disease and has a barrel chest, use the lower third level of the lateral chest in locating the right atrium. This then establishes the reference position prior to each subsequent CVP measurement and reading. These maneuvers are essential because an accurate reading is vital.

If the patient cannot tolerate a flat supine position because of orthopnea with left-sided heart failure, he may sit at a 45° angle with the zero point of the manometer adjusted to the level of the right atrium in the sitting position. This then becomes the established reference position. Between measurements the patient may lie and sit in any position of comfort.

### 3. *Measurement of Pressure.*

a. After the catheter has been properly positioned by the physician and the reference position is established, the nurse regulates the fluid from the flush bottle to run directly through the catheter into the vein ("solution arm" to "delivery arm" in diagram), in order to maintain the patency of the system.

b. By turning the stopcock from "solution arm" to "manometer arm," the manometer is then filled to a level of 20 to 25 cm.

c. The stopcock is then turned from the "manometer arm" position to "delivery arm" position for the actual pressure reading. With each respiration, the meniscus of the column of water in the "manometer arm" fluctuates. The reading is taken at the maximum level the meniscus reaches after it attains an average level in the column, indicating equal pressure in the manometer and the vena cava.

d. To keep the system open for subsequent readings, the stopcock is returned to its original position ("solution arm" to "delivery arm") and the flow is controlled by a microdrip method.

e. It is essential that the patient be relaxed at the time measurement is made, because straining, coughing, or any other activity which increases the intrathoracic pressure will cause spuriously high measurements. When CVP is measured while the patient is receiving mechanical respiratory assistance, the respirator must be temporarily disconnected to obtain a meaningful reading.

4. *Precautions.*

a. The nurse should ascertain at frequent intervals that the connections between the catheter and its attachments are secure. If the catheter becomes disconnected from the remaining system, it may become clotted, and a possible source of air embolism exists.

b. If the original reference position was established with the patient in a flat position, it is necessary that this position be resumed at the time of pressure reading. Even slight elevation of the head of the bed can result in false determinations.

c. If the CVP shows a significant change in either direction during repeated readings, the nurse should inform the physician promptly of this variation.

For example, an elderly patient who had sustained significant blood loss had a CVP of 3 cm water before receiving 1000 cc of blood and 1000 cc of saline solution. The nurse, noting that the CVP has risen from 3 to 5 to 8, then to 11 cm of water within two hours, should advise the physician of this increase, since it may reflect overloading of the cardiovascular system and forewarn of impending pulmonary edema. Conversely, failure of the CVP to increase after fluid replacement might indicate additional blood or fluid loss.

# ENDOCRINE GLAND SURGERY

Operation upon the glands of endocrine secretion may be followed by life-threatening complications which result fundamentally from loss of essential hormones. The propensity for complication is further enhanced by the basic endocrine disease which necessitated surgery and which may have engendered a profound metabolic disturbance prior to the operation.

## ADRENAL GLAND SURGERY

### THE PROBLEM

The adrenal glands consist of a cortex and medulla. The cortex secretes steroids which affect carbohydrate and protein metabolism (glucocorticoids) and mineralocorticoids which regulate salt and water balance. Aldosterone, a separate steroid, is also secreted by the adrenal cortex and influences electrolyte balance in conjunction with the mineralocorticoids. The glucocorticoids and mineralocorticoids are essential to life, and replacement therapy with these particular hormones must be instituted after adrenalectomy to prevent vasomotor collapse and death. Aldosterone, as such, apparently is not vital for survival after total adrenalectomy, provided the cortical hormone, cortisone (which contains both glucocorticoids and mineralocorticoids) is given. Similarly, replacement therapy for the many other steroids produced by the adrenal cortex, including the sex hormones, is not required after surgery. Most patients following total adrenalectomy can be maintained by small doses of cortisone itself.

The adrenal medulla secretes the catecholamines, epinephrine and norepinephrine, which participate in the maintenance of vasomotor function, particularly during periods of stress. Neither of these hormones is essential to life or needs to be replaced after extirpation of the adrenal glands. A more detailed description of the adrenal glands and of medical emergencies related to their dysfunction is found in Chapter VI "Metabolic Crises."

Adrenalectomy is performed in most instances for disturbances that result in hyperfunction of hormonal activity. The classical indication for such surgery is Cushing's syndrome, a disease in which the amount of circulating corticosteroids is markedly increased because of an adrenal tumor or hyperplasia. This overproduction of cortical steroids leads to faulty protein synthesis, severe disturbances in carbohydrate metabolism manifested by diabetes, and the retention of sodium and water with resultant hypertension. Whether the patient has surgical extirpation of a single gland (because of a functioning tumor) or total adrenalectomy for bilateral adrenal hyperplasia, preoperative preparation with parenteral administration of steroids is necessary.

Adrenalectomy is also performed for functioning tumors of the adrenal medulla (pheochromocytoma). As stated, the hormones secreted by the medulla, epinephrine and norepinephrine, do not have to be replaced after total adrenalectomy. However, in the presence of pheochromocytoma, where the vascular tone has become dependent on these vasoactive amines, temporary replacement with norepinephrine is usually required. When the tumor is removed, the patient is suddenly deprived of the vascular support of these catecholamines and his vasomotor tone is abruptly decreased. This event results in dilatation of the vascular tree with pooling of the circulating blood volume and vascular collapse, a catastrophe which can be avoided by the careful administration of norepinephrine.

Bilateral adrenalectomy is sometimes undertaken as part of the total treatment program for metastatic cancer of the breast. The rationale of this surgery relates to the beneficial effect of total depletion of estrogens on the rate of growth of metastatic breast lesions achieved by total oophorectomy and adrenalectomy.

The major problem associated with adrenal surgery is the complication of resulting adrenal insufficiency that may develop if the replacement dosage of cortisone is inadequate to meet body needs. Normally, the maintenance dosage can be established without difficulty and presents no problem. However, during periods of increased stress postoperatively, such as illness or trauma, the dosage of cortisone must be increased because the body is unable to produce the additional amount of steroid hormone demanded by these circumstances.

## ASSESSMENT OF THE PROBLEM

The earliest symptoms of adrenal cortical insufficiency are lassitude and easy fatigability, followed by anorexia, increased thirst, cramping abdominal pain, and fever. If the condition remains untreated, the patient may develop hypotension and shock and die in coma.

Surgery for removal of pheochromocytoma is usually associated with marked vasomotor instability, both during surgery and in the immediate postoperative period. Manipulation of the gland during the surgical procedure may cause a sudden rise in blood pressure and precipitate serious ventricular tachyarrhythmias. Postoperatively, hypotension may develop unless norepinephrine is administered at this time.

## PRINCIPLES OF TREATMENT

Replacement therapy with cortisone is usually initiated on the day of surgery in the following manner:

*during surgery*—hydrocortisone sodium succinate, 100 mgm I.M.,

*four hours after* the initial dose, 50 mgm I.M.,

*every six hours* thereafter, 40 mgm I.M.,

*first postoperative day*—hydrocortisone sodium succinate, 50 mgm I.M. every 8 hours,

*second postoperative day*—hydrocortisone sodium succinate, 25 mgm I.M. every 6 hours; or cortisone acetate, 25 mgm orally every 6 hours,

*third postoperative day*—cortisone acetate, 25 mgm orally every 8 hours; desoxycorticosterone acetate, 2 mgm I.M., if no edema or heart failure,

*fourth postoperative day*—cortisone acetate, 12.5 mgm orally every 6 hours; desoxycorticosterone acetate, 2 mgm I.M.,

*fifth postoperative day*—cortisone acetate, 12.5 mgm every 8 hours orally, and

*sixth postoperative day*—through *tenth postoperative day*—long-acting desoxycorticosterone trimethylacetate at appropriate dosage levels.

The adequacy of the dosage schedule can be estimated by

assessing the patient's symptoms and by measurement of blood sugar, electrolytes, blood pressure, and body weight.

In the event of acute adrenal insufficiency, emergency treatment consists of the rapid correction of the insufficient steroid blood level by the intravenous injection of 100 mgm of hydrocortisone. During periods of obvious stress the maintenance dosage of cortisone must be increased to circumvent the possibility of acute insufficiency.

During and after the removal of pheochromocytoma, vascular tone must be preserved by the administration of norepinephrine. The drug should be given through a catheter that lies within a large vein, since extravasation of this drug, which is a powerful vasoconstrictor, may cause localized ischemia and even necrosis of subcutaneous tissue and skin. The rate of administration of norepinephrine is regulated to maintain the blood pressure near the range of 120/80. Excessive amounts of this drug may lead to an alarming increase in blood pressure and the production of a cerebrovascular accident. Norepinephrine may be required for 24 to 72 hours postoperatively, the dosage being gradually decreased until the patient's cardiovascular system has adapted to the sudden low level of circulating amines induced by removal of the tumor.

## THE NURSING ROLE

The major nursing care following adrenalectomy involves careful observation of the patient for signs or symptoms of acute adrenal insufficiency. Specifically to be noted are:
- a. blood pressure and pulse rate,
- b. temperature elevation,
- c. loss of appetite,
- d. increased thirst,
- e. abdominal pain,
- f. drowsiness and lassitude,
- g. daily body weight.

Patients receiving norepinephrine should have continuous ECG monitoring and frequent blood pressure determinations. In the event of frequent premature ventricular beats or the development of ventricular tachycardia, the infusion rate should be decreased and the physician notified promptly. (See pages 67–69 regarding these arrhythmias.)

## THYROID GLAND SURGERY

Partial or subtotal thyroidectomy is the most common form of endocrine surgery and is usually performed without complication. Total ablation of the thyroid gland, however, may lead to two potentially life-threatening complications.

1. Vocal cord paralysis and airway obstruction secondary to recurrent laryngeal nerve injury. The recurrent laryngeal nerve may be injured or even severed during thyroid surgery. This nerve innervates the cricothyroideus muscle, which tenses the vocal cords and affects the tone of the voice. If the nerve has been damaged during thyroidectomy, the vocal cords relax and cause obstruction of the larynx. This complication can often be immediately identified by the anesthesiologist as he withdraws the endotracheal tube. The vocal cords in this situation are drawn to the midline and are immobile. Vocal cord injury also can be recognized early in the postoperative period by a characteristic inspiratory stridor or "crowing" sound which is indicative of airway obstruction. In this circumstance the patient will use accessory muscles of respiration, but will be unable to maintain an adequate airway. An immediate tracheostomy is required as a life-saving measure.

2. Removal of the parathyroid glands during the thyroidectomy presents a serious complication. (See pages 207–209 regarding role of parathyroid glands.) The surgeon should always inspect excised thyroid tissue for the presence of parathyroid glands. If they are found, they should be re-embedded into the muscles within the neck. In some instances hypoparathyroidism after thyroidectomy is the result of trauma or devascularization of the parathyroid glands and may be transient in nature.

Loss of parathyroid function can be recognized from signs of hypocalcemic tetany. This hyper-irritability of the neuromuscular system can be demonstrated by:

a. Chvostek's sign (see page 207), in which twitching of the corner of the mouth occurs in response to gentle tapping just anterior to the lower lobe of the ear.

b. Trousseau's sign, palmar turning of the hand because of spasm of the muscles within the forearm, elicited by obstructing the blood flow to the arm with a blood pressure cuff (see page 207).

The resultant hypocalcemia that follows parathyroid gland removal can easily be ascertained by measuring blood calcium levels. Calcium levels below 8.5 mgm per cent are very suggestive of parathyroid insufficiency. Prompt therapy with calcium salts must be given (1 gram of calcium gluconate intravenously at first and then 10 grams of calcium chloride orally each day thereafter). If uncorrected, hypocalcemia may lead to convulsions, cardiac arrhythmias, and death.

Postoperative hemorrhage may occur suddenly and cause severe laryngeal edema and closure of the glottis. This bleeding is frequently caused by dislodgement of ligatures in the heavily vascularized thyroid remnant, resulting from swallowing.

## THYMUS GLAND SURGERY

The precise physiologic function of the thymus gland, other than its role in immunologic control, is still uncertain. However, it is known that certain patients with myasthenia gravis enter states of remission after thymectomy.

Myasthenia gravis is characterized by progressive weakness of the voluntary muscles. The defect producing this weakness lies in either a lack of release of acetylcholine at the motor end plate of striated muscle or an excessive amount of the enzyme cholinesterase at this site, which inactivates acetylcholine. The treatment is only symptomatic, rather than curative, and consists of administration of acetylcholine (or one of its stable esters) or of parasympathomimetic drugs which have an anticholinesterase effect, such as neostigmine (prostigmine) or pyriodostigmine (mestinon).

Hyperplasia of the thymus gland occurs in more than one-half of patients with myasthenia gravis; however, some patients without myasthenia gravis have tumors of the thymus gland (thymomas) which produce muscle weakness and other symptoms similar to myasthenia gravis.

Thymectomy is performed when patients do not respond to medical treatment. The procedure appears valuable in many instances, and it has been shown that remissions occur in a high percentage of patients undergoing this operation.

The immediate postoperative period may be marked by profound muscle weakness occurring most significantly in the muscles of respiration. Patients generally experience great difficulty in clearing the respiratory tract of mucus and fluid, and a tracheostomy with constant ventilation on a respirator is usually required. The problem may be exaggerated by difficulty in swallowing and nasal regurgitation of fluid. If the volume of secretions cannot be controlled despite the use of cholinergic drugs, bronchoscopy may be required to prevent, or treat, the atelectasis that results from mucus plugs.

Because the thymus gland is located within the mediastinum, the postoperative care is similar to that involving any thoracotomy. (See pages 355–371.)

## PITUITARY GLAND SURGERY

Removal of the pituitary gland (hypophysectomy) is performed most often to control progression of metastatic breast cancer. Some clinicians also advocate hypophysectomy to combat progressive diabetic retinopathy. Excision of this master gland results in the cessation of stimulating hormones that influence function of the other endocrine glands. Thus, hypophysectomy reduces production of both adrenal and ovarian estrogens by removing the follicle-stimulating hormone (FSH) from the ovary and adrenocorticotrophic hormone (ACTH) from the adrenal. The resultant depletion of estrogen impedes growth of metastatic breast carcinoma. At the same time and in the same manner, removal of the pituitary creates thyroid and adrenal insufficiency, as well as inhibiting male and female sex hormone production. A profound disturbance in water balance (diabetes insipidus) may follow hypophysectomy because of the lack of antidiuretic hormone (ADH), previously produced by the posterior lobe of the pituitary. Therefore, following ablation of the pituitary, patients must receive thyroid and adrenal steroid replacement and usually antidiuretic hormone (pitressin) as well.

Hypophysectomy is performed through a right frontal craniotomy, after which the hypophyseal stalk is divided and the gland removed by curettage and exposure of the sella turcica to Zenker's solution.

The postoperative period is usually uncomplicated except for some disturbance of water and electrolyte balance related to the reduction of pitressin. Most patients are ambulatory 24 to 48 hours after surgery, with a total hospitalization of 10 days. Hormonal replacement consists of maintenance therapy of cortisone and dessicated thyroid, orally.

Nursing care involving frontal craniotomy has been described in Chapter X "Head Injuries."

Complications that may occur are loss of vision, visual field defects, neurologic changes, and infection. Occasional patients have rhinorrhea for a short period of time.

## HEAD AND NECK SURGERY

### THE PROBLEM

Patients undergoing extensive surgery in the head and neck region, including radical neck, mandible, and tongue dissections, occasionally present special problems in postoperative management.

**Upper Airway Obstruction.** Obstruction to the airway may result from hemorrhage into the tracheobronchial tree from occlusion of the airway entrance by soft tissue which has been made flaccid by the operative procedure itself, or from injury to tissue nerve supply.

All members of the intensive care team must be trained to recognize upper airway obstruction. Typical findings include:

    a. Stridor. This early sign is characterized by a coarse, high-pitched sound on inspiration and can be recognized near its onset by placing a stethoscope over the trachea.

    b. Labored respiration. This more advanced sign is manifested by retraction of the supraclavicular and intercostal spaces during inspiration, and the use of the accessory respiratory muscles. These signs are the result of increased negative intrathoracic pressure secondary to the obstruction to the inflow of air.

c. Hypoxia. Restlessness, and, later, cyanosis may develop as a result of inadequate tissue oxygenation. With advanced hypoxia, significant $CO_2$ retention is to be anticipated and cardiac or respiratory arrest may occur in this circumstance.

If airway obstruction exists, an endotracheal tube must be inserted immediately, either through the nose or mouth. If respiratory distress is marked, an airway must be established by tracheostomy.

**Hemorrhage.** A less frequent complication of radical head and neck surgery is hemorrhage into one of the extravascular spaces of the neck. This bleeding produces angulation or direct compression of the trachea. Such obstruction may be difficult to recognize early in its course, particularly when large, bulky dressings are present. Bloodstained dressings should be cause for suspicion that hemorrhage has occurred, and the operative site should be examined in this circumstance. If bleeding is identified within the closed spaces of the neck, the area must be drained and operative control of the bleeding point established.

A late and catastrophic complication of radical neck dissection is necrosis and hemorrhage from the carotid artery. During neck dissection, this artery, which lies just beneath the skin, is usually freed of surrounding connective tissue and fat. Carotid hemorrhage results from necrosis of the skin flaps which have been found during operation to expose the underlying tissues. Immediate hemostasis can best be obtained by direct pressure over or just below the site of hemorrhage. Carotid bleeding demands immediate surgical intervention.

**Pneumothorax.** An additional pulmonary complication, unrelated to upper airway obstruction, is pneumothorax, caused by injury to the apical pleura in the inferior extent of neck dissection. This complication is not accompanied by stridor, but can be recognized by signs of respiratory distress and the absence of breath sounds over the involved hemithorax. If this diagnosis is suspected, it can easily be confirmed by chest x-ray. Immediate aspiration of the chest in the second intercostal space anteriorly with the patient in a sitting position provides prompt relief of this potentially serious complication, while simultaneously confirming the diagnosis.

## THE NURSING ROLE

Patients who have had head and neck surgery require careful observation to ascertain the earliest signs of airway obstruction or hemorrhage. During the immediate postoperative period it is a wise practice to specifically seek the presence of stridor by listening over the trachea with a stethoscope periodically. Dressings should be checked frequently to rule out hidden bleeding.

Because of pooling of oral secretion, suctioning of the oropharynx is usually required. Care must be given to protect the operated areas and the intraoral suture lines during suctioning.

Communication may be difficult for many of these patients, especially those with hemiglossectomy. The nurse can resort to patient's nonverbal communication in this circumstance. She should also provide the patient some means for writing (e.g., a slate or tablet) during the recovery period.

Because the sight of the patient with a tracheostomy, suction equipment, catheters, etc., is particularly disturbing to family and visitors, the nurse should advise visitors of how the patient will appear in order to minimize their emotional reactions.

## *APPENDIX TO CHAPTER IX*

### BREATHING EXERCISES

I. *Indications*
   1. All patients age 50 or more on bed rest or admitted for surgery.
   2. All patients at any age with cough, sputum, shortness of breath, or wheezing.
II. *Position*
   Assist the patient to relax in the proper position to facilitate maximum expansion of the thorax. He may lie supine or on either side in a position of comfort with the head and neck in a neutral position. If he lies flat on his back with his knees flexed, the abdominal muscles become relaxed, permitting maximal excursion of the diaphragm.
III. *Diaphragmatic-Abdominal Breathing*
   Instruct the patient to inhale quietly through the nose, using

the diaphragm by ballooning the upper abdomen, and to exhale through the mouth by contracting, or sinking in, the abdominal muscles. In learning this maneuver, patients often find it helpful to place one hand on the mid-abdomen. After learning in supine-knees flexed position, the patient should practice diaphragmatic breathing in sitting and standing positions.

## THE SEGMENTAL BRONCHI

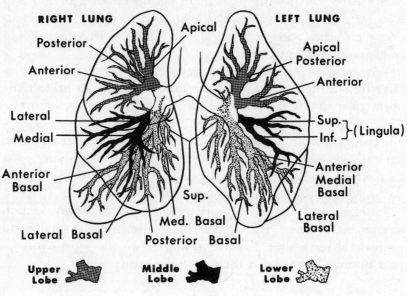

Fig. 3

## Treatment procedure, postural drainage, positions, clapping, and vibrating

I. *Treatment Procedure*

Position the patient, clap for 1–2 minutes, then vibrate during 3–4 exhalations and complete the cycle by having the patient cough. An effective cough is produced by deep exhalations; use abdominal muscles for deep coughing. A short period of rest should follow each cycle. Treatments should be scheduled before meals and at bedtime.

II. *Postural Drainage Positions*

These positions are used to promote drainage from the lung by using the force of gravity to move secretions to the main bronchi, where they can be coughed up.

III. *Clapping, cupping, or tapping* causes air to dislodge secretions and moves them to the main bronchi for expulsion. This is done with the hand in a cupped position by flexion and extension of the wrist; clap the chest wall over the involved lung area. The percussive action produced by tapping helps to dislodge mucus plugs and thick secretions. Clapping is done gently with both hands; clap the same areas with alternate hands or one hand at a time for one or two minutes.

IV. *Vibrating* is done by placing one hand on top of the other hand or placing one hand on each side of the patient's rib cage. The nurse contracts and tenses her shoulder muscles (deltoids and pectorals), and compresses and gently vibrates the patient's chest wall *as the rib cage moves inward on exhalations*. In vibrating, move upward with rib cage during *exhalations only*. This is done during 3–4 exhalations with periods of rest and relaxation.

Clapping and vibrating are indicated in bronchiectasis, bronchitis, emphysema, and cystic fibrosis. Contraindications to clapping and vibrating are hemorrhage and pain.

## LOBES AND AREAS TO BE DRAINED

| I. *LOWER LOBES* | *Specific Location* | *Positions* |
|---|---|---|
| a. Apical Segment | a. Right and/or Left Superior Bronchus | Patient lies in a prone position with a pillow under the abdomen. |
| | | *Clap* the lower ⅓ posterior rib cage on the affected side for 1–2 minutes; *vibrate* the same area clapped during 3–4 exhalations. |
| b. Anterior Basal Segment | b. Right and/or Left Anterior Basal Bronchus | The foot of the hospital bed is elevated to about 45° by turning the gatch. The patient lies in a supine and Trendelenburg position with two pillows placed under his hips, and he flexes both knees to relax the abdominal muscles. |
| | | *Clap* the lower ⅓ of the anterior rib cage on the affected side; *vibrate* the same area. |

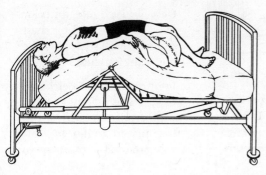

| | | |
|---|---|---|
| c. Lateral Basal Segment | c. Right and/or Left Lateral Basal Bronchus | Same as I-b except the patient lies on his unaffected side. |

*Clap and vibrate* lower ⅓ of the lateral rib cage on the affected side.

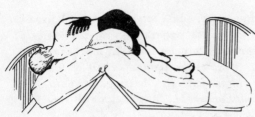

| | | |
|---|---|---|
| d. Posterior Basal Segment Median Basal Segment | d. Right and/or Left Posterior Basal Bronchus | Same as I-c except the patient lies in a prone position, with one or two pillows under the abdomen and hips. |

*Clap and vibrate* lower ⅓ of the posterior rib cage on the affected side.

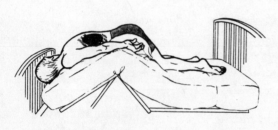

## II. *MIDDLE LOBE*

| | | |
|---|---|---|
| a. Right Middle Lobe | a. Medical or Lateral Bronchus | Same as I-b. Place a pillow from the right axilla to the right side; the patient turns ¼ to the left side. The left shoulder is abducted 90° and the left elbow is flexed 90°; both arms may be left on the sides. |

*Clap and vibrate* anterior and lateral right chest from the axillary fold to the mid-anterior chest.

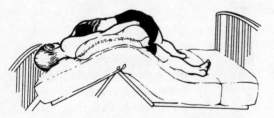

## III. *LINGULA*

| | | |
|---|---|---|
| a. Left Upper Lobe | a. Superior and/ or Inferior Lingular Bronchus | Foot of the bed is elevated to 45°. The patient lies in a supine position with a pillow placed under his left side from the shoulder to |

his hip to maintain a ¼ turn to the right and he flexes his knees.

*Clap and vibrate* from left axillary fold to the mid-anterior chest.

IV. *UPPER LOBES*

| | | |
|---|---|---|
| a. Upper Lobes | a. Right and/or Left Apical Bronchus | Patient sits with a slight variation according to the location of the lesion; he leans forward to drain the posterior lobe and backward to drain the anterior lobe.<br><br>*Clap and vibrate* upper back between the base of the neck and the left and/or right shoulder with the fingers extending over the clavicles. |
| b. Anterior Parts | b. Right and/or Left Anterior Bronchus | Patient lies in a supine position with a pillow under his knees for relaxation.<br><br>*Clap and vibrate* the chest anteriorly below the left and right clavicle and above the nipple to the level of the sternal end. |
| c. Posterior Right | c. Right Posterior Bronchus | Patient lies in a prone position with a ¼ turn to the right, and he places his left arm toward his back. His head and shoulders are elevated 45° on three pillows.<br><br>*Clap and vibrate* over the right shoulder blade. |

| d. Left Pos-<br>terior | d. Left Posterior<br>Bronchus | Patient lies in a prone posi-<br>tion with 1/4 turn to the left<br>with his right arm out-<br>stretched toward his back.<br>His head and shoulders are<br>elevated 45° on three pil-<br>lows. |
|---|---|---|

*Clap and vibrate* over the left shoulder blade.

Prepared by:

Charles Carman, M.D.
Assoc. Prof. of Medicine
In Charge of Respiratory Diseases

Katherine Smutko, R.P.T.
Department of Physical Therapy

Marie Kurihara, R.N., M.A.
Medical-Surgical Nursing
Instructor School of Nursing

Wayne Emery, Medical Illustrator
Audio Visual Aids Department

University of California Medical Center
San Francisco, California

## Bibliography

ARTZ, C. P. and HARDY, J. D., (eds.): *Complications in Surgery and Their Management,* Second edition, W. B. Saunders Co., Philadelphia, 1967.

BEAL, J. M., (ed.): *Manual of Recovery Room Care.* Second edition, The Macmillan Co., New York, 1962.

BECKMAN, HARRY: *Pharmacology,* W. B. Saunders Co., Philadelphia, 1961.

BEESON, PAUL and MCDERMOTT, WALTER: *Textbook of Medicine,* Philadelphia, W. B. Saunders Co., 1963, pp. 133–137.

BLAND, J. H.: *Clinical Metabolism of Body Water and Electrolytes,* W. B. Saunders Co., Philadelphia, 1963. pp. 133–137.

BURGESS, R. E.: Fluids and Electrolytes. *Amer. J. Nursing,* 65:90–95, October 1965.

CARMAN, C. T.: Diagnosis and Treatment of Respiratory Acidosis. *Anesthesia and Analgesia,* 45:126–132, January–February 1965.

DAVIS, L. E., (ed.): *Christopher's Textbook of Surgery,* Seventh edition, pp. 711–713. W. B. Saunders Co., Philadelphia, 1960.

FRENAY, SR. M. AGNES CLARE: A Dynamic Approach to the Ileal Conduit Patient. *Amer. J. Nursing,* 64:80–84, January 1964.

GALANTE, M. and FOURNIER, D. J.: Adrenalectomy for Metastatic Breast Carcinoma. *J.A.M.A.* 163:1011–1016, March 23, 1957.

GLENN, F. and MANNIX, H., JR.: The Surgical Management of Pheochromocytoma. *Surg. Gynec. Obstet.,* 116:613–622, 1963.

GLENN, F. and BEAL, J. M., (eds.): *Surgical Clinics of North America.* 44 (2):303–573, 1964.

GLENN, F.: Surgical Treatment of Biliary Tract Disease. *Amer. J. Nursing,* 64:88–92, May 1964.

HARVEY, A., McG.: Myasthenia Gravis. In: Cecil-Loeb *Textbook of Medicine.* P. B. BEESON and W. McDERMOTT, (eds.). Eleventh edition, pp. 1455–1460. W. B. Saunders Co., Philadelphia, 1963.

HENDERSON, L. M.: Nursing Care of Acute Cholecystitis. *Amer. J. Nursing,* 64: 93–96, May 1964.

HERRMAN, C., JR.: Myasthenia Gravis: Brief Guide to Diagnosis and Management. *California Med.,* 106:275–281, 1967.

HOCKSTEIN, ELLIOT and RUBIN, ALBERT: *Physical Diagnosis,* pp. 328–332. McGraw-Hill Book Co., New York, 1964.

KURIHARA, MARIE: Postural Drainage, Clapping, and Vibrating Techniques. *Amer. J. of Nursing,* 65:76–79, November 1965.

*Manual of Recovery Room Care.* 2d ed. New York Hospital, Department of Surgery, N.Y., The Macmillan Co., 1962.

NORRIS, W. and CAMPBELL, D.: *Anesthetics, Resuscitation and Intensive Care.* The Williams and Wilkins Co., Baltimore, 1965.

PEARSON, O. and RAY, B. S.: Results of Hypophysectomy in the Treatment of Metastatic Mammary Carcinoma. *Cancer* 12:85–92, January–February 1959.

ROE, B. B.: Myasthenia Gravis Secondary to Thymic Neoplasm. *J. Thoracic Surg.,* 33:6:770–775, June 1957.

SAFAR, P.: *Respiratory Therapy.* F. A. Davis Co., Philadelphia, 1965.

SMITH, D. R. and GALENTE, M.: The Use of the Bricker Operation in Urology. *Am. J. Surg.* 96:254–263, August 1958.

Symposium on Intensive Care Nursing. *Nursing Clin. North America* 3:1–93, 1968.

# Chapter X

# Head Injuries

FRANK E. NULSEN, M.D.

M. ARLENE MARTIN GARDNER, R.N., M.A.

## THE PROBLEM

Head injuries are of two types: those which penetrate the skull and brain, and those which do not. These latter are designated as *closed* type head injuries.

Certain anatomical and physiological considerations are important to an understanding of how the brain can be affected, both initially and subsequently, from *closed head* injury. In such injuries, the brain shows evidence of bruising after the head has been subjected to a decelerating force (e.g., the sudden arrest of movement after falling downstairs or striking the auto dashboard after collision). Less severe closed injuries to the brain are likely when an individual is beaten or struck on the head than in situations in which the head leads in decelerating the entire moving body.

Because the brain is enclosed in a tight bony box and is held suspended in a thin cushion of fluid, external forces diffusely affect its entire contents. Although some parts of the brain can undoubtedly suffer greater bruising or tearing stresses than others, the injury due to impact is never limited to only one focal area. Therefore, in a closed head injury, purely focal signs, such as weakness of an arm or leg or speech disturbance, are not seen without associated diffuse effects upon cerebration (i.e., the level of consciousness, orientation, sensorium, and/or responsiveness). Since normal cerebration involves proper function of multiple brain areas, the patient's mental state (particularly his degree of responsiveness) is always the best determinant of the existence and severity of initial brain injury.

A second consequence of the rigid confinement of the brain within a rigid bony box is that the volume available for the brain becomes reduced in the event of intracranial bleeding (hematoma). This compression of brain volume produces both focal and diffuse effects, with the ultimate catastrophe being uncal or cerebellar herniation. Of lesser concern is the restriction which the bony box imposes on the anticipated swelling of the brain (reactive edema) following trauma. Such edema may last from 48 to 60 hours after injury, and, until it subsides, is associated with increasing impairment of brain function.

A final consideration in head injuries is the high susceptibility of the intracranial contents to infection whenever bacteria from the external environment can gain access to the brain either through direct introduction (perforating wounds) or indirectly through a basilar skull fracture where bacteria harbored in air sinuses can invade the meninges.

**Cerebral concussion.** The mildest form of traumatic insult to the head is termed *cerebral concussion,* in which the patient momentarily loses consciousness at the time of injury. If such a "blackout" does *not* occur following the initial trauma, the likelihood of brain injury is minimal. (*But* the possibility of subsequent brain damage from intracranial bleeding still exists, whether or not loss of consciousness occurs.)

The neurological examination and mentation of patients after concussion are normal. Lumbar puncture is not usually indicated in this circumstance, but if it is performed, the cerebrospinal fluid (CSF) is clear and the pressure is near normal (about 150 mm of water).

The exact mechanisms involved in this sudden disturbance of consciousness, with total reversibility, are poorly understood. It is thought that mechanical agitation in some way results in a release of enzymes which interfere with electrical conduction of nervous impulses for a brief period. The enzymes are then metabolized, after which total recovery follows. Brain function returns to normal in all respects after a simple cerebral concussion.

**Cerebral contusion or laceration.** When actual bruising of the brain occurs, associated with temporary or permanent structural damage, the injury is described as a *cerebral contusion.* The degree of injury is reflected by alterations of the patient's mental state. With a minimal contusion, the return of consciousness is not as prompt as with a cerebral concussion and there is impaired recall of events prior to the injury (retrograde amnesia). In its mildest form, this amnesia is manifest only by a loss of the precise details of events occurring immediately before the impact; in its more pronounced forms, the amnesia may extend for a period of hours before the accident occurred. Patients with this latter type of memory loss often have some disorientation, slowness of reaction, headache, vomiting, and other mild neurologic abnormalities.

More severe contusions are paralleled by increasing disturbances in responsiveness in the following progression: (1) disoriented, but able to make appropriate response to commands; (2) out of contact, but still muttering and moving purposefully; (3) inert and responding only to *strong* stimuli; (4) no reponsiveness, or *decerebrate* thrusting (in the now critically damaged brain). These gross disturbances in cerebration are accompanied by major abnormalities in neurologic and autonomic function.

In general, the degree of brain contusion is reflected by the amount of blood extravasated from the brain surface into the surrounding subarachnoid fluid. In a mild contusion the CSF may be overtly clearly, with perhaps 100 red blood cells being found on microscopic examination. Moderate injuries may be suspected from grossly pink fluid. and severe injuries from bloody red CSF. The CSF pressure is increased in most instances of cerebral contusion.

Some clinicians prefer to classify severe contusions as *cerebral lacerations.* This categorization refers only to the degree of injury and is not a distinct entity, such as concussion vs. contusion.

Even when the initial brain insult is not further complicated, the clinical course of patients with severe cerebral contusion is inherently difficult for the following reasons:

1. Because of the helplessness of the patient, along with decreased reflexes, secretions may accumulate in the tracheobronchial tree, causing airway obstruction. This interference with breathing not only results in decreased tissue oxygenation, but also leads to

an increase in venous pressure. This combination of venous congestion and anoxia further compromises the injured brain.

2. Patients with cerebral contusions have a high propensity for focal seizures which may become generalized and continuous. If not recognized and treated at their onset, such seizures may exhaust the patient and aggravate an already critical picture.

3. Imbalance of the autonomic nervous system frequently accompanies injuries to the base of the brain (hypothalamus). This derangement is manifested by marked *overactivity* of the autonomic system with increased temperature (to 40°–41° C), rapid pulse rate, and tachypnea. This uncontrolled overdriving effect can result in exhaustion, myocardial infarction, pulmonary edema, or secondary brain damage.

4. In the obtunded patient, serious injuries of the trunk or extremities are sometimes overlooked. In some instances, patients with brain injury, capable of recovery, develop hypotension and tachycardia which are erroneously attributed to the head injury rather than to their true cause, which may be blood loss into the chest or abdomen. Because the patient offers no complaint, a considerable delay may intervene before the correct diagnosis is established and as a result definitive treatment is delayed.

5. Disorientation, even in the awake, conscious patient, poses problems. During periods of confusion these individuals may attempt to climb over protective bed rails, and thus sustain limb fractures or further head injuries.

**Intracranial hematoma.** About 5% to 15% of patients with head injuries, treated in general hospitals, develop intracranial hematoma after either contusion or concussion. The bleeding, which usually occurs between the brain and the skull, is readily accessible to surgical intervention. There are two types of intracranial hematoma:

1. *Epidural.* This type of bleeding may result when a branch of the middle meningeal artery is torn at the point of a skull fracture in the bony groove between the skull and the dura. The hematoma, fed by this small artery, grows rapidly to bring a patient to extremis in one to six hours after the injury. Occasionally, the hematoma will require 24 hours to manifest itself.

2. *Subdural.* Subdural bleeding is more common than epi-

dural hematoma. It usually arises from a tear in a vein passing from the surface of the brain to the sagittal or lateral venous sinus. It is believed that while the venous bleeding usually stops by self-tamponade compression, a resulting jelly clot in the compartment between the dura and the arachnoid continues to swell or grow by imbibing fluid from surrounding tissues. The acute subdural hematoma develops slightly more slowly than the epidural hematoma, with manifestations of worsening usually beginning in the first few hours after injury.

(Although not relevant to the present discussion, it is important to distinguish *acute* from *chronic* subdural hematomas. The latter may develop *weeks* after a seemingly trivial injury by fluid osmosis into a small subdural clot.)

Normally, the first examination of the patient can be used to assess the degree of brain dysfunction referable to the original insult, as well as serving as a baseline for future comparisons.

A patient with an enlarging hematoma will show worsening in one or all of four directions during the period of observation:

1. *Responsiveness.* Responsiveness of the patient clearly deteriorates as compared to the baseline examination. For example, a disoriented, combative patient who requires restraint may gradually become "peaceful" and difficult to waken. This change by itself is sufficient to call for prompt intervention. (The obvious danger of giving morphine or barbiturates to agitated patients of this type is clearly apparent because of the serious diagnostic dilemma that results.) Alteration of cerebral function develops because the growing hematoma (the size of a large pancake which may cover at least two-thirds of a cerebral hemisphere) compresses a large area of brain and displaces midline structures under the falx.

2. *Vital signs.* As a result of the hematoma, changes may occur in cerebral regulation of blood pressure, pulse, and respiration. The increasing volume of hematoma with rising intracranial pressure reduces cerebral vascular blood flow by increasing resistance to perfusion. Vasomotor centers in the medulla, responding to the resulting reduction in oxygen supply and the increase in carbon dioxide accumulation, activate vasoconstrictor mechanisms throughout the body to raise systemic blood pressure in

an attempt to improve perfusion. The pulse rate *slows* at about the same time because of increasing intracranial pressure. Despite these compensating factors, cerebral perfusion becomes increasingly inadequate. In this setting, the respiratory center shows evidence of progressive failure manifest by a *periodic* pattern of abnormal respiration (fast, deep breathing alternating with apnea, designated as Cheyne-Stokes breathing). Ultimately the center fails and breathing ceases. Because the respiratory center is more resistant to anoxia than most other brain areas, this latter disturbance, signaling terminus, usually appears late in the clinical course after obtunding of the patient is extreme. Artificial respiration for a patient whose breathing has stopped as a final evidence of brain dysfunction is rarely a useful measure. This anoxia to the respiratory center is enhanced by an additional anatomic factor, namely, the proximity of the bony ring of the foramen magnum to the base of the brain. Increased intracranial pressure forces the cerebellar tonsils into the spinal canal and focal compression of the adjacent medulla occurs.

In the brain-injured patient, it is extremely important to realize that the warning signs of *increasing* blood pressure and *slowing* pulse are the *opposite* of those customarily anticipated with shock. It takes special emphasis in teaching the nursing and house staff to achieve concern about the seriousness of a slow, strong pulse in the brain-injured patient. These changes may occur only *after* the patient has passed a point of no return and cannot be considered sole criteria for urgency of surgical intervention.

**3. *Changes in focal motor ability.*** Changing function of one part of the body under direct motor control by the brain is usually a less striking manifestation of growing hematoma than changes in general responsivenes and in pulse and blood pressure. Nevertheless, such motor changes may be the first sign of a definite worsening in the patient already obtunded by brain contusion or may occasionally represent the first evidence of new intracranial insult in an individual who may be quite alert after head injury.

Usually the first sign of focal cerebral hemispheric dysfunction is hemiparesis. The comparative ability to move the two sides of the body is one of the few evaluations easily made even in the uncooperative patient. Because there may well be some degree of hemiparesis from the initial brain contusion, the significance of this finding resides in quantitative *changes* during the period of observation.

A growing hematoma can cause progressive hemiparesis by two mechanisms: (a) pressure upon the cortical areas of the brain controlling movement can reduce motor function, probably through local interference of the blood supply. This pressure affects movement on the side of the body *opposite* (contralateral) to the hematoma; or (b) in some instances, the *entire* brain can be displaced to the point where the midbrain (through which cerebral impulses are transmitted outward to the body) is thrust against the sharp edge of the tentorial ring of fibrous dura in which it is enclosed. Thus, a right-sided hematoma can gently displace brain toward the left so that the midbrain is then thrust against the sharp edge of the tentorium on the left. As a result the *left* cerebral peduncle and midbrain, carrying impulses for the contralateral side of the body, is mechanically compressed and a hemiparesis results on the *same* side of the body as the hematoma.

Thus, progressing hemiparesis can reflect a hematoma on *either* side of the brain (ipsilateral or contralateral). While this uncertainty of site is of concern to the surgeon, the practical point is that increasing hemiparesis should be recognized as evidence of a growing hematoma. Finally, movement of the arm, face, or leg either voluntarily or in response to a pain stimulus may *seem* to improve in certain circumstances where painful stimuli not previously causing withdrawal of arm or leg now cause it to thrust in extension toward the stimulus. *Actually,* this response is a sign of further worsening of the patient, since it indicates in fact no more than a primitive reflex. It implies that the cerebral hemisphere which had already lost its ability to control contralateral body movements has finally lost its ability to inhibit these primitive reflexes which have gained independent activity because of compression incurred at the level of the midbrain.

4. *The pupils.* Pupillary inequality represents another area of focal neurological change. Minimal difference in pupillary size can exist as a variation of normal. Marked enlargement of one pupil can result from bruising and bleeding within the orbit, in the absence of brain damage. But whenever a pupil approaches full dilatation while its partner remains constricted, uncal hernia-

tion must be presumed in a patient already obtunded from head injury.

In addition to herniation of the cerebellum through the foramen magnum previously described, another site for herniation is through the ring formed by the fibrous tentorium and its lateral bony insertions. (The ring accommodates the connecting isthmus of the midbrain.) That portion of the cerebrum immediately overlying the gap between the tentorial ring and the midbrain is the uncus (the most medial portion of temporal lobe). When the uncus is forced through the ring by hematoma in or above the cerebral hemisphere, the oculomotor nerve (the third cranial nerve) which bridges this aperture between the midbrain and the tentorial edge, is compressed. The resulting nerve dysfunction produces palsy of the muscles which turn the globe of the eye and open the lid. However, pupillary dilatation (i.e., loss of pupillary constrictor innervation) is the most obvious evidence of CN III nerve dysfunction in the obtunded patient.

Loss of CN III nerve function, although not disabling by itself, is a sign of impending catastrophe. If it is caused by a hematoma that has displaced the uncus into the tentorial ring, the next event (often within 15 minutes) is the development of decerebration. This terminal event reflecting compression of the midbrain by the adjacent uncal herniation is accompanied by marked reduction of the blood supply and secondary hemorrhage into this vital brain tissue. All connections between cerebrum and brainstem are interrupted at this stage, and the body is governed only by brainstem reflexes. The first evidence of decerebration is the extensor thrust of an extremity which, on previous stimulation, withdrew purposefully or showed paralysis. It is important to realize that this type of brain death may occur (depending on the site of the hematoma) before a generalized increase in intracranial pressure and cerebellar herniation begin to affect blood pressure, pulse, and breathing. Nevertheless, pupillary inequality precedes decerebration, as do changes in responsiveness and movement, which occur even earlier. Emergency surgical intervention is always indicated, without further observation, when a patient is admitted to the hospital with a dilated pupil; it can be assumed that the earlier signs of worsening have already occurred outside the hospital.

**Intracerebral hematoma.** While intracranial hematoma formation following head injury usually occurs between the skull and the brain, a contusion of the brain can produce an *intracerebral hematoma,* usually in a temporal lobe. A small intracerebral hematoma ordinarily undergoes spontaneous resorption, but a large one (4 or 5 cm in diameter) can gradually enlarge further by imbibing fluid to produce pressure effects, even in the absence of further bleeding. In this situation focal hemiparesis, as well as speech difficulty, is evident particularly when the dominant temporal lobe is involved. These findings are superimposed on the diffuse changes in responsiveness seen with ordinary cerebral contusion. When observed in terms of the four parameters mentioned above, worsening in responsiveness and motor ability become evident over a period of hours or days. These patients then become candidates for either early or late surgical intervention, as in the case of a subdural or extradural hematoma.

**Cerebral edema.** Cerebral contusion, like any contusion elsewhere in the body, is followed by a degree of reactive edema. In the brain this swelling (or cerebral edema) usually reaches its peak at about 60 hours after the initial insult, and then begins to recede. This edema, by itself, can generally be expected to cause a much milder and more gradual deterioration than that seen with actual hematoma formation. The increase in intracranial fluid content is usually safely tolerated and becomes reversible after 60 hours if the patient does not also harbor a hematoma or a widespread cerebral contusion. On rare occasions, when there is marked edema of the brain but no hematoma is present, surgical decompression over the most contused area of the brain may be necessary as a life-saving procedure. Medical measures designed to reduce reactive brain swelling after trauma are discussed subsequently.

**Skull Fracture.** Skull fracture is primarily important when it carries a serious risk of infection. A comminuted fracture underlying a scalp wound contains devitalized tissue and contaminated bone fragments. Careful surgical debridement is required to control this source of infection. A basilar skull fracture which permits CSF to leak from nose or ears demands prophylactic use of antibiotics to prevent meningitis. The resulting dural defect usually heals, but occasionally late surgical repair is necessary if a permanent fistula develops. A clean depressed skull fracture, under intact scalp, may require surgical elevation on the theory that bone pressure on the cortex could set up a seizure focus. The actual intracranial volume occupied by such a depression is insignificant, unless further complicated by hematoma formation.

For these reasons, a skull fracture as such is not usually a serious threat to life; furthermore, it is important to realize that there is no clear correlation between skull fracture and underlying brain contusion after closed-head injury. Large fractures may exist without any accompanying brain contusion or subsequent intracranial bleeding. Conversely, rapidly developing subdural hematomas or serious initial contusions may occur in the absence of a skull fracture.

The site of skull fracture is not a reliable guide for localizing the exact area of brain damage. In some instances the point of maximal contusion can underlie the area of skull fragmentation; but the injury is as likely to be on the opposite side of the head (contrecoup contusion) or to exist primarily in the temporal lobes or hypothalamus because of shearing stresses provided by the configuration of the base of the skull.

On this basis, skull x-rays are of much less significance than careful observation in the management of patients with serious head injuries. Even when x-rays show lateral displacement of a calcified pineal gland from the midline, suggestive of the presence of a hematoma, clinical findings have often already raised this suspicion.

## ASSESSMENT OF THE PROBLEM

**In the emergency ward.** Prior to being admitted to an intensive care facility, most patients with head injuries will first have been examined in an accident ward where emergency treatment is normally instituted. After securing an adequate airway, establishing an intravenous infusion, measuring vital signs, and drawing blood for laboratory testing, specific notation should be made concerning initial neurologic findings. The patient's responsiveness should be described in terms of his behavior, with special note of any changes induced by examination or treatment procedures (such as change in position upon suctioning, venipuncture, etc.). Pupillary inequality must be ascertained immediately, since a unilaterally enlarged pupil is an indication for emergency surgery without awaiting further observation.

**History.** Only after the patient's emergency needs are attended to, and a baseline for subsequent observation established, should time be dedicated to obtaining the history from witnesses. Ideally, another member of the team should obtain the history while emergency treatment is being administered. Particular emphasis is given to the details of the trauma as well as to the patient's behavior since the time of injury. If it can be elicited that the patient awoke temporarily following the blow to his head, but that he is now out of contact again, the presumptive diagnosis of expanding intracranial hematoma can safely be made from this fact alone.

The past history should include facts pertinent to CNS symptoms, diabetes, known vascular disease, and the use of drugs or alcohol. Because of the frequent use of long-term anticoagulant therapy among large numbers of patients with previous myocardial infarction, it is especially important to ascertain the usage of these drugs among patients with head injury. In the event of a history of such therapy, close observation is mandatory, because intracranial hematomas can expand with incredible rapidity in the presence of drug-induced decreased prothrombin activity. In this circumstance a patient may pass from a near normal level of brain function to a point bordering on extremis, within a period of 20 minutes. Immediate administration of Vitamin $K_1$ oxide should be initiated after laboratory evaluation of the impaired clotting mechanism has been demonstrated.

**Physical examination.** As noted, all patients with head injuries should be examined completely to detect concomitant trauma which may be obscured by limited responsiveness. The possibility of intrathoracic or intra-abdominal injury should specifically be considered. The extremities should be examined to ascertain fractures or injuries to nerves or arteries.

**Neurologic examination and subsequent observation.** The major indices of the severity of head injury are:

    a. responsiveness,

    b. motor ability,

    c. vital signs,

    d. pupillary inequality.

Because of their constant attendance at the bedside, nurse members of the team are in a key position to evaluate these parameters. (The specific methods for such evaluation by nurses are described in the nursing role.)

**Trephining the skull.** In the event of either a dilated pupil or changes in responsiveness, motor ability, or vital signs suggesting an intracranial hematoma, the most important diagnostic step involves trephining of the skull and the opening of the dura at the frontal, posterior, and temporal locations bilaterally. If a hematoma is discovered between the brain and the skull, its consistency will determine whether drainage through the multiple skull openings will be sufficient or whether a large bony window must be removed to permit access to a solid clot.

The frontal and occipital trephine openings are used for ventriculography in the event that a surface hematoma is not encountered and further diagnostic information is required.

**Radiological examination.**

    a. *Skull x-rays.* As mentioned previously, skull x-rays are of limited value in assessing the severity of head injury. While the demonstration of a skull fracture may increase the suspicion of hematoma, the only valid evidence for the diagnosis of an intracranial mass is displacement of the pineal gland. Even this radiographic landmark has limited usefulness, since the pineal gland must be calcified to be visualized. Unfortunately, the gland is calcified in only approximately 30% of patients over the age of 45, and rarely in younger persons.

    b. *Arteriography.* The value of x-rays can be enhanced by the use of contrast studies with radiopaque material. The procedure involves the injection of an opaque contrast medium through either the common carotid or the right brachial artery, which permits identification of intracranial blood vessels by x-rays taken at half-second intervals after the injection. Displacement of intracranial arteries and veins will outline a large hematoma and define whether it is intracerebral or extracerebral.

Cerebral arteriography is employed most often in patients who gradually or questionably become drowsier, although reponsive to simple commands.

Perhaps the major disadvantage of cerebral angiography is the time required to complete the study. Depending on the sophistication of available personnel and equipment, angiography may consume 30 to 60 minutes. In the progressively deteriorating patient who has reached a point of poor responsiveness, this time luxury cannot be afforded.

   c. *Ventriculography and pneumoencephalography.* When skull trephination has not revealed a hematoma, and time is a vital factor, a suspected intracranial mass can often be localized by ventriculography. A needle is placed in the ventricle through the previously made trephine opening and the cerebrospinal fluid withdrawn. The volume of CSF is then replaced by air, which casts a radiolucent shadow. A mass lesion displaces or distorts the ventricles from their normal shape and position and can be identified.

The same visualization of the ventricles can be accomplished by pneumoencephalography, where air is introduced into the lumbar *spinal canal* to fill the ventricles. The procedure is normally performed in a sitting position and is stressful to an already sick patient. Therefore, this last test is rarely employed in a patient with acute head injury.

**Lumbar puncture.** Lumbar puncture (LP) yields little information of value in the management of a patient with head injuries. While the puncture may reveal an elevated CSF pressure and the presence of red blood cells, these findings do not define the need for possible surgical intervention. Furthermore, the procedure of LP is not without risk, and sometimes there is a dramatic worsening in neurologic function soon after the test. In most instances the deterioration is related to altered intracranial dynamics that encourage herniation of the cerebellum or uncus. Despite these possible dangers, LP is nevertheless justifiable in diagnostic problems where patients are found unresponsive, and the possible role of trauma is uncertain.

**Echoencephalography.** Although this special test is still in a developmental stage, it offers considerable diagnostic promise. By the reflection (echo) of ultrasound waves it is possible to estimate whether normally midline structures are significantly displaced to one side. This ability to identify midline displacement has the same diagnostic importance as visualization of the pineal gland. The incidence of false negative and false positive results obtained in most medical centers today precludes the use of echo studies as the sole criterion for management decisions.

**Brain scan.** By systematically measuring radioactivity over the surface of the head following the intravenous administration of a short-lived radioactive isotope, certain pathologic changes within the skull can be identified. The "tracer" isotope is usually linked to an albumin compound which reaches diseased brain tissues in high concentration. Both inflammatory processes and a localized increase in vascularity can disturb the blood-brain barrier and result in abnormal concentrations in radioactivity. The test is most useful for defining the location and extent of a brain tumor or abscess. It is also beneficial in detecting a chronic subdural hematoma that occurs weeks after a trivial head injury (not associated with brain contusion). The test does not appear of value in the diagnosis of acute head injuries, because contused areas of the scalp and underlying muscle often show increased radioactive uptake which may be confused with an intracranial hematoma.

## PRINCIPLES OF TREATMENT

**1. Control of pain and of hyperactivity.** In the early stages of observation, where change in responsiveness of the patient is a major factor in assessment, it is important that cerebration not be impaired by narcotics. Pain must be managed by the judicious use of codeine or other mild analgesics. Morphine is likely to depress the patient's responsiveness severely and at the same time to cause pupillary constriction which interferes with this important parameter of observation. For these reasons morphine is to be avoided in patients with acute head injuries.

Severe restlessness or hyperactivity is best managed by the use of short-acting agents, as sodium amytal intramuscularly, or paraldehyde. A cautious small dose of these drugs is used initially and increasing amounts are given thereafter as necessary. Patients with serious complications who are severely agitated or extremely uncooperative and noisy should not be sedated simply because their behavior is disturbing to others. Ideally, combative patients should be kept in an isolated soundproof room and managed by an intelligent combination of limited sedation and carefully applied restraints (when absolutely necessary).

**2. Control of convulsions.** Anticonvulsant therapy may be used *prophylactically* when the nature of the brain injury is such that seizures are anticipated. Once a seizure has occurred, anticonvulsants are *always* used, as additional seizures are to be expected; these will complicate future assessment and management of the patient. The usual program for maintenance therapy includes phenobarbital (32 mgm t.i.d.) and Dilantin (100 mgm t.i.d.). In case of repeated major seizures the dosages of these drugs may be increased and supplemented with short-acting agents such as sodium amytal.

**3. Control of cerebral edema.** When cerebral edema is associated with a gradual worsening of the patient's condition, the problem is best managed by the use of the cortical steroid, dexamethasone. With a marked degree of cerebral edema, the full dosage of this steroid is 10 mgm intravenously initially and 4 mgm intramuscularly every 6 hours thereafter. Disadvantages of steroid therapy include the possibility of poor wound healing, lowering of resistance to infection, and the reactivation of peptic ulcer disease. Customarily, steroids are used only briefly during the acute phase, and the dosage is reduced rapidly as circumstances permit.

Both intravenous urea and mannitol often produce a dramatic reduction of brain swelling. Although the use of these compounds is unfortunately followed by a rebound effect, both agents are nevertheless considered indispensable for temporarily controlling a rapidly deteriorating intracranial situation until surgical intervention can be accomplished. The value of low molecular weight dextran for improving brain perfusion and treating edema has not been clearly established to date.

**4. Prevention of stress ulcers.** Acute ulceration of the stomach and duodenum commonly develop after head injury. Atropine has been used to prevent this complication. By inhibiting vagal impulses this drug theoretically reduces the risk of stress ulcers, which presumably occur from autonomic imbalances associated with the injury. At the same time it may be appropriate to employ nasogastric tube feedings and antacid therapy, provided there is adequate peristalsis and that no significant abdominal distention or gastric retention develops after the feedings.

**5. Control of infection.** Antibiotics are often used prophylactically for head wounds associated with drainage of CSF. In general, however, it is good practice to reserve antibiotics for specific infections and to use them aggressively and effectively at that time. Criteria for antibiotic treatment include the development of pneumonia and atelectasis in the obtunded patient, and urinary tract infections related to catheter drainage.

**6. Control of respiratory insufficiency and metabolic disturbances.** Among patients with severe cerebral contusion, respiratory insufficiency is a common complication. This results from a combination of factors, including reduced or absent spontaneous activity and decreased responsiveness. Ventilatory assistance by means of tracheostomy and a mechanical respirator is usually required. It is essential that adequate oxygenation be maintained and that blood $O_2$, $CO_2$, and pH be determined at regular intervals. It is important to recognize that cerebral anoxia from inadequate respiratory exchange is a leading cause of death in head injuries (Mayfield and McBride).

Furthermore, the obtunded patient will likely suffer imbalance in hypothalamic-endocrine control of water and electrolyte balance. Monitoring of blood levels of BUN, pH and electrolytes, and assay of urinary electrolyte output and concentration become temporarily necessary to support the patient within safe levels of chemical balance by proper direction of fluids administered.

**7. Use of hypothermia.** In some medical centers, the induction and maintenance of prolonged hypothermia has achieved popularity as a therapeutic measure capable of contributing to the survival of patients with severe brain contusions. In principle, the brain suffering from contusion, edema, and arterial spasm (all of which reduce perfusion) is more likely to survive the ischemic period if its metabolic needs are reduced. Specifically, the brain's metabolic requirements appear to be reduced about 6.5% with each degree of body temperature reduction. Thus, at a hypothermic level of 32° C the brain's oxygen requirements are 33% lower than at normothermic (37° C) levels. Equally significant, the metabolic requirements at normal temperature are 20% lower than those existing with a *hyperthermic* level of 40° C.

While there is attractive experimental evidence in animals to suggest that induced hypothermia reduces the reaction to brain injury, the evidence regarding human head injuries is less clear. The uncertainty relates to the inherent difficulty of treating comparable cases (no two head injuries are entirely alike), with and without hypothermia, to prove the true efficacy of treatment. Hypothermia is *not* frequently selected as a therapeutic measure, because its long-term use creates many problems and these disadvantages must be weighed against the anticipated beneficial effect. For example, when the temperature is reduced below 35° C, both responsiveness and motor ability of the patient are reduced; at still lower levels of 32° or 33° C, even the monitoring of vital signs becomes difficult. The clinical picture is further confused by the need for autonomic blocking agents to control shivering and vasoconstriction. These drugs can produce hypotension and undesirable degrees of sedation, and for these reasons the usual assessment of brain function in terms of responsiveness, motor ability, and vital signs is interfered with. Thus, during hypothermia, the elevation in blood pressure anticipated with a hematoma may be obscured by the antagonistic effect of autonomic blockers. Similarly, the significance of pulse rate is lost because of the cardiac slowing created by this artificial hibernation. With the loss of these indices, a new intracranial event may not be recognized until the final, near-terminal signs of unilateral pupillary dilatation or Cheyne-Stokes breathing have occurred.

The principle of body cooling is primarily valuable in achieving *normothermia* in patients with hypothalamic injury where disturbances of the temperature mechanisms create hyperthermic body temperatures of 40° C or higher.

## THE NURSING ROLE

**General considerations.** The goals of care during the acute phase of illness in patients with head injuries are shared by the physician-nurse team. The major aims are twofold: (1) *to recognize promptly the early manifestations of worsening intracranial status* and to plan for immediate appropriate surgical intervention when indicated; the patient with head injury is particularly vulnerable to rapid intracranial changes which can lead to irreversible neurologic damage or death if undetected and untreated; and (2) *to provide measures of care for the helpless patient which will sustain and maintain* physiologic function until self-sufficiency returns. In effect, this second goal is directed toward minimizing complications and promoting recovery.

**Clinical observations.** Because the extent and progress of head injury are best assessed by comparing the clinical condition at periodic intervals, it is essential that nurse specialists be trained to recognize pertinent findings which reflect the patient's status.

Assessment is conducted in the following manner:

1. *Responsiveness.*

a. Does the patient respond to questioning? This fact can be one of the most important indications of severity of brain damage. It is important to ascertain and specifically record the patient's orientation to person and environment.

b. If he does not respond to questioning, can he follow commands? The ability to follow commands indicates that a degree of responsiveness remains. In order to compare subsequent observations, it is important that an established procedure be followed by all personnel in describing the patient's ability to respond to command. A suggested routine for this purpose should include procedures which also test motor ability at the same time (e.g., protrusion of tongue, elevation of arms, etc.).

c. Is the patient unresponsive to questioning and command and thus out of contact? Assessment of the totally unresponsive patient should include the following type of observations: Does he move in a purposeful and appropriate manner (either spontaneously or in response to a change in body position)? Is he increasingly agitated or increasingly inert?

The response to painful stimuli applied to each foot and hand should be specifically noted in patients out of contact. The intensity of stimulus required to evoke a response reflects the general level of consciousness, while the character of movement (i.e., a failure to withdraw, purposeful withdrawal, or reflex thrust toward the stimulus) is an index of focal motor ability.

2. *Motor ability.* Changes in motor ability can readily be detected in the conscious patient by simple testing:

a. The patient is directed to show the examiner his teeth. The facial expression on both sides of the face should be observed during this maneuver to detect any signs of asymmetry of the facial muscles.

b. The patient is asked to lift his arms halfway to the vertical plane and to hold them in this position. A downward drift or wobbling of one arm is a sensitive index of beginning weakness and is usually a more valuable guide than comparison of hand grip (which is prone to subjective interpretation).

c. Strength of dorsiflexion of the feet and toes is tested against the resistance of the observer's hand (patients with multiple injuries may experience pain on lifting the entire leg from the bed but can dorsiflex the toes without discomfort). This test affords a simple means of ascertaining leg strength.

3. *Vital signs.* The pulse rate, blood pressure, rate of respiration and temperature must be recorded at frequent intervals. Classically, intracranial hematomas produce slowing of the pulse and elevation of the blood pressure (the systolic pressure increases while the diastolic pressure remains essentially the same).

Unfortunately, these changes in vital signs are often *late* consequences of head injury; they follow the earlier warning changes found in the degree of responsiveness.

4. *Pupillary inequality.* The detection of a major difference in pupil size after head injury has unique significance in the assessment of the problem. Unlike variations in responsiveness, vital signs, and motor ability, all of which can be appraised only on the basis of repeated observation, the finding of a unilaterally dilated pupil is strong evidence for the mechanical effects of intracranial hematoma. This sole finding usually demands immediate surgical intervention, and further observation for progression (in this case, to irreversible decerebration) is distinctly ill-advised.

Pupillary inequality is best determined by comparing the pupils *simultaneously* in an equal light of sufficient intensity. This technique is more accurate than examination of the pupils individually with a bright flashlight. In a cooperative patient the pupillary size can be simply observed during the course of a conversation. If the patient will not (or cannot) open his eyelids, the examiner should simultaneously lift both lids and examine the pupil size, using a light of comfortable intensity. When swelling of the lids prevents visualization, a decision must be made whether observation of the pupils is of sufficient importance to merit the injection of proteolytic enzymes (e.g., Wydase) into the lids to reduce swelling.

5. *Drainage of cerebrospinal fluid from nose or ear.* Just as any dressing applied to a wound must be examined for the amount and character of drainage, the patient with head injury must be observed for signs of leakage from the nose or ears. When a communication exists between the intracranial contents and the exterior, a mixture of blood and CSF will be recognized. It is important to distinguish blood draining from local trauma (e.g., a fractured nose) and bloody CSF. In the latter instance, blood-CSF mixture produces a watery, pale ring surrounding a bloody center on a gauze pad.

When a clear nasal discharge exists, the fluid may be either CSF or merely watery mucus. These fluids can be distinguished by the use of Testape, which gives a positive sugar reaction with CSF and a negative reaction to mucus.

CSF drainage from the nose or ear should not be controlled

by packing. The fluid should be collected in a loosely slung external bandage and the amount of drainage estimated periodically. Similarly, the ear and nose should not be suctioned to clear these fluid contents, because of the threat of introducing infection.

CSF leakage usually stops spontaneously and is not a serious complication of head injury in its own right, provided that it is recognized and treated (by prophylactic antibiotics).

**6. *Seizures.*** The nurse must be keenly aware of the possibility of seizures following head trauma, and should be prepared to observe and record these events as they occur. It is important that the nurse-observer realize that she may be the only person to witness a seizure and her description of the event assumes great importance because it may define the site of injury; obviously, seizure activity cannot be repeated at will. The nurse should include the following in her description of a seizure:

a. How was the patient positioned at the time?

b. Were the movements of a repetitive jerking character (clonic seizure) or did they involve stiffening (tonic seizure)?

c. What was the behavior of all four extremities and face?

d. In what direction did the head turn?

e. What was the position of the eyes?

f. Was the patient incontinent of urine or feces?

g. Was breathing adequate during the seizure or did cyanosis result from breath-holding?

h. What was the duration of seizure movements?

i. What was the interval before the patient returned to his previous level of responsiveness? (Post-ictal depression).

**Temperature Control Technique.** Currently, the use of hypothermia is employed less and less in patients with head injuries and intracranial surgery (see following pages). Rather, the aim of temperature control is that of maintaining *normothermia*. Nursing measures employed to combat hyperthermia and resultant further brain damage include the standard use of aspirin, tepid sponging, placement of ice bags to the groin and axillary areas, and reduction of the patient's environmental temperature. An electrically controlled cooling mattress, popularly referred to by its misnomer "ice mattress," is frequently utilized for this same purpose of maintaining normothermia. Principles of nursing care in temperature reduction are listed below and are selectively applicable to the promotion of either aim—the maintenance of normothermia or the induction and use of hypothermia.

1. Temperature reduction can be accomplished with an electrically controlled cooling mattress. One type of mattress includes a dorsal and ventral layer which enables the patient to be completely encased in the cooling coils. Other lightweight and flexible mattresses are designed to cover just the trunk and as such are perhaps the most adaptable for routine use, particularly since their use prevents weight on the patient's chest area, which may depress respiration.

A light blanket or a sheet should be placed between the patient and the cooling mattress when hypothermia is initiated.

2. The hypothermic equipment is designed to achieve and maintain a desired body temperature. This requires continuous monitoring of the body temperature, either with an esophageal or a rectal thermometry system.

3. The body's response to cold is that of peripheral constriction and shivering. In effect, shivering represents a mechanism for *producing* heat, and this muscular activity must be controlled if a lowered body temperature is to be achieved. Herein rests the fallacy of ice vs. tepid water sponging. The former can produce shivering and promote the very feature, unwanted heat, which it has been employed to reduce. Furthermore, shivering, if prolonged, can induce the added hazards of metabolic acidosis and myocardial irritability. Shivering can usually be prevented (or at least controlled) by the use of chlorpromazine (Thorazine), or promethazine HCl (Phenergan).

4. The collection of clinical data and their interpretation can be complex (in a hypothermic individual). For example, low blood pressure per se should not be accepted at its face value and interpreted as a sign of shock. In some instances there is an apparent decrease in blood pressure because of peripheral vasoconstriction (secondary to chilling) which gives spuriously low readings on auscultation. Secondly, Thorazine, in the dosages required to prevent shivering, is capable of producing profound hypotension in a patient with brain damage (Bloor).

5. A major objective of nursing care is to maintain the desired reduced body temperature. This aim is sometimes difficult to achieve when employing hypothermia, especially in obese patients, in whom downward "drifting" below the desired level may occur. In this circumstance, fat deposits (along with the skin and muscles) continue to cool blood, resulting in peripheral temperatures several degrees lower than that recorded in the esophagus or rectum. This feature of "drifting" requires that the machine be turned off at a point two degrees before the desired temperature is reached; otherwise the patient's temperature may continue to drop further after the cooling is discontinued. More sophisticated hypothermic equipment includes combined systems for cooling and warming, with the patient's temperature controlling a thermostatic device which automatically regulates the temperature at a predetermined level.

6. If the physician should direct control of temperature below normothermic levels, it is mandatory that continuous electrocardiographic monitoring be utilized once the body temperature is reduced below 35° C. At this level cardiac arrhythmias are common and sudden death may occur. The nurse should observe the monitoring system to detect the occurrence of premature ventricular contractions which ordinarily precede the onset of fatal ventricular fibrillation. Equipment for defibrillation should be at the bedside whenever hypothermia is employed.

7. Prolonged use of cooling devices can result in frostbite. It is essential that the electrical thermometry system be occasionally checked against a standard clinical thermometer, because these instruments are not foolproof, and dangerously low temperatures can be inadvertently reached by machine malfunction.

It is important to lubricate the body at the onset of hypothermia and periodically thereafter. This protection, along with frequent inspection of the total body surface, is a necessary component of nursing management.

Areas of the body distal to the heart, particularly hands and feet, require special attention in order to guard against prolonged effects of cold and reduced circulation. Together with frequent inspection, boots and mitts can be improvised for purposes of additional protection.

## THE NURSING ROLE: A CASE PRESENTATION

Various facets of the nursing role in the management of the patient with head injury can best be demonstrated by the following case history:

**History and initial course.** A 22-year-old college student was brought to the hospital emergency ward approximately 20 minutes after involvement in an auto accident. The history obtained from fellow passengers is as follows: the patient was riding in the right front seat and had neglected to fasten his seat belt. Road conditions were slippery and the auto ran head-on into the rear of a halted car at an intersection. The impact and sudden deceleration were sufficient to throw the patient forward, causing his head to strike the dashboard. He seemed out of contact for perhaps half a minute, but then began to moan and clutch his head. On the way to the hospital he seemed confused, but was fully cooperative while awaiting emergency care in the examining room.

Physical examination revealed that he was bleeding vigorously from a left frontal scalp laceration; the bleeding was temporarily controlled by a pressure bandage. The patient complained of generalized headache and looked uncomfortable. He remembered nothing of the accident and had retrograde amnesia; his last memory was of being in a theatre he had left three hours previously. His recall resumed at the point of being helped out of the car at the hospital. Except for this interval of amnesia, his mental status and orientation appeared intact.

The vital signs were all normal. There was no loss of motor ability of face, arms or legs. Two observations were of concern: on plantar stimulation of the left foot, extension of the left great toe was noted (Babinski's sign), and there was mild involuntary resistance to forward flexing of the neck and to flexing the extended legs at the hip (Kernig's sign).

The original clinical impression was that the patient had sustained more than a simple concussion and that a mild cerebral contusion was present. The basis of this conclusion was the presence of amnesia, the fact that the patient was confused after recovering consciousness, his reflex abnormality (Babinski's sign), and the signs of meningeal irritation indicative of the leakage of blood from the contused surface into the CSF (Kernig's sign).

In view of the patient's good condition, skull x-rays were obtained to rule out a comminuted fracture underlying a skull laceration. (In the absence of a laceration, skull films would probably not have been obtained. If a comminuted fracture exists, the contaminated bone fragments must be removed before suture of the scalp incision.) The radiographic examination showed no fracture and, as anticipated in a young man, there was no pineal gland calcification to serve as a guidepost to the presence or absence of a still asymptomatic intracerebral hematoma.

As the laceration was being closed under local anesthesia, the patient complained bitterly of an increasing headache, and he vomited. Physical examination showed that the patient was still oriented and that motor performance and vital signs remained normal. Because of the increasing headache and the occurrence of vomiting (a more important prognostic sign in adults than in children, who often vomit after trivial concussion), the patient was transferred to the intensive care area.

**Admission to the intensive care area.** Assessment of the patient's condition was made immediately by the physician-nurse team. Baseline observations were recorded as follows:

*Responsiveness:* "He complains of headache and acts as if he does not want to be disturbed. He knows the name of the hospital, the day, and the approximate time."

*Motor ability:* "He can hold his arms extended without drift. The tongue is extended and there is a symmetrical grimace of the facial muscles. Dorsiflexion of the toes shows equal strength bilaterally."

*Vital signs:* "Temperature was 37.2° C; blood pressure 130/80; pulse rate 96. Respirations are even and slightly hurried at a rate of 24 (probably because the patient is uncomfortable)."

*Pupil size:* "The pupils are equal."

Subsequent observation and recording of these parameters was scheduled at 15-minute intervals thereafter.

**Plan of care.** The following plans were established by the team:

1. The nurse will observe the patient and notify the physician immediately if there is any significant worsening in any of the four parameters of observation.

2. Blood is to be drawn for hematocrit, white blood count, and cross match for 3 units of blood in the event surgical intervention becomes necessary.

3. Because of the possibility of surgery and the fact that the patient has vomited, an intravenous infusion consisting of 2.5% dextrose and saline solution is to be started and allowed to drip slowly at a rate of 75 cc per hour.

4. When the patient's parents arrive, they may visit with the patient briefly and should remain to talk to one of the house staff. As a kindness to an anxious family, the physician will ask the nurse member of the team to explain the situation before they see the patient. The family can be advised that the patient shows evidence of having sustained a mild bruise to the brain and that full recovery may be expected. In the meantime he is being observed closely in the intensive care unit for the possible development of a blood clot which would require surgery.

5. The only drug to be used is 32 mg of codeine for headache. This dosage should give partial control of pain without contributing to the obtundation of the patient.

**Initial clinical course.** The vital signs and pupillary size were checked every 15 minutes and recorded on a flow sheet. Observations, made by the nursing team, were recorded as follows:

12:00 Midnight—Volunteers that his headache is severe; oriented to time and place; cooperates for motor testing; no motor deficit found.

12:05 a.m.—Blood drawn. Intravenous started.

12:15 a.m.—Urine specimen obtained. Moaning frequently and complains of headache. Remains oriented to time and place. Cooperates grudgingly to motor testing; questionable slight drift of left arm (Fig. 1), but drift disappears when patient is asked to try harder.

12:25 a.m.—Brief emesis of 20 cc bile-colored fluid. No airway problem. Still oriented, but questions must be repeated to get response. Dr. Jones notified in operating room and intern called.

12:30 a.m.—Intern examined patient, agreed that left arm drift is present. The intern then called the neurosurgical resident, who instructed him to prepare a unit of urea for use and to advise the blood bank that transfusions might be needed. He then notified the operating room and the anesthesia department to mobilize

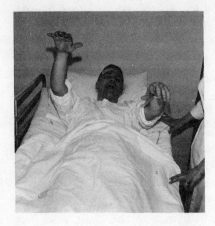

Fig. 1. Drift of left arm as the cooperative patient attempts to lift arms equally.

Fig. 2. Patient now lifts only right arm on command to lift both.

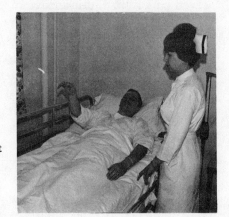

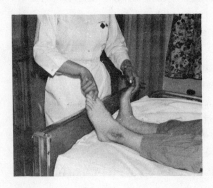

Fig. 3. The examiner detects definite weakness in left toe dorsiflexion.

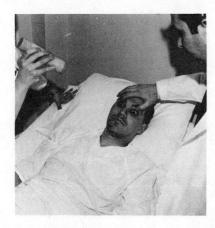

Fig. 4. The right pupil is now larger than the left.

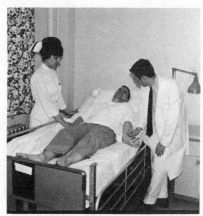

Fig. 5. The left arm, not moved voluntarily, responds to pin stimulus by extension of elbow and flexion of wrist and fingers.

personnel for craniotomy. (The family was also advised of the likely need for surgery in view of the changing clinical picture.) 12:40 a.m.—Emesis 30 cc. No airway difficulties. Patient now only mutters in response to questions; will not lift arm from bed (Fig. 2), but right arm moves normally. Slight weakness of left face and left toes now apparent (Fig. 3). Urea infusion started by intern.

12:45 a.m.—On repeated command patient moves right arm and leg, but cannot move left arm or leg. Right pupil *now slightly larger than left* (Fig. 4). Neurosurgical resident here. (In addition to confirming the nurse's observations, the resident stimulated the left arm and foot with a pin. Instead of a hoped-for purposeful withdrawal from the stimulus, the patient responded by thrusting the left arm with flexion of the wrist and fingers (Fig. 5) and by the thrusting of the left leg rather than withdrawing from the stimulus. This pattern suggested uncal herniation and the onset of decerebration. Compression of the midbrain was suggested by the enlargement of the right pupil, indicating third-nerve impingement.)

12:50 a.m.—Foley catheter was inserted and 20 cc of urine obtained. Atropine—0.6 mgm given I.M. Patient transferred to OR for craniotomy.

Skilled nursing observation, with understanding of the implications of the changing clinical course, permitted prompt surgical intervention as soon as an intracranial emergency was suspected. It is important to recognize the significance of careful observation in assessing a worsening course. Vital signs, by themselves, would not have suggested a changing status until a much later time (12:40 a.m., or 25 minutes after the nurse first noticed left arm drift). Reliance on vital signs alone might well have resulted in irreversible changes or death.

**Surgical intervention.** As the patient's head was being shaved in the operating room, a rapid urinary output was noted along with a temporary improvement in his intracranial situation as a result of the dehydrative effect of the urea. Responsiveness improved to the point where the patient demanded the doctors stop shaving his head. His right pupil returned to an equal size with the left, and he was able to move his left arm and leg weakly on command. The blood pressure returned to a more normal level of 130/80.

Under light general anesthesia administered through an endotracheal tube, a right coronal trephine was performed and revealed a solid blood clot between bone and dura. A small amount of clot forced its way through the bony opening. In view of the now established diagnosis of epidural hematoma with the probability of continued active bleeding from a torn artery on the dural surface, a large temporal bony opening was created. A solid blood clot about 4 cm in thickness was removed. Active bleeding welled up from beneath the remaining clot. The dura was then rapidly freed from the inner table of the skull down to the floor of the middle fossa, where the point of arterial bleeding was visualized and controlled. Following this, the remainder of the clot was removed, after which the muscle and scalp incisions were closed.

The patient awoke promptly on discontinuation of the anesthesia, answered questions with few words, cooperated in commands, but was not oriented. He was barely able to lift his left arm and left leg from the stretcher and still showed obvious weakness of these extremities. The pupils were equal and vital signs were at their pre-emergency level. He was returned to the intensive care unit at 2:45 a.m.

**Postoperative course.** The physician-nurse team discussed the immediate program of care. Two major threats existed. (1) A possibility existed (about 5%) that bleeding from a small dural surface vessel could resume insidiously and re-form an intracranial hematoma. (2) Cerebral edema was to be anticipated. This swelling results from the insult of the original brain contusion and the later brain compression by the hematoma.

*The basic orders* included:

1. Observation of the previously described parameters every 15 minutes.

2. Careful measurement of I.V. fluid intake and urinary output.

3. Prevention of postoperative atelectasis by turning the patient hourly, and deep breathing and coughing exercises.

4. Prophylactic anticonvulsant therapy (phenobarbital and Dilantin) because of the strong possibility of seizures following removal of hematoma.

5. Codeine for headaches if the patient is alert enough to demand relief of pain.

6. Portable skull x-rays, to be used as a baseline to identify the initial position of the silver clips tagged to the dura during surgery. In the event of a recurrence of a hematoma, subsequent x-rays will show a change in the position of these markers, indicating that a mass has again developed between the skull and the dura.

During the first three hours significant improvement was apparent, with a full recovery of the left hemiparesis and the return

of orientation. The nurse noted that the patient now had a retrograde amnesia for the hospital period prior to surgery. He was
alert and inquired about the surgery and about the probable
length of his hospital stay. He remained in good condition
through the next 12 hours, although he appeared somewhat more
sluggish in his behavior and complained about his headache.
Temperature elevation to 38° C developed.

The nursing note, 12 hours after surgery, indicated the following: "There was twitching of the left hand which, after 5
seconds, spread to involve the left face and left leg. The head and
eyes turned to the left after which there was a brief generalized
convulsion, with breath holding but no cyanosis. The patient
awakened promptly and was oriented, but slightly lethargic. Some
drifting of the left arm is noted. The neurosurgical resident was
called promptly."

The question was whether this episode represented intracranial worsening or whether the dosage of anticonvulsant medication was inadequate to control the seizures. The left-arm drift was
explainable on a post-ictal basis. Close serial observation was essential to rule out the possibility of a fresh hematoma. The physician
chose to increase the dosages of phenobarbital and Dilantin, and
additional amounts were given intravenously at once. A syringe
containing 250 mgm of sodium amytal was placed in readiness at
the bedside.

Twenty minutes later twitching resumed in the left hand, followed by turning of the head and eyes to the left; the patient remained in contact. At this point the physician injected the sodium
amytal, which controlled the seizure within 10 seconds, before it
became generalized. Four similar focal seizures occurred within
the first 24 hours, but they were confined to the left hand, with
no loss of consciousnes. No additional seizures were noted thereafter.

At 36 hours postoperative a very gradual worsening in responsiveness was apparent. The nursing note stated, "He sleeps
when not disturbed. He did not know the time, the day, or his
whereabouts. He would say, 'My headache is not too bad.' He follows commands. There is a moderate drift of the left arm. The
vital signs have been stable except for a temperature elevation to
38.5° C and a pulse rate of 92."

The increasing fever, the worsening in responsiveness, and the left-arm drift were of concern. Physical examination by the physician showed no signs of atelectasis or pneumonia to account for the fever. Urine analysis disclosed no white cells. It was felt that the fever was likely the result of meningeal irritation due to disintegration of blood within the cerebrospinal fluid ("chemical meningitis"). However, because of stiff neck a lumbar puncture was done to rule out bacterial meningitis. The fluid was deeply yellow, showed normal sugar content, 400 wbc (and subsequent negative culture).

Regardless of the cause of the fever, its progression must be halted because of the increased metabolic demands it creates in an already injured brain. Normally, the temperature should be controlled below 38° C. In this case the original approach involved use of aspirin every 3 hours by mouth and exposure of the body to air-conditioning. In the event of higher temperatures, regulation of body heat to normothermic levels may have to be achieved with hypothermic equipment.

It was concluded that the changes in responsiveness and motor ability were the result of cerebral edema. Nevertheless, repeat skull x-rays were obtained and showed the silver clips at their original position against the skull wall.

Recognizing that cerebral edema would progress for perhaps another 24 hours, corticosteroid therapy was initiated. Ten mgm of dexamethasone was given intravenously initially and 4 mgm I.M. ordered every 6 hours thereafter. Since the average dose of phenobarbital used to control seizures may contribute to obtundation, the dosage was reduced to ordinary maintenance levels.

The patient remained sluggishly responsive for another 24 hours and then rapidly became alert and regained full arm strength. He was transferred from the ICU to standard hospital quarters on the fourth postoperative day and discharged home on the eighth day.

This true life example is presented to contrast the sudden acute developments requiring early recognition and surgical intervention with the gradual postoperative evolving problems of seizures, fever, and cerebral edema which were properly differentiated from postoperative hematoma formation and appropriately treated.

## Bibliography

ALEXANDER, D. M. and SIMON, M. D.: Cerebral Angiography. *Nursing Times,* 57:116–117, 123–124, January 27, 1961.

BROOKS, H. L.: The Golden Rule for the Unconscious Patient. *Nursing Forum,* 4:12–18, March 1965.

BLOOR, B. M.: Intracranial Bleeding, in *Current Therapy,* pp. 492–493. H.F. COON, (ed.), W. B. Saunders Co., Philadelphia, 1963.

CAVENESS, W. F., WALKER, A. E., (ed.): *Head Injury Conference Proceedings.* Lippincott Co., Philadelphia, 1966.

CHESNEY, D. N.: Echoencephalography. *Nursing Times,* 62:498–500, April 15, 1966.

DOONAN, K. A.: Extradural Hematoma. *Canadian Nurse,* 58:828–834, September 1960.

EVANS, J. P.: Acute Trauma to the Head. *Postgraduate Medicine,* 39:27–30, January 1966.

EVANS, J. P., et al.: Experimental and Clinical Observations on Rising Intracranial Pressure. *Archives Surgery,* 63:107–114, July 1951.

FRY, O. M.: Aspects of the Postoperative Care of Neurosurgical Patients. *Amer. J. Nursing,* 35:16–18, January 1935.

GAUTIER-SMITH, P. C.: Hazards of Lumbar Puncture. *Nursing Mirror,* 121:xiii–xvi, October 22, 1965.

GIBSON, J.: Mental Effects of Head Injury. *Canadian Nurse.* 55:1118–1119, December 1959.

GIBSON, R. M.: Subdural Haematoma. *Nursing Times,* 57:267–269, March 3, 1961.

GLEASON, A. M.: Cerebral Edema: Care of the Patient. *Amer. J. Nursing,* 61:93–94, March 1961.

GURDJIAN, ELISHA S. and WEBSTER, JOHN E.: *Mechanisms, Diagnosis and Management of Head Injuries.* Little, Brown, Boston, 1958.

HARDIMAN, M.: Intracerebral Haematoma. *Nursing Times,* 56:308–310, March 11, 1960.

HICKEY, M. C.: Hypothermia. *American Journal of Nursing,* 65:116–122, January 1965.

HOUSEPIAN, E. M.: Current Problems in the Surgical Management of Pain. *AORN,* 3:70–75, September–October 1965.

LEAK, W. N.: Body Temperature and Hypothermia. *Nursing Times.* 53:374–376, April 5, 1957.

LOCKHARDT, P.: Social Rehabilitation Following Severe Head Injuries. *Nursing Mirror,* 118:48–50, April 17, 1964.

MAYFIELD, FRANK H. and McBRIDE, BERT H.: Craniocerebral Trauma. In *Neurological Surgery of Trauma,* Arnold M. Meirowsky (ed.),

Office of the Surgeon General, Department of the Army, Government Printing Office, Washington, D.C., 1965.

MEIROWSKY, ARNOLD M., (ed.): *Neurological Survey of Trauma,* Office of Surgeon General, Department of the Army, Washington, D.C., 1965.

MULLAN, SEAN: *Essentials of Neurosurgery,* Springer Publishing Co., Inc., New York, 1961, pp. 137–158.

New Radiographic & Isotopic Procedures in Neurological Diagnosis. *JAMA,* 188:524–529, May 11, 1964.

*Neurological Surgery of Trauma,*
Prepared and published under the direction of Lt. Gen. Leonard D. Heaton; Editor-in-Chief, Colonel John Boyd Coates, Jr.; Editor, Arnold M. Meirowsky; Office of the Surgeon General, Dept. of the Army, Washington, D.C., 1965. Supt. of Documents, U.S. Gov. Printing Office, Washington, D.C.

PENNYBACKER, J. B.: Abscess of the Brain—I. *Nursing Mirror,* 95:239–241, June 13, 1952.

PENNYBACKER, J. B.: Abscess of the Brain—II. *Nursing Mirror,* 95: 267–268, June 20, 1952.

POOL, J. LAWRENCE and POTTS, D. GORDON, *Aneurysms and Arteriovenous Anomalies of the Brain,* Harper and Row, New York, 1965.

POTTER, J. M.: Complications of Head Injury. *Nursing Times,* 61:892–893, July 2, 1965.

POTTER, J. M.: Nursing Observations of Patients with Head Injuries. *Nursing Times,* 58:1310–1313, October 19, 1962.

RAMEY, R. B.: The Minor Concussion. *Amer. J. Nursing,* 57:1444–1445, November 1957.

RADLEY-SMITH, E. J.: Abscesses of the Brain. *Nursing Mirror,* 117:i–iii, December 6, 1963.

RAMSAY, A. M.: Infections of the Central Nervous System 2 Acute aseptic meningitis, meningo-encephalitis and acute encephalitis. *Nursing Mirror,* 114:iii–vi, xii, August 3, 1962.

REGAN, M.: The Nursing of Intracranial Cases. *Amer. J. Nursing,* 30:695–701, June 1930.

ROB, C.: Diagnosis and Treatment of Extracranial Arterial Occlusion. *Am. Assoc. Industr. Nurses J.,* 12:6–9, July 1964.

ROWLAND B.: Neurosurgery and Hypothermia. *Canadian Nurse,* 56: 697–701, August 1960.

RUSSELL, W. R.: Some Reactions of the Nervous System to Trauma. *Brit. Med. J.,* 2:403–407, August 15, 1964.

SHERWOOD, T.: Surgery in the Treatment of Pain. *Nursing Times,* 57:1129, September 1, 1961.

SLOBERG, P. S.: Medical Management of Intracranial Aneurysm. *The Heart Bulletin,* Michigan Heart Association, July–August, 1962, pp. 73–77.

STEPHENS, C. M.: Drugs for Patients with Severe Head Injuries. *Nursing Times,* 59:1510, November 29, 1963.

STEPHEN, C. R.: Current Status of Hypothermia. *Anesthesia and Analgesia,* 54:97–103, January–February, 1964.

SYMONDS, C. P.: Concussion and Its Sequelae. *Lancet,* 1:1–5, 1962.

TASKER, R. R.: Increased Intracranial Pressure. *Canadian Nurse,* 61: 207–208, March 1965.

TOLLEFSRUD, V. E.: When a Patient Has Chemosurgery. *Amer. J. Nursing,* 59:1414–1416, October 1959.

YOUNG, J. F.: Recognition, Recording, Significance of the Signs of Increased Intracranial Pressure. *Canadian Nurse,* 61:209–212, March 1965.

*Film:* "Essentials of the Neurological Examination." Smith, Kline and French Laboratories, Philadelphia, Pa., 1962.

# CHAPTER XI

# Chest Surgery

JEAN MAC VICAR, R.N., M.S.
HARVEY J. MENDELSOHN, M.D.

## THE PROBLEM

Patients who have undergone surgical procedures, or sustained injuries, involving the chest wall, pleura, lung, mediastinal structures, and/or diaphragm may develop important and dangerous physiological and biochemical alterations postoperatively. These problems are caused basically by inadequate pulmonary ventilation and/or inadequate pulmonary or systemic blood circulation.

When ventilation is inadequate, the patient will become hypoxic from lack of oxygen, and/or hypercapneic or acidotic from retention of carbon dioxide in the arterial blood. These disturbances may produce a variety of clinical symptoms and signs, or may exist only in a subclinical form, becoming apparent shortly before catastrophic respiratory and/or cardiac arrest.

Inadequate circulation of blood to the lungs and peripheral tissues usually results from blood loss with low cardiac output. The reduction in circulation contributes to generalized hypoxia and acidosis; it also may lead to ischemia of such vital organs as the brain, heart, kidneys, or liver. These latter changes may be irreversible if not quickly corrected. The end effects of circulatory and respiratory insufficiency are interrelated, and their relative significance is frequently difficult to evaluate independently in a critical situation.

The fundamental aim of care is to prevent the occurrence of inadequate ventilation and circulation, if possible, and to recognize and treat these disturbances if they have already occurred. These goals can be accomplished only with an understanding of the origin of the problems.

**The basis of inadequate ventilation.** The primary pulmonary physiologic derangement that produces *hypoxia* and *hypercapnia* is *alveolar hypoventilation,* which results in a lowered *ventilation-perfusion* ratio. (Adequate blood perfusion to the lung is, of course, essential to maintaining a normal ratio, and therefore circulatory failure must be recognized and treated before the symptoms of alveolar hypoventilation occur, if possible.)

*Alveolar ventilation* is defined as that part of the total amount of air breathed or exchanged per minute (*tidal ventilation*) that reaches the alveoli. The portion not reaching the alveoli is the air within the *dead space* (which consists of the oropharyngeal airway, trachea and conducting portion of the bronchial tree. In the normal adult the dead space contains about 150 cc). Alveolar ventilation or volume plus dead space ventilation make up *tidal ventilation.* The normal adult requires 2000 cc of alveolar ventilation per minute per square meter of body surface area to meet his metabolic needs for oxygen and to permit elimination of carbon dioxide.

Following a thoracic surgical procedure or a thoracic injury, hypoventilation may be caused by the following processes:

1. *Obstruction of the airway* by retained secretions is probably the most frequent cause of hypoventilation; this produces *atelectasis* if allowed to persist. (*Atelectasis* is defined as airlessness of all or part of a lung; in this instance it results from obstruction of the airway leading to an anatomical unit after which the air in the obstructed segment is absorbed and the alveoli collapse.) Such atelectasis may be widely distributed in small patchy areas, creating the so-called "wet lung" syndrome, or the collapse may involve segments, lobes, or an entire lung.

2. *Pain* obviously will reduce voluntary mechanical ventilation; this hypoventilation is a restrictive phenomenon.

3. The *central nervous system may be obtunded* by anesthetic agents, sedatives, narcotics, and muscle relaxants given during operation; these depressants reduce the respiratory drive and muscular power mediated by the central nervous system. Any pre-

existing neuromuscular or skeletal disease involving the thoracic cage will further contribute to hypoventilation.

4. *Compression of lung tissue* by intrapleural air (*pneumothorax*) or blood (*hemothorax*) decreases ventilation quantitatively.

5. *Paradoxical respiration,* which occurs when the rib cage is made unstable by multiple rib fractures or rib removal (as in thoracoplasty), may quickly produce serious degrees of hypoventilation and lead to further retention of secretions because of ineffectiveness of the patient's coughing ability.

6. *Gastric dilatation and abdominal distention* may compress the lungs and decrease ventilation by pushing the diaphragm upward.

7. *Bronchiolar spasm,* or narrowing, may seriously obstruct ventilation. This state may be caused by allergy or intrinsic disease, or by irritation, edema, and infection from retained secretions. Spasm of this type seriously lowers ventilation-perfusion ratios.

**The basis of circulatory insufficiency.** The most likely cause of circulatory insufficiency among postoperative patients is blood loss or fluid depletion resulting in hypovolemia. Beyond a critical point cardiac output is affected and the shock syndrome ensues.

Cardiogenic factors, by themselves, may result in a markedly reduced cardiac output. Patients with underlying myocardial disease may develop arrhythmias, hypotension, or myocardial infarction during the course of surgery, complications which reduce effective perfusion of the lung and disturb the ventilation-perfusion ratio.

Hypotension that is *not* due to hypovolemia or primary cardiac disease may result from neurogenic causes. Particularly important in this category is pain-induced hypotension. Relief of severe pain with morphine or a nerve block is frequently followed by a rise in blood pressure.

**Common thoracic operative procedures.** The common thoracic operative procedures and the diseases for which they may be performed are as follows:

A. *Exploratory thoracotomy with lymph node biopsy, lung*

*biopsy, or wedge resection.* This operation consists of a major incision, usually intercostal, through a posterolateral parascapular approach through the 4th, 5th, 6th or 7th intercostal space. An anterior approach through the 3rd, 4th, or 5th intercostal space is occasionally used. The pleura is opened and the ribs spread to gain wide exposure of the lung and entire hemithorax. There is usually less pain and disability from the anterior approach. Exploratory thoracotomy with biopsy is usually performed to rule out carcinoma. Therefore no additional procedure is required because the lesion is either benign or else a nonresectable diffuse carcinoma is found. The thorax is usually drained by a tube placed through an intercostal space.

B. *Lung resection.* This procedure may involve either a *lobectomy*—removal of one complete lobe; *pneumonectomy*—removal of an entire lung; *segmentectomy*—removal of one or more segments of a lobe; or *wedge resection*—removal of any portion of a lobe. The surgical approaches are the same as described for exploratory thoractomy. A chest drainage tube is not usually used after pneumonectomy, but is always used for the other resections. Lung resections are done for bronchogenic carcinoma, bronchial adenoma, solitary pulmonary metastases, bronchiectasis, tuberculosis of the lung (which has not been healed by medical treatment), lung abscess, localized chronic pulmonary infection, undiagnosed solitary pulmonary lesions, congenital or acquired pulmonary cysts, and congenital lobar emphysema.

C. *Resection of mediastinal cysts or tumors.* This procedure is usually done through a posterolateral thoracotomy incision on the side, and at the level, of the lesion. Occasionally, when the lesion is clearly anterior, it is best approached through an anterolateral intercostal or a median sternal-splitting incision. Mediastinal masses are usually cysts or neoplasms and may be benign or malignant. Other structures in the mediastinum approached in the same way are vascular lesions including patent ductus, double aortic arch, and aneurysms of the aorta or great vessels. In these procedures, a single chest tube is usually used for drainage.

D. *Repair of diaphragmatic hernia.* The most common surgical repair is for the correction of a hiatus hernia. The incision in this circumstance is usually left posterolateral in the 8th intercostal space. Traumatic hernias are repaired through this same approach.

Congenital and anterior parasternal hernias are often repaired transabdominally. Chest tube drainage is usually, but not always, employed.

E. *Esophageal surgery.* These procedures may include esophagectomy for carcinoma, extramucosal myotomy for achalasia (Heller procedure), resection of diverticulum, and repair of tracheoesophageal fistula. They are performed through posterolateral incisions at the appropriate level. The resections may or may not include a procedure to immediately reconnect the remaining esophagus to the stomach by esophagogastrostomy or bowel interposition. Chest tube drainage is usually used.

F. *Thoracoplasty; major resection of ribs for tumor; or repair of funnel chest.* These extensive procedures are done through regional approaches with the aim of remaining outside the pleural cavity. Frequently, however, the pleura is entered inadvertently and tube drainage or aspiration is then required to expand the lung. These procedures may be accompanied by considerable pain; in addition, if much of the rib cage is removed, instability and a paradoxical motion of the chest wall may result. Thoracoplasty is seldom performed today for the treatment of cavitary pulmonary tuberculosis. Occasionally, this surgery is employed to close a chronic empyema space. Correction of funnel chest deformities (pectus excavatum) involves removal of most of the costal cartilage on each side of the sternum to free the sternum, which is then brought forward.

G. *Decortication.* This procedure is designed to free a lung that has been trapped and constricted by an organized clot or by an infection. Many lung leaks are usually created during surgery, and drainage, by at least two chest tubes, is always carried out. Rapid and complete re-expansion of the decorticated lung is essential for success.

H. *Other thoracic procedures, such as lung biopsy, pleural biopsy, or drainage of empyema.* Patients subject to these procedures usually do not require intensive care.


## ASSESSMENT OF THE PROBLEM

1. Detection of Hypoventilation, Hypoxia, and Hypercapnia
   A. *Quantitative methods.* It is clear that these derangements

of respiration cannot accurately be assessed by clinical evaluation alone, since such observation is merely qualitative. To obtain a definitive picture of respiratory insufficiency, quantitative measurements of arterial blood gases, as well as ventilatory exchange studies, are ultimately required.

Desired information in this regard includes the obtaining of the following data:

### 1. BLOOD GASES

a. Is there sufficient oxygen in the arterial blood? This fact is determined by measurement of the partial pressure of oxygen in arterial blood ($pO_2$). Normal $pO_2$ in room air is about 100 mm Hg.

b. Is there adequate elimination of carbon dioxide as measured by its partial pressure ($pCO_2$)? Normal $pCO_2$ is about 40 mm Hg.

c. Is the patient acidotic from progressive accumulation of $CO_2$, as determined by the pH of arterial blood? Normal pH is 7.4.

Arterial $pO_2$, $pCO_2$, and pH can be readily and rapidly determined with the use of the electrode method of measurement of these parameters. Blood is collected in a heparinized syringe with an 18 or 20 gauge needle from a femoral or brachial artery puncture. The syringe, packed in ice, is sent to the laboratory for immediate analysis of the blood gases and pH.

### 2. VENTILATORY EFFICIENCY

Is ventilatory exchange adequate? Quantitative assessment of ventilatory efficiency is achieved by measurement of the tidal ventilation. The technique involves the use of a spirometer from which the volume of air expired per breath and per minute is determined. The measurement is quite simple among patients in whom cuffed tracheotomy or endotracheal tubes are in place. Without these conduits a mouthpiece with a nose clip, or a face mask, can be used but the procedure is more difficult in such cases because of the need for patient cooperation.

The estimated minimal tidal ventilation required in a given

individual can be calculated from a nomogram which correlates tidal volume with height and weight.

**B. *Clinical observations*.** The above measurements do not obviate the need for clinical assessment of respiratory insufficiency; they merely enhance diagnostic accuracy.

Clinical assessment of hypoventilation, hypoxia, and hypercapnea include the following (see Chapter I, "Respiratory Insufficiency and Failure," for additional details):

1. rate of respiration;
2. blood pressure and pulse rate;
3. the appearance of decreased respiratory excursion;
4. dyspnea, labored respiration or stridor;
5. rales or rhonchi;
6. retraction of rib cage;
7. observation of skin color for cyanosis; and
8. cerebral effects including the presence or absence of restlessness, irritability, disorientation, and, ultimately, stupor and coma.

Cerebral effects are the most significant evidence for hypoxia and hypercapnea. Unfortunately, all of the other clinical signs mentioned above are variable, and hypoxia and hypercapnea may remain undetected for long periods of time, with an insidious progress to a sudden respiratory or cardiac arrest. For example, cyanosis is an unreliable sign of hypoxia and is frequently unrecognized when present in small degree. It may be obscured by peripheral vasoconstriction or may not be recognized in patients who are anemic, despite the presence of profound hypoxia. Similarly, reliance cannot be placed on the pulse rate or blood pressure. The pulse may be elevated or abnormally slow with hypoxia, and the blood pressure is usually elevated until the late stage of cardiac decompensation when it falls precipitously. Physical examination may be of limited benefit in estimating the degree of hypoventilation unless obvious airway obstruction exists or breathing is very shallow. For these reasons early or intermediate degrees of hypoventilation can seldom be detected by clinical observation alone, and the use of objective measurements previously described becomes essential to accurate diagnosis.

## 2. Detection of circulatory inadequacy

As noted, circulatory failure among postoperative patients, manifested by decreased cardiac output, is usually the result of blood loss, underlying cardiac disease, or neurorganic reflexes. If uncorrected, hypotension and shock develop, which result in decreased pulmonary and central perfusion, with tissue hypoxia and acidosis. Each of these possibilities must be investigated in evaluating the cause of hypotension and shock.

**A.** *Blood loss.* An increasing pulse rate or a drop in blood pressure (beyond the preoperative level) is cause for suspicion of blood loss; therefore, frequent measurement of the blood pressure and pulse rate is essential in the postoperative period. More advanced hypovolemia will be reflected by progressive oliguria or anuria, as well as changes in the sensorium.

Hypovolemia may be estimated grossly by comparing preoperative and postoperative hematocrit values and by replacing the volume of blood loss during and after the operation with transfused blood, plasma expanders, and other fluids given intravenously.

More accurate assessment of hypovolemia (and the adequacy of fluid replacement) can be made by periodic determination of blood volume, using radioactive albumin or dye-dilution techniques. A practical and simple method for controlling fluid replacement for hypovolemia involves continuous monitoring of central venous pressure (see pages 293–295).

**B.** *Underlying cardiac disease.* Every effort must be made to evaluate carefully the cardiovascular system prior to surgery, because a high percentage of these patients may have independent cardiac disease (particularly coronary heart disease) which can affect the postoperative course. The usual history, physical examination, as well as electrocardiography and radiographic examination of the chest (for heart size) should be performed before surgery is undertaken.

In the postoperative period patients may develop arrhythmias or even myocardial infarction which seriously affect cardiac efficiency. Continuous electrocardiographic monitoring is particularly valuable in high-risk cases following surgery.

**C.** *Neurogenic hypotension.* Hypotension that cannot be explained on the basis of blood loss, volume depletion, or cardiac disease is sometimes the result of neurogenic reflexes due to pain or chest trauma. This entity, when suspected, can often be verified by the return of normal blood pressure after adequate control of the pain stimulus.

## PRINCIPLES OF TREATMENT

The basic aim of care in the postoperative period, as stated, is to obtain and maintain respiratory and circulatory efficiency and to prevent physiological and biochemical alterations that may result from inadequate pulmonary ventilation and tissue perfusion. The methods of achieving this state of equilibrium are described in detail in the following section on the nursing role in chest surgery.

## THE NURSING ROLE

**Admission.** Most patients admitted to the intensive care unit after chest surgery have been in the recovery room until their condition has sufficiently stabilized to permit transfer. The patient may or may not be conscious, may or may not have an airway, tracheostomy, or endotracheal tube in place, and may or may not have one or more thoracotomy drainage tubes in place.

Unfortunately, most patients are not known to the intensive care nursing staff until they reach the facility. Therefore, it is important that the surgical and nursing staffs discuss the diagnosis, the surgical procedure, the operative findings, and related problems that may be anticipated, as soon as possible after admission. (Ideally, a nurse from the intensive care division should accompany the anesthesiologist or surgeon on rounds the evening before surgery, in order to obtain a more complete picture of the problem.)

The initial responsibilities of the nurse are to ascertain that the airway is patent; to institute oxygen therapy if indicated; to attach thoracotomy tubes to the suction apparatus; to check the dressing for bleeding or drainage; and to determine the blood pressure, pulse, and rate of respiration. These findings should be carefully recorded (Fig. 1) for comparative purposes.

While performing these functions, the nurse should greet the

Fig. 1. Intensive Care Nurses Notes

NAME_____HOSPITAL No._____

Date: _____ Operation: _____ Returned from O.R.: _____

Pre-Op Blood Pressure _____ Blood Loss: _____ Received in O.R.: Blood _____ Fluids. _____

| TIME | | | | | | | | |
|---|---|---|---|---|---|---|---|---|
| PULSE & RESPIRATIONS | | | | | | | | |
| BLOOD PRESSURE | | | | | | | | |
| SPUTUM | | | | | | | | |
| COUGH | | | | | | | | |
| TRACHEAL SUCTION | | | | | | | | |
| MEDICATIONS | | | | | | | | |
| TEMPERATURE | | | | | | | | |
| OXYGEN LF/M | | | | | | | | |
| THORACOTOMY TUBES AND DRAINAGE | | | | | | | | |
| EXERCISES | | | | | | | | |
| REMARKS: POSITION DRESSING EMPHYSEMA (SUBCUTANEOUS) COLOR MONITOR (ECG) OTHER | | | | | | | | |
| SIGNATURE | | | | | | | | |

356

patient by name, chat with him, and carefully observe his general appearance. In this way the nurse becomes aware of the patient's level of consciousness while establishing social contact, and at the same time ascertains his manner of breathing, tenseness of body position, color and texture of skin, etc.

**Subsequent care.** While specific care and nursing responsibilities from this point are dictated by the patient's particular circumstances, there are certain orders and procedures common to all patients who have had thoracic surgery.

1. *Check airway and respiratory exchange.* If the airway is occluded, stridor, cyanosis, or inadequate chest and lung expansion may be apparent. If in doubt, quick auscultation with a stethoscope will confirm this possibility. If obstruction is not relieved immediately by positioning of the head and jaw or by suctioning of the pharynx, endotracheal tube, or tracheostomy tube, then emergency help from the nearest physician should be obtained. A laryngoscope, endotracheal tubes, and tracheostomy sets should obviously be available in the intensive care unit, in a designated place. In the event of unexpected respiratory arrest, mouth-to-mouth resuscitation or bag breathing is instituted by the nurse until the patient has been properly intubated. (An Ambu type bag which uses room air should be available.) If cardiac arrest occurs, closed chest heart massage must be instituted immediately until the resuscitation team arrives.

2. *Institute oxygen therapy.* The catheter or cannula methods for delivering oxygen are preferred for thoracic surgical patients, rather than masks, because of the need to have the patient cough up secretions at frequent intervals. Oxygen flow is set at 7–10 liters/min. unless otherwise ordered. (Methods of oxygen administration are described in Chapter I, "Respiratory Insufficiency and Failure.") An oxygen tent is *not advisable* because high levels of oxygen are difficult to achieve and because frequent observation and treatment of the patient are distinctly impeded by the tent.

3. *Take vital signs every 15 minutes until patient is conscious; then every hour until stabilized.* A general criterion for stability is the restoration of the preoperative blood pressure and pulse rate. The actual frequency of observation is dependent on

the variation between the preoperative and current findings. A persistently low blood pressure should arouse suspicion and may indicate insufficient circulating fluid volume, hemorrhage, hypoxia, pain, or cardiogenic causes, as discussed above. While it is routine to record the blood pressure, pulse rate, respiratory rate, and temperature, it is also expected that the nurse will concurrently make other observations which may prove to be of equal or greater importance than the vital signs. These include ease of respiration; color of the skin, nail beds, and mucous membranes; state of sensorium; movement, or lack of movement, of extremities and facial muscles; presence of stridor; and retraction of chest with respiration. These qualitative observations are also recorded on the Intensive Care Nurses Notes (Fig. 1). The use of the summary type form gives a better "evaluation at a glance" than the more extended (and usual) "nurses' notes."

4. *Keep the patient flat in bed until consciousness returns* (*unless symptoms of shock indicate otherwise*). The supine position is usually the position of choice following thoracic surgery. In the Trendelenberg position, the abdominal organs may impinge upon the diaphragm, thereby restricting in varying degrees the movement of the lungs. In addition, pressure on the mediastinal structures may result in decreased venous return, with a consequent diminution in cardiac output. This latter possibility should be considered when hypotension is present, in which case a slight elevation from the supine position may enhance venous return and improve cardiac output. Venous pooling in the lower extremities may also be contributory to hypotension. Elevation of the legs without elevating the hips or application of elastic bandages to the extremities may be helpful in this circumstance.

5. *Change position frequently.* The basic principle in positioning the post-thoracic surgery patient is the prevention of alveolar hypoventilation. This results primarily from restriction in the movement of the thorax, which reduces the ability of the underlying lung to expand to its potential. The aim of positioning is to avoid this type of restriction.

The position of the patient will depend on the surgical procedure performed. For example, after a lobectomy, full lateral turning on both sides should be employed, inasmuch as there is lung parenchyma on the operated, as well as the unoperated, side.

However, patients with pneumonectomy should be turned only one-quarter of the full lateral position, because the mediastinum is no longer confined. Extreme lateral turning allows the mediastinum to move too widely and may cause compression of the remaining lung, or create traction or torsion phenomena on the vena cava. Nevertheless, lying on the side is permissible for short periods of time, certainly long enough for usual back care. Twenty-four hours postsurgery the patient may be turned on either side, provided he tolerates this, as evidenced by stability of pulse and blood pressure.

Shifting of the mediastinum can be suspected from deviation of the position of the trachea in the neck, and from change in position of maximum impulse of the heart beat (either medially or laterally from its normal position in the fifth interspace near the midclavicular line).

When there is question about a shift of the mediastinum, x-ray examination of the chest is helpful, or the intrapleural pressure can be measured directly with an open-end "U" manometer.

**6. *Encourage clear airway by coughing and deep-breathing exercises.*** Because hypoxia and hypercapnia (the major complications of thoracic surgery) are most often due to atelectasis resulting from obstruction of the airway by retained secretions or blood, it is essential that a clear airway be maintained during the postoperative course. This is one of the primary responsibilities of the intensive care team.

The simplest means for maintaining a clear airway are deep-breathing and coughing exercises initiated immediately after the operation. The success of this plan depends on the full cooperation of the patient. To achieve this, careful preoperative instruction in coughing and deep-breathing exercises is essential. Before the operation the team should inform the patient about the site of his incision, and also that he will have fairly severe postoperative pain and that, despite the pain, he will have to breathe deeply and cough (with assistance) to clear his secretions.

The following method of instruction for breathing and coughing exercises has proved effective:

With the patient in a sitting position, the nurse holds her hand approximately two inches in front of the chest wall and instructs the

patient to breathe in (and expand the rib cage) until the chest wall
reaches the nurse's hands. At the same time the patient is directed to
"billow out the abdomen" by relaxing abdominal muscles. On expiration the patient should cough while tightening the abdominal muscles
and consciously constricting the rib cage.

These exercises should be started as soon as the patient has
regained consciousness after surgery and should be repeated *every
hour* (or more often if necessary) for the first 24 hours. The
assistance of a thoracic physiotherapist is particularly valuable in
this regard. Even with this help the nurse should not abdicate
her responsibilty for carrying out this vital postoperative procedure.

The frequency of exercises after the first 24 hours is dependent primarily on the degree of cooperation of the patient and his
ability to cough up secretions without assistance. This cooperation
is influenced by several factors, the most important of which are
pain and fear. The effect of pain is to restrict movement of the
thoracic cage, with subsequent reduction of the mechanical bellows action. Although it is obviously necessary to use narcotics and
analgesics to control pain the dosage must be minimized in order
to avoid the undesirable effect of obtundation and subsequent loss
of patient cooperation. Many patients restrict essential thoracic
cage movement because of fear of tearing the incision, or fear
that the lung will "pop out" through the incision site.

These anxieties can be lessened by supporting the incision
during the coughing procedure. Proper manual support of the
incision does, in fact, decrease stretching of it, and thereby lessens
pain; in addition, it permits the nurse to assist in depressing the
thoracic cage during the expiratory phase of respiration. The
position of the nurse's hands during this procedure is dictated by
the following anatomical considerations: there is more flare of the
lower rib cage than of the upper rib cage, because the last five
pairs of ribs are not attached anteriorly to the sternum; the
sternum elevates on inspiration and the diaphragm flattens out.
Inasmuch as the diaphragm contributes more than 50% to the
respiratory process, its movement must not be restricted.

The correct and the incorrect positions of the nurse's hands
in supporting the patient are shown in Figs. 2 and 3. The two
significant points are: do not hold the chest with a viselike grip

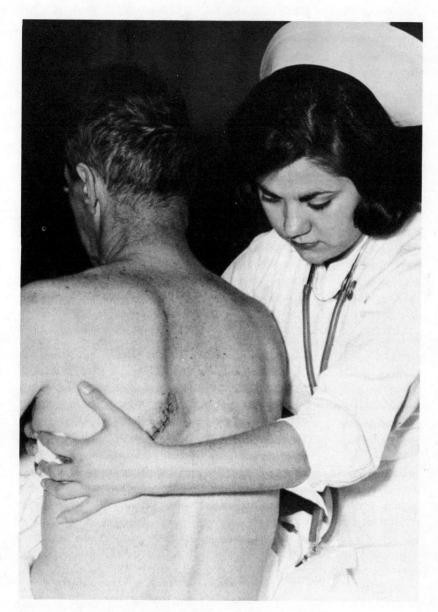

Fig. 2. Correct Positioning of Hands.

Note that nurse's head is behind patient. Her face is away from the spray of the cough and at the same time she is in a position to "listen" to the sound of the respirations.

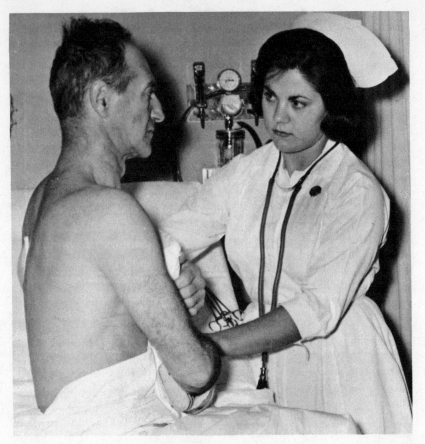

Fig. 3. Incorrect Positioning of Hands.

Incision is not supported: nurse receives full effect of cough: pillow across the chest cage restricts expansion: nurse is not in position to "listen" to respirations or assist in mechanics of expiration. (Note clamps for thoracotomy tubes.)

across the sternum, and do not hold the patient at the lower portion of the rib cage. Both of these latter maneuvers are unsound anatomically. It is important that the nurse (and the patient) be reminded of the need for the repetitive performance of the procedure. The inexperienced nurse may "feel sorry" for the patient and, attempting to be kind to him, allow him to sleep for three or four consecutive hours. This is not in the patient's interest during this stage of recovery from surgery.

If a patient develops atelectasis postoperatively, it is usually due (except in rare instances) to a lapse in nursing care. The most common cause of atelectasis is the plugging of a bronchus or a bronchiole with mucus, a problem which can be prevented in almost every instance by following the principles outlined above.

While performing deep-breathing and coughing exercises, an occasional patient may develop syncope. This momentary loss of consciousness may be caused by two factors: (a) the exercises may increase the intrathoracic pressure, which in turn impedes the venous return to the heart. The decreased venous filling subsequently reduces the output of the heart and may result in cerebral ischemia; (b) large amounts of carbon dioxide are "blown off" during the process of rapid, deep breathing (hyperventilation). This pulmonary loss of carbon dioxide causes sudden reduction in the amount of the gas in the blood, resulting in unconsciousness. Syncope is usually self-limiting, and the patient recovers in minutes.

**7. *Initiate tracheal suctioning.*** If the patient fails to clear secretions, despite coughing and deep breathing, other methods must be employed to preserve an unobstructed airway.

Nasotracheal suction is usually the first procedure attempted in this circumstance.

The criteria for employing nasotracheal suction are the presence of stridor, rhonchi, and "wet" cough (which is either nonproductive or fails to clear the lung). Suspected airway obstruction should be verified by auscultation with a stethoscope (while the patient breathes deeply and coughs) as well as by x-ray examination of the chest. Portable chest films should be taken regularly (usually daily) while the patient is in the intensive care unit. These films will demonstrate the presence or absence of intrapleural air or fluid and pulmonary atelectasis or infiltration.

The principles of tracheal suctioning have been previously described in the Chapter I, "Respiratory Insufficiency and Failure." Reviewing the technique, tracheal suctioning is best performed with the patient in the sitting position, with the catheter introduced through the nares. If difficulty is encountered, the tongue should be pulled forward. It has been found that after the catheter is in the trachea, turning the patient's neck sharply to the unoperated side will assist in directing the catheter down the bronchus of the operated side. Caution must be exercised in performing deep tracheal suctioning in instances where a suture line may be traumatized by the catheter.

Although there are several methods that can be used to promote effective cleaning of the tracheobronchial tree when properly used, we do not employ them routinely. They are as follows:

a. INHALATION OF HIGH CONCENTRATIONS OF CARBON DIOXIDE results in forced deep breathing. This, in turn, induces coughing, which loosens retained secretions and permits the expansion of collapsed alveoli. These concentrations of carbon dioxide can be achieved by direct administration of the gas from a tank via an anesthetic mask or, more easily, by having the patient rebreathe into a Dale-Schwartz tube through a mouthpiece while the nose is occluded. This rebreathing raises the carbon dioxide level sufficiently to produce the same effect as direct carbon dioxide inhalation, and is better controlled and tolerated than the older method of simply rebreathing into a paper bag.

b. TWO POPULAR METHODS FOR PRODUCING PULMONARY EXPANSION are the use of intermittent positive pressure breathing (IPPB) and blow bottles. We consider both of these methods ineffective. Traver found that "at the 0.5 level a significantly greater proportion of the subjects exhibited a productive cough while using the rebreathing tube (.55) than while using the IPPB apparatus (.25)." We use IPPB solely to administer aerosol medications, as bronchodilators or antibiotics, rather than to expand the lung. In our experience, the blow bottle is not effective in encouraging proper techniques, and we do not recommend its use, because there is a tendency to substitute this simple, but inefficient, procedure for effective coughing and deep-breathing exercises.

c. TRACHEAL INSTILLATION OF SOLUTIONS through a percutaneously placed small plastic tube has been described by Webb (1962). The tube is inserted into the trachea by way of a thin-walled needle passed through the skin immediately after surgery. A small amount of saline (with or without mucolytic agents) instilled into the trachea at regular intervals results in involuntary coughing. Additionally, the instilled solution thins secretions by dilution and chemical action.

d. INHALATION OF AEROSOL MIST generated by a nebulizer is an effective way of keeping the tracheobronchial secretions thin and permitting the mucus to be cleared by the ciliary mechanism and cough. The droplet size of the mist is important. The fine droplet, 2–4 microns in diameter, is carried down to the smallest and most distal bronchiole. Larger droplets become impacted on the surfaces of the trachea and the larger caliber bronchi and cause thin secretions at these levels. We have found that the ultrasonic nebulizer which generates a normal saline mist consisting of fine droplets is effective at all levels in the tracheobronchial tree. One must be careful, in using this mist, not to run it at high density for long periods, because it may produce excessive irritation that can be tolerated only intermittently. Mist generators, their conducting tubes and reservoirs, and the solutions used must be maintained in sterile condition and changed every 24 hours. Failure to do this has resulted in dissemination of serious tracheobronchial and pulmonary infection.

Mist therapy may be administered either by mask or in a mist or oxygen tent. The mask method is preferable, since it allows closer observation of the patient and avoids the "caged-in" feeling engendered by the tent. The mist is delivered for 5 to 20 minutes every hour by way of the mask. When a tent is used, the patient is kept in the tent and out of it for 30-minute periods. For patients with tracheostomy the mist can be directed into a tracheostomy mask, using oxygen or compressed air at a flow of 2 to 7 liters per minute.

Therapy is discontinued when the patient is able to bring up secretions with ease. Because patients produce sputum easily and effectively with this form of treatment, it is often necessary to "wean" them from this therapy gradually, as their ability to bring up secretions unaided returns.

**8. Check drainage bottles and thoracotomy tubes frequently.** The nurse should be responsible for noting the drainage through the thoracotomy tubes. Specifically, the nurse must observe and record the type and volume of fluid drainage (e.g., frank blood, pink color, mucopurulent). In addition, careful check must be kept on the rate of air return from the chest tubes to the collection bottle. This amount of air leak from the lung is of vital importance. If the bubbling in the water-sealed bottle is rapid, a considerable loss of air is occurring and the physician should be notified promptly, so that the amount of negative pressure (suction) can be increased to prevent collapse of the lung, or shifting of the mediastinum produced by the air leak within the chest.

The usual suction pressure within the system, about 20 to 30 centimeters of water, can be achieved by the use of various types of pumps or wall suction regulators. The amount of suction can be increased as necessary, and pressures up to 90 cm of water have not proved harmful in our experience. It is recommended that each drainage tube be connected to an individual water-sealed bottle. In this way the air and fluid drainage from each tube can be monitored and a non-draining tube can be removed without interfering with the remainder of the system. Normally, thoracotomy tubes are left in place for 24 hours after all air drainage and significant fluid drainage has ceased. Early removal of these tubes facilitates increased activity by the patient without encumbrance and frequently relieves some of the chest pain.

*In the event that one of the thoracotomy tubes becomes disconnected during the period of necessary suctioning, it is essential that the tube be clamped immediately.* Two Kelly (or similar) clamps should be available at the bedside at all times for this purpose, and all personnel in the unit should be fully aware of the grave danger that an open tube may pose (e.g., collapse of the lung or shift of the mediastinum).

9. *Observe patient for evidence of subcutaneous emphysema.* It is not unusual to note the presence of air in the subcutaneous tissue of the neck and chest after chest surgery. This collection results from leaks in the lung or bronchi which permit air to escape into tissue planes and reach the subcutaneous area. This subcutaneous emphysema is usually not of serious consequence and merely causes a grotesque, bloated appearance. In infants, however, there is danger that the vena cava or trachea may be compressed by the air-distended tissues.

If the amount of subcutaneous emphysema increases progressively, it may be assumed that the thoracotomy tube is not effectively draining air from the pleural space, and insertion of a new tube may be required. Very rarely, drainage of the mediastinum or a tracheostomy may be necessary.

The nurse should estimate the progression of subcutaneous

emphysema by measuring the circumference of the neck at frequent intervals and by marking the extent of air spread in the chest wall with a skin-marking pencil. Explanation and reassurance that the emphysema is anticipated should be given to the patient and his family.

In patients with pneumonectomy (where thoracotomy tubes are not used routinely), subcutaneous emphysema is limited to the amount of air left in the hemithorax at the time of closure. Progressive emphysema in these patients may indicate a serious leak in the bronchial stump. This is a serious complication and the nurse should be particularly cognizant of extending emphysema in these patients; the surgeon should be notified promptly in this event.

**10.** *Permit fluids by mouth post-nausea and record intake and output.* The nurse should encourage fluids by mouth as a means of assuring adequate hydration. Optimal hydration is essential in these patients as a means of preventing increased viscosity of mucus. Elimination of bronchial and tracheal secretions is accomplished with greater facility in patients receiving adequate fluids.

Accuracy in measuring and recording fluid intake and output, always important in the postsurgical patient, is of particular significance in the management of patients with pneumonectomy. The pulmonary circulatory system is reduced by removal of a lung and therefore overloading of the vascular tree becomes a threat. Overzealous administration of intravenous fluids can lead, rather rapidly, to acute pulmonary edema, with its sequelae. The possibility of developing pulmonary edema is further enhanced by the increased permeability of capillaries resulting from hypoxia.

**11.** *Check dressings frequently for bleeding.* When checking dressings, the nurse should obviously note the amount of saturation. It is pertinent to note whether the drainage is frank blood or more serosanguinous in nature. If the dressing is dry, the time of this observation should be recorded in order to define the onset of subsequent bleeding.

**12.** *Patient activity.* Once the vital signs have stabilized, the patient should be "dangled." Progressive ambulation should be started on the first postoperative day. During this period of activity the chest tubes may be clamped and disconnected if they are not draining secretions. If air drainage exists, obviously the drainage tubes should not be clamped. While the patient is out of bed, the drainage bottles must be maintained at a level 18 inches lower than the chest.

Passive exercises should be started four hours after the patient recovers from anesthesia. The goals of the physical therapy procedures (MacVicar), of which passive exercises are only a small part, are to preserve symmetrical body alignment, to re-educate muscles transected or contused during the surgical procedure, to maintain normal range of joint motion, and to maintain maximum pulmonary function. Here, again, nursing notes (prior to transfer to the ICU) concerning any factor which would preclude effective range of motion of the shoulder girdle or upper extremity on the operated side are helpful to the intensive care unit nurse.

Passive exercises are performed by having the nurse support the patient's arm and assist in abduction, adduction, forward flexion, and internal and external rotation of the extremity on the operated side. These exercises are done twice every four hours on the day of the operation and on the first postoperative day, after which the patient should be ready to exercise on his own. Any activity, e.g., encouraging the patient to reach for his glass of water and to comb his own hair, constitutes other worthwhile means of beginning active exercising.

**Complications.** The members of the intensive care team should be completely familiar with those complications commonly seen during the immediate postoperative period. The two most frequent complications, atelectasis and subcutaneous emphysema, have been previously discussed. Other problems are as follows:

1. *Pneumothorax.* When air reaches the free pleural space (the potential space between the two layers of the pleura), a pneumothorax is said to exist. Such air may reach the free pleural space from openings in the lung, which may occur spontaneously or result from surgery or trauma. When there is communication between the pleural space and the outside of the body, the pneumothorax is classified as "open" or "sucking." The more common type, the "closed" pneumothorax, is not accompanied by an external communication, and the air reaches the pleural space directly from the lung.

The classic symptoms of pneumothorax are sudden shortness of breath and chest pain, associated with a rapid pulse rate. The signs are decreased or absent breath sounds over the collapsed lung, hyper-resonance over the affected hemithorax, and (with a large pneumothorax) displacement of the mediastinum to the unaffected side. The diagnosis can be confirmed by x-ray examination of the chest, which demonstrates the amount and position of air in the pleural space.

When the volume of the pneumothorax is small, the air may be resorbed without therapy, but in postsurgical pneumothorax, which is usually of significant size, intervention is necessary. The usual treatment is to remove the air from the pleural space by means of an intercostal tube passed through a trocar under local anesthesia. The tube is then connected to a water-sealed drainage system with or without suction. Aspiration of air with a needle may be adequate if the leak from the lung has ceased. Expansion of the lung usually follows these procedures.

Persistent air leak may be troublesome even to the experienced surgeon, and requires various maneuvers.

**2. Hemothorax.** Bleeding into the intrapleural space from the lung or severed vessels may occur after operation or injury. If the blood is unable to escape from the pleural space, a hemothorax is produced. Hemothorax uniformly compresses the lung (except in pneumonectomy), and can be expected to shift the mediastinum to the opposite side if the amount of blood is sufficiently large. Frequently, pneumothorax and hemothorax exist together and the effects are compounded by the combined volumes of air and fluid. Hemothorax should be suspected when the patient becomes dyspneic or when the pulse and respiratory rates increase while blood pressure decreases. Dullness and decreased-to-absent breath sounds over the affected hemithorax, along with shift of the mediastinum, as evidenced by deviation of the trachea and the point of maximal cardiac impulse toward the opposite side, are signs of fluid in the chest. An upright portable chest film will show a diffuse opacity with mediastinal shift toward the opposite side. A fluid level will be present in the upright film if there is associated pneumothorax. Treatment consists of thoracentesis or intercostal tube drainage. If these procedures do not succeed in emptying the pleural cavity, either because of persistent bleeding or because of clotting or loculation, surgical evacuation of the blood and clot with direct control of bleeding is usually indicated.

**3. *Gastric dilatation.*** The complication of gastric dilatation following surgery has been previously described in Chapter IX, "The Complications of General Surgery." In the postoperative thoracic patient this problem may be especially dangerous because of the additional respiratory embarrassment it creates. Dilatation of this type is more common with left-sided surgical procedures and occurs in the immediate postoperative period. It may be related to the insufflation of anesthetic gases into the stomach during the period of anesthesia. Gastric dilatation can be detected by percussion over the stomach, and the diagnosis is confirmed by an upright chest film. Since such films are usually obtained a few hours after surgery, this possibility should be a definite consideration when viewing the films. Treatment consists of gastric decompression by way of a nasogastric tube.

**4. *Cardiac arrhythmias.*** The development of abnormal cardiac rhythm after thoracic surgery is not infrequent. Atrial fibrillation is the most common arrhythmia occurring during this period, but any type of rate and rhythm disturbance may occur. These arrhythmias most often have significant hemodynamic consequences, and must be controlled. The likelihood of development of arrhythmias is highest in patients with pre-existing cardiovascular disease and in the elderly. It has become a common practice to monitor the electrocardiogram during the early postoperative period, particularly among high-risk candidates. The treatment of the most serious arrhythmias has been considered in Chapter II, "Acute Myocardial Infarction."

**5. *Acute pulmonary edema.*** Failure of the left ventricle as a consequence of chest surgery is uncommon except in patients with previous congestive heart failure or in patients with pneumonectomy. The latter complication has been described and is related to overloading the vascular tree. Monitoring of central venous pressure (pages 293–295) appears to be a worthwhile procedure to minimize the threat of inducing acute pulmonary edema. The treatment of acute pulmonary edema is found in Chapter III, "Circulatory Emergencies."

**6. *Infection.*** Pleural and pulmonary infections are no longer common problems in thoracic surgery. The incidence of infection has been greatly reduced, even among patients having surgery for infectious diseases, by maintaining proper preoperative and postoperative bronchopulmonary toilette along with definitive antibiotic therapy. (We do not use antibiotics routinely for "clean" cases where rapid and complete lung expansion is anticipated, nor do we employ prophylactic antibiotics unless infected areas have been entered during the operative procedure.) When a bronchopulmonary wound or a pleural or other infection is present, the antibiotic to which the organism is sensitive is used. Aerosol antibiotics for tracheobronchial infections may be helpful. Purulent collections should be drained surgically.

**Psychological Needs of the Patient and His Family.** The patient's psychological response to chest surgery is often profound, because the surgery involves a vital organ of the body, and this should be appreciated by the patient-care team. Understandably, all patients have some concern about death or becoming a "respiratory cripple." This creates special needs in both the preoperative and postoperative periods. Medical and nursing personnel must feel confident that the patient was prepared emotionally to the maximum extent possible for the operation. Physiological effects of psychological turmoil should be recognized. For example, in one investigation (Dumas and Leonard, 1963) it was shown that patients who were emotionally distressed preoperatively tended to vomit more frequently postoperatively than those who were originally relatively free of such distress. A sound approach to the problem is a permissive demeanor by the entire team, which allows the patient to verbalize his feelings.

Reliance should not be placed merely on the fact that explanation of the surgical procedure has been given the patient. In this regard, Streeter noted a surprising lack of knowledge by the patient of his disease, which was unexpected "because of the extent of instruction of the patient by doctors and nurses." This finding emphasizes the need for careful attention to what the patient "understands."

Far more attention should be directed toward the attitudes of families as well as patients. Helping a sick patient to recover calls for the well-timed, well-chosen, well-balanced supportive and disciplinary components of the therapeutic process; and the ministrations of *both* the doctor and the family as well as the nursing personnel. Although visiting periods must be brief to protect the efficiency of the intensive care unit, it is important that team members have an awareness of the value of these visits to patient and family.

## Bibliography

American Hospital Association: The Law in Brief. *Hospitals, J.A.H.A.,* 39:118–119, December 1, 1965.

American Hospital Association: The Law in Brief. *Hospitals, J.A.H.A.,* 39: 111–112, March 1, 1965.

COMROE, J. H.: *Physiology of Respiration.* Year Book Medical Publishers, Chicago, 1964.

DALE, W. A.: Rebreathing Tube for Prophylaxis and Treatment of Atelectasis. *The American Journal of Surgery,* 98: 20–24, July 1959.

DEVINCENTI, M. J., KOENING, M. B., CARMODY, M. M.: Some Reactions of Cardiac Patients to Visitors. *Nursing Outlook,* 8: 693–695, December 1960.

DUMAS, R. G., LEONARD, R. C.: The Effect of Nursing Care on Postoperative Vomiting. *Nursing Research,* 12:12–15, Winter, 1963.

GEORGOPOLOUS, B. S., MANN, F. C.: *The Community General Hospital.* The Macmillan Co., New York, 1962.

HARDY, J. D.: *Pathophysiology in Surgery.* Williams and Wilkins Co., Baltimore, 1958.

HERSHEY, N.: A Nurse's Liability for Negligence in Supervision. *American Journal of Nursing,* 62: 115–116, May 1962.

HORTY, J. F.: What Are Legal Issues in Special Care? *The Modern Hospital* 104: 56–58, January 1965.

JACKSON, J. K.: The Role of the Patient's Family in Illness. *Nursing Forum,* 1: 118–128, Summer, 1962.

JOHNSON, J., KIRBY, C. K.: *Surgery of the Chest.* Year Book Medical Publishers, Chicago, 1964.

KOREY, R. C., BERGMANN, J. C., SWEET, R. D., SMITH, J. R.: Comparative Evaluation of Oxygen Therapy Techniques. *Journal American Medical Association,* 179: 767–772, March 10, 1962.

LIKERT, R.: *New Patterns of Management.* McGraw-Hill, New York, 1961.

MACLEAN, L. D., DUFF, J. H.: Central Venous Pressure as a Guide to

Volume Replacement in Shock. *Diseases of the Chest,* 48:199, August 1965.

MacVicar, J.: Exercises Before and After Thoracic Surgery. *American Journal of Nursing,* 62:61–63, January 1962.

Pace, W. R.: *Pulmonary Physiology.* F. A. Davis Co., Philadelphia, 1965.

Richardson, H. B.: *Patients Have Families.* Commonwealth Fund, New York, 1945.

Sagath, E. E.: Using a Pleural Pump Postoperatively. *American Journal of Nursing,* 62:102–103, May 1962.

Seeman, M., Evans, J. W.: *Stratification and Hospital Care: The Performance of the Medical Interne.* Engineering Experiment Station, The Ohio State University, Columbus, Ohio, 1961.

Streeter, G. A.: Phantasies of Tuberculosis Patients. *Psychosomatic Medicine,* 19:287–292, July–August 1957.

Trail, I. D., Monke, J. V.: Psyche Sequelae of Surgical Change in Body Structure. *Nursing Forum,* 3:14–23, 1963.

Webb, W. R.: Clinical Evaluation of a New Mucolytic Agent. *Journal of Thoracic and Cardiovascular Surgery.* 44:330–343, September 1962.

# Chapter XII

# Heart Surgery

JEAN A. YOKES, R.N., M.S.N.
WILLIAM A. REED, M.D.

## THE PROBLEM

The postoperative care of patients undergoing cardiac surgery is influenced by several factors:

1. frequent co-existing disease,
2. impairment of cardiopulmonary function as the result of:
   a. decreased myocardial efficiency,
   b. residual organic disease,
   c. effects of perfusion,
3. psychological effects of cardiac surgery.

Existing pathological alterations in the heart, lungs, liver, and kidneys resulting from the cardiac disease which necessitated surgery require special care designed to maintain function in these damaged organs during the postoperative period. This dysfunction is frequently aggravated by the use of medications prior to surgery which in themselves may cause alterations of body constituents, especially blood electrolytes.

Other potential complications involve the effects of general anesthesia, extracorporeal circulation (ECC), and the degree of restoration of circulatory function following the surgical repair.

Although specific operative procedures are not considered here, it is important that those responsible for the postoperative patient care have some basic understanding of the different surgical operations. For example, few problems would be anticipated in a young patient following repair of an atrial septal defect, in contrast to the prognosis for an elderly patient with severe mitral valve disease in whom multiple complications may develop because of the chronicity of the disease, as well as the decreased ability of the elderly to tolerate surgical procedures.

Usually within the first few hours following recovery from anesthesia the course of the patient's recovery, as well as the nature of ensuing complications, can be predicted. In our experience, most of the immediate complications occur in the post-anesthesia recovery room (PARR), but complications such as arrhythmias or heart failure may develop in the intensive care unit (ICU). Obviously, the management of therapy is essentially the same in either physical area.

## ASSESSMENT OF THE PROBLEM

Pertinent facts about the patient's medical history that the intensive care team should be aware of in caring for the cardiac patient postoperatively include a knowledge of the following:

**Past history**

1. Age; sex of patient; duration of disease.
2. Previous operative procedures.
3. Previous illnesses, particularly when they may predispose to complications, e.g., pulmonary embolus, phlebitis, pneumonitis, bacterial endocarditis, allergies, asthma, abnormal bleeding, mental illness, hepatic or genitourinary diseases.

**Present illness**

1. Reason for surgery.
2. Degree of preoperative impairment of cardiac function.
   a. Class I:    asymptomatic.
   b. Class II:   symptomatic with normal activity, but controlled with medication.
   c. Class III:  symptomatic with limited activity and medication.
   d. Class IV:   symptomatic with bed rest and medication.
3. Is surgery expected to be curative, partially corrective, or palliative?
4. Does the patient have coexisting pulmonary problems?
5. Will the proposed operation be associated with further impairment of the cardiorespiratory function (even though temporary)?

**Laboratory and diagnostic tests used for preoperative patient assessment.** In our institution the following information is obtained prior to surgery and discussed by a team of surgeons, cardiologists, and the nurse specialist, in a preoperative conference.

1. *Hemoglobin* and *hematocrit* determination as a baseline for reference and to indicate the need for correction of anemia, if present, before surgery.
2. *Urinalysis* to determine the presence of urinary tract infection or renal impairment, problems which could complicate surgery.
3. *BUN* to determine renal impairment.
4. *Bilirubin* to determine liver impairment which could complicate surgery.
5. *Transaminase* to determine liver impairment.
6. *Electrolytes* to determine the extent of electrolyte imbalance due to the use of diuretics and/or the presence of congestive heart failure.
7. *Chest x-rays* to evaluate the presence of cardiac abnormalities as well as coexisting pulmonary pathology.
8. *ECG* to evaluate chamber enlargements, coronary heart disease, and those changes associated specifically with abnormalities for which the patient is to be treated, such as left ventricular hypertrophy.
9. *Phonocardiogram* to supplement clinical auscultatory findings.
10. *Vectorcardiogram* to supplement the ECG findings.
11. *Cardiac catheterization* to quantitate the severity of the lesion.
12. *Prothrombin time, bleeding and clotting times,* and *platelet count* to rule out a bleeding diathesis.
13. Specific *pulmonary function studies,* in selected circumstances, e.g., for bronchiectasis associated with mitral stenosis.

## PRINCIPLES OF TREATMENT

**Preoperative care.** Preoperative preparation is given to the patient by the team. The preparation should consist of the following:

a) An explanation of the proposed surgery and the reason it is being performed.

b) The anticipated postoperative period, including the restriction of oral fluids, relief of pain, ambulation, etc.

c) The need for intermittent positive pressure breathing apparatus (IPPB) and deep breathing and coughing exercises to prevent pulmonary complications.

d) A description and explanation of the equipment that will be connected to the patient in the postoperative period, i.e., chest drainage tubes, high humidity oxygen apparatus, indwelling uri-

*Table 1*

NURSES' CHECKLIST FOR PREOPERATIVE PREPARATION
OF HEART SURGERY PATIENTS

Patient's name _____ Diagnosis _____

| Explanation of, or instruction in: | Date | Nurses' Initials |
|---|---|---|
| 1. Intake and output (stress accuracy) .................. | | |
| 2. Void in A.M. before surgery or insertion of Foley catheter ............................................. | | |
| 3. Practice deep abdominal breathing and coughing ...... | | |
| 4. Practice use of IPPB (Bennett) for thoracic surgery cases | | |
| 5. Recovery Room or Intensive Care Unit Regime | | |
|    a. frequent vital signs ........................... | | |
|    b. chest tubes for thoracic surgery patients .......... | | |
|    c. croupette or oxygen catheter for thoracic surgery patients ...................................... | | |
|    d. intravenous feedings; fluids by mouth withheld .... | | |
| 6. O R permit signed ................................ | | |
| 7. Private duty nurse request signed, if ordered, and given to coordinator ...................................... | | |
| 8. Skin preparation ................................. | | |
| 9. Laboratory reports on chart ........................ | | |
| 10. Removal of hairpins, jewelry (wedding ring taped), fingernail polish and dentures or artificial eye ....... | | |
| 11. Preoperative medication given ..................... | | |

Encourage expression of feelings as a way of preventing resignation. Submission leads to helplessness and despair; it consumes energy, often to the point of immobilization. Encourage patient's own powers to deal actively with threats. Help patients use own powers to gain control of self and situation.

nary catheter, intravenous tubing, and monitoring devices.

e) A demonstration of range of motion exercises.

The method and extent of this instructional program will, of course, depend on the emotional and physical condition of the patient, as well as his age and intelligence. A preoperative check list of the explanation given the patient is placed on the front of his chart, so that all nursing personnel become aware of the content of what has already been discussed (Table 1). This information may then be supplemented as required. An important area in need of nursing research is the kind, amount, and appropriate time for preoperative preparation of the patient.

**Postoperative Care and Complications.** Following cardiac surgery the fundamental aim of treatment is to achieve an optimal physiologic state while healing occurs. This involves the maintenance of adequate respiratory and cardiac function along with control of fluid and electrolyte balance.

Despite careful preoperative planning and precise operative treatment, complications may occur in the postoperative period. For this reason, the recognition and immediate treatment of these complications becomes an important part of the postoperative management of heart surgery.

The most common complications following heart surgery are:
1. Postoperative hemorrhage.
2. Cardiac tamponade.
3. Respiratory insufficiency.
4. Cardiac arrhythmias.
5. Heart failure due to
   a. Overhydration.
   b. Electrolyte imbalance.
   c. Inadequate function of the myocardium.
   d. Inadequate repair.
   e. Effects of operative manipulation on cardiac function.
   f. Malposition or malfunction of prosthesis.
6. Shock.
7. Infection.
8. Alterations in body temperature.
9. Renal depression or anuria.

10. Neurologic malfunction due to:
   a. Organic pathology.
   b. Psychologic effects of organic or emotional nature.
11. Liver malfunction.

Some of these complications are more common with one type of corrective surgery than with others, and it is important that those caring for postoperative cardiac patients be familiar with the relative frequency of the specific complications. (Table 2.)

*Table 2*

|  | Mitral stenosis | Mitral insufficiency | Aortic stenosis and/or insufficiency | Combined aortic and mitral valve disease | Ventricular septal defects | Atrial septal defects | Cyanotic heart disease |
|---|---|---|---|---|---|---|---|
| Hemorrhage | − | − | − | + | − | − | + |
| Arrhythmias | − | − | ∓ | ± | + | − | − |
| Respiratory | + | − | − | + | ± | − | − |
| Heart failure | − | ∓ | − | + | LATE (4–5 days) | − | ± |
| Neurologic | − | − | + | ++ | − | − | − |

## Specific Complications

1. *Postoperative hemorrhage.* All patients drain blood from the thoracic cavity following cardiac surgery; the amount varies from patient to patient. Amounts in excess of 5 ml/kg/hr should be considered excessive blood loss. The drainage is measured hourly (unless excessive bleeding occurs) by observation of the blood level in a calibrated cylinder. A gradually decreasing hourly drainage may reflect cessation of bleeding and may be considered a good prognostic sign. (In assessing the hourly rate it is important to ascertain that drainage is not obstructed from clots, etc., and it is imperative that the drainage tubes be maintained in a patent condition by frequent manipulation and milking.)

Since all patients who have had open-heart surgery receive anticoagulants during surgery, the clotting mechanisms must post-operatively be restored to normal. This is accomplished by the neutralization of heparin with protamine sulfate, and the elimination of abnormal clot lysis by the administration of epsilon aminocaproic acid. (EACA, a competitive inhibitor of enzymatic activation of plasminogen, prevents the destruction of fibrin).

Other blood abnormalities, particularly platelet depression resulting from extracorporeal circulation (ECC), are usually self-limiting and are corrected by the patient's own homeostatic mechanisms after a few hours. Other clotting abnormalities may be related to poor liver function (commonly seen in patients with chronic congestive heart failure), and require the administration of Vitamin K and/or fibrinogen. If bleeding persists in the post-anesthesia recovery-room period, the use of protamine sulfate and EACA are repeated. (These drugs, along with calcium gluconate have been previously given in the operating room following the completion of surgery.) Failure to control bleeding with these agents may necessitate the use of fresh blood, platelets, or fibrinogen.

Clotting abnormalities such as decreased platelets, decreased fibrinogen, increased fibrinolysis, and prolonged bleeding time are most commonly seen in patients with severe polycythemia, which is a sequela of hypoxemia associated with cyanotic heart disease. A second situation in which bleeding may occur in the postoperative period involves patients who required prolonged periods of cardiopulmonary bypass. Increased fibrinolysis caused by destruction of the formed elements of the blood and decreased liver function can cause alterations in the normal blood-clotting mechanism.

Fibrinolysis is recognized as a major contributing cause of postoperative hemorrhage. The euglobulinlysis assay is a reproducible method of evaluating fibrinolytic activity. A lysis time of less than forty-five minutes is usually associated with increased bleeding.

A program for maintaining hemostasis in the cardiac surgery patient can be outlined as follows:

1. Neutralization of heparin by protamine sulfate when extracorporeal circulation is employed. Ordinarily, protamine sulfate is given in a dosage that is 1.5 times the initial heparin that has been used (3 mg/kg). This amount does not include the amount of heparin contained in the blood used to prime the

pump oxygenator. Protamine titrations are not routinely done, but facilities should be available to perform the determination, if required.

2. Administration of EACA in a dosage of 150 mg/kg of body weight: one-fourth of the dosage given immediately after ECC and the remainder given over a four-hour period if the euglobulinlysis time is abnormal.

3. Careful surgical technique, of course, reduces the threat of bleeding.

4. Leaving the pericardium open allows for drainage of blood into the previously opened right hemithorax.

5. Transfusion of whole blood.

Patients should generally be transfused until a normal central venous pressure is attained. Blood transfusions are usually safe, from a standpoint of volume, if the central venous pressure is below 15–20 cm of water. In a patient with a low blood pressure, a low urinary output, and a low venous pressure, blood is given until correction of the blood pressure and urinary output or venous pressure is increased, whichever occurs first. A determination of left atrial pressure may be used in selected patients as a guide to blood replacement. If only the central venous pressure increases (above 20 cm) other causes for hypotension and a decreased urinary output must be sought. Blood replacement is thereafter determined by the amount of blood lost and by the clinical picture. As mentioned previously, careful measurement of blood loss is made hourly unless such loss is excessive. The amount of loss should be related to the size of the patient. Tubes must be cleared carefully to prevent accumulation within the chest cavity. Gradual decrease in the rate of bleeding is to be expected and, in uncomplicated cases, very little blood loss occurs after about six hours postoperatively. Sudden cessation of chest drainage, increase in venous pressure and/or a decrease in systemic pressure, respiratory embarrassment, and a decreased urinary output all may indicate intrathoracic or intrapericardial bleeding with accumulation, and must be recognized and treated promptly.

Laboratory studies helpful in assessing hemorrhage are prothrombin time, euglobulinlysis time, serum fibrinogen, and hematocrit and hemoglobin. However, careful observation of clinical changes in the patient's circulatory status should serve as the major guide, and the laboratory results are considered only as an adjunct to the proper determination of therapy.

**2.** *Cardiac tamponade.* Recognition of cardiac tamponade is a second major problem. It is important for the nurse to know whether the pericardium was completely sutured and whether the mediastinal pleura was incised to allow for drainage of blood into the thoracic cavity and the chest tubes. That the pericardium was left open does not entirely eliminate the possibility of cardiac tamponade, since fibrin may form over the epicardium anteriorly (where it was left open), while blood accumulates posteriorly (unless a posterior incision was made in the pericardium).

Cardiac tamponade may be suspected when there is an *increase* in venous pressure (usually above 15 cm of water), associated with *decreased* systolic blood pressure (and narrowed pulse pressure) in a patient with signs of bleeding. Decreased urinary output and signs of systemic shock may also be present. Recognition of cardiac tamponade demands immediate corrective measures in the form of aspiration of the pericardial space or operative drainage, usually the latter.

**3.** *Respiratory insufficiency.* Postoperative respiratory complications are seen commonly in those patients undergoing surgery for correction of defects associated with abnormal pulmonary blood flow and mitral valve disease. In addition, temporary impairment of gas exchange across the alveolar membrane occurs to varying degrees in most patients after extracorporeal circulation. Several factors give rise to this change. Patients with long-standing mitral valve disease, chronic bronchitis, pulmonary emboli or pulmonary congestion also tend to have poor pulmonary function, and postoperative respiratory insufficiency becomes likely. The problem is aggravated when the valvular surgery does not completely correct all the hemodynamic defects.

Although some authors have suggested that most patients should have continuous respiratory assistance via tracheostomy or endotracheal tube following open-heart operations, such assistance has not been routinely necessary in our experience. The following specific measures are taken to promote and maintain adequate pulmonary function:

a. Judicious use of muscle relaxants during surgery and adequate reversal of their actions postoperatively.

b. Careful observation of the patient until he is fully recovered from anesthesia with assisted ventilation during this period.

c. Blood gas measurements at completion of the operative procedure (and subsequently as indicated) with correction of abnormal pH and $pCO_2$.

d. Croupette, isolette, or open-top tent with high humidity until respiratory pattern is normal and mucus secretions no longer are a problem.

The management of patients requiring ventilation assistance is described in detail in Chapter I, "Respiratory Insufficiency and Failure."

Small children and infants generally have more secretions following surgery than adults and may require frequent nasotracheal suction. If the bronchial tree is not kept free of secretions, the risk of respiratory arrest is high. Laryngeal edema and laryngospasm may occur in children following removal of the endotracheal tube. Great care must be exercised in tracheal suctioning of infants, as bradycardia followed by cardiac arrest can result. It may be advisable to obtain the services of the anesthesiologist or surgeon for this procedure.

**4. *Cardiac arrhythmias.*** As with other complications, cardiac arrhythmias after heart surgery are influenced by the specific lesion treated and on how completely physiologic function has been restored to normal by surgery. The following rhythm disturbances are of special concern in the postoperative period:

a. HEART BLOCK

Heart block may follow operative procedures for ventricular septal defects, atrial septal defects (of the septum primum type), or subaortic stenosis and transpositions of the great vessels, all of which involve manipulation in the upper portion of the ventricular septum or outflow portion of the left ventricle. On the other hand, heart block is *uncommon* following aortic and mitral valve replacement.

Continuous postoperative monitoring of electrical activity of the heart (ECG) is essential in all patients who have demonstrated heart block, transient or otherwise, during the operative procedure. Prior to leaving the operating room it is probably wise to insert a transvenous pacing catheter or direct epicardial electrodes (which can be removed later) in any patient with heart block. The treatment of heart block and monitoring techniques are described in Chapter II, "Acute Myocardial Infarction."

b. VENTRICULAR TACHYCARDIA

This represents a distinct warning of the possibility of ventricular fibrillation. Any patient with ventricular tachycardia should remain on a cardiac monitor with all resuscitative equipment at the bedside. See Chapter II, "Acute Myocardial Infarction."

C. ATRIAL FIBRILLATION

Prior to surgery, all patients with mitral valve disease who have a normal sinus rhythm are given quinidine in an attempt to prevent atrial fibrillation. The usual dosage is 200 mgm every six hours, but the dosage is best determined by serum quinidine levels. (In the occasional patient with a persistent atrial arrhythmia due to long standing mitral valve disease, electrical cardioversion is the best method of management.) See Chapter II, "Acute Myocardial Infarction."

5. *Heart failure.* The most common cardiac problem after surgery is myocardial failure (low cardiac output), resulting from pre-existing pathology as well as the stress of surgery. Since many operative procedures, especially those for tetrology of Fallot, ventricular septal defects, and aortic valve replacement involve intermittent coronary artery perfusion, the likelihood of myocardial hypoxia is obviously increased. A compromise must be reached between the maintenance of normal myocardial blood flow and the deprivation of flow to obtain good exposure for repair. Hypoxia results in impairment of myocardial contractile force, the degree depending upon the health of the myocardium and the length of hypoxic periods. Some patients who require coronary artery perfusion or who have had periods of hypoxic arrest have

moderate hypotension lasting for six to twelve hours postoperatively. It is important to distinguish such hypotension from cardiogenic shock. With simple hypotension the patient will be alert, have dry skin, good peripheral color, and normal central venous pressure, and will produce 30 ml/hr or more of urine. The hypotensive patient in shock is vasoconstricted, clammy, anuric, and restless. Hypotension itself requires very little treatment while shock must be vigorously treated. (See Chapter IV, "Shock.")

There is a high incidence of fluid and electrolyte disturbances in patients with acquired heart disease which contributes to the development of heart failure. Care must be taken to avoid overloading the cardiovascular system in the postoperative state, and for this reason intravenous fluids should be restricted in this period. For the first three days after surgery, 500–700 cc per square meter body surface per 24 hours (including oral intake) is usually sufficient; Ringer's lactate solution or dextrose in water is the usual fluid used. Use of parenteral fluids containing sodium should be minimized as a precautionary measure against the development of sodium overload.

Digitalis preparations are withheld 24 to 48 hours prior to the operative date. The drug is resumed in the postoperative period and ordered daily, depending upon the patient's requirement. Heart failure is common following total repair of tetrology of Fallot and acquired valve disease, and is usually treated by digitalization on the day of operation, care being taken to avoid intoxication. Digoxin is used in most patients, because of fewer problems with toxicity. A Lead II ECG is done each day. If digoxin is given twice a day or more frequently, a Lead II ECG is done prior to each dose. A short strip is placed in the progress notes, and the total dosage of drug administered is recorded.

6. **Shock.** Although the problem of shock has been considered in Chapter IV, certain aspects of therapy peculiar to postoperative cardiac patients are pertinent here.

a. Blood volume is restored until the central venous pressure is normal. A small, #15, plastic catheter inserted into the inferior vena cava in the operating room is used to measure central venous pressure. Blood may be given until the venous pressure is elevated to 20 cm $H_2O$ if necessary. Further transfusions will probably not improve cardiac output once the venous pressure is at this level, and other causes for shock must be investigated.

b. Morphine sulfate is given in small doses intravenously for relief of pain and anxiety. Patients rarely require large dosages. The intravenous method of administration is preferable because the absorption of the drug by other routes is unpredictable.

c. Oxygen therapy administered by equipment used for ventilation may be necessary if the restoration of blood volume (step "a") does not improve the cardiac output. Pressures used to deliver the proper tidal volume and gas mixtures must be determined by individual circumstances. One hundred per cent oxygen is not ordinarily required; over a period of time this concentration can produce signs and symptoms of oxygen toxicity.

d. Isoproterenol (Isuprel) may be used to improve myocardial contractility; it is given as a continuous drip if the patient does not have a tachycardia or ventricular arrhythmia. The use of isoproterenol in these circumstances, however, may precipitate a dangerous increase in heart rate. This drug also has some peripheral vasodilator action. The rate of administration of isoproterenol is regulated by the need of the patient and the response to treatment.

e. Vasopressors are rarely used. In a hypotensive, but not vasoconstricted patient, pressor agents may occasionally be added to the intravenous fluid.

Such patients may have good myocardial contractility, warm, dry skin, and a systolic blood pressure of 70–80 mm Hg. Under these circumstances the patient would probably maintain himself, but use of a vasopressor would boost the blood pressure 10–20 mm Hg and promote a little better renal function. Metaraminal bitartrate (Aramine) in small doses (10–50 mgm in 1000 cc intravenous fluid) is the drug of choice. In small doses, it produces a less intense peripheral and renal vasoconstrictive effect. Intravenous or intramuscular doses of metaraminal do not cause tissue slough.

**7. *Infection.*** Infection is an ever-present potential hazard with heart surgery. Septicemia usually results in death among patients with intracardiac prostheses, and great care must be taken to avoid this complication. Good evidence exists to support the prophylactic use of antibiotics in the immediate preoperative and early postoperative period. These agents are administered via an intravenous catheter for 48 hours, after which intramuscular routes are used for three to five days. Prophylactic therapy is then discontinued. (Using this approach, wound infection and septicemia have decreased from 15% to 1.8% in this institution.)

Most infections after surgery are due to staphylococcus; therefore, the drugs of choice are penicillin and staphcillin. If patients are allergic to penicillin, chloroamphenicol and erythromycin are used as substitutes.

**8. *Alterations in body temperature.*** With closed-heart surgery there is very little disturbance of body temperature unless complications are present. On the other hand, open-heart procedures are followed by an elevation of body temperature in the majority of patients. Characteristically, the rectal temperature spikes to 39° C in the early postoperative period and usually persists at this level for three to four days. Chills are not common during this febrile period. The exact cause of this disturbance in body temperature is not explainable, but bacterial infection must always be ruled out. (In more than 300 cases, routine blood cultures were positive in only two persons.)

When the patient's temperature reaches 37° C in the postoperative period, the bed covering should be minimal. If the temperature reaches 38.5° C or above, aspirin is administered rectally.

In infants and children, elevated body temperature is best controlled by ice bags in preference to the hypothermia blanket. Adding to the discomfort of the treatment, shivering, in response to cooling with the thermal blanket, causes an increase in metabolism and leads to a rise in body temperature. Ice bags are often satisfactory for lowering the body temperature of adults as well. However, for some adult patients the use of the hypothermia blanket may be indicated if body temperature is difficult to control. Methods of controlling body temperature while preventing trauma and providing comfort for the patient are an area of nursing practice in need of research.

9. *Renal depression or anuria.* Renal function may be depressed following cardiac surgery primarily for the following reasons:

a. decreased cardiac output;

b. the lower nephron syndrome developing after multiple transfusions;

c. increase in plasma hemoglobin due to breakdown of red blood cells during ECC;

d. the stress of surgery on pre-existing renal disease.

An indwelling bladder catheter should be used in all patients until normal renal function is re-established (as evidenced by BUN, creatinine, and adequate hourly urinary output).

The judicious use of mannitol is perhaps warranted in the presence of low cardiac output states, but there is little reason to use other drugs. Improvement in cardiac output is usually followed by return of renal function.

10. *Neurologic disturbances.* A patient should normally awaken within an hour or two after cardiac surgery. If he does not, the following possibilities should be considered: embolic damage, hypoxia, and previous brain damage.

In closed mitral valvulotomies, a thrombus or calcium deposit from the valve is usually the agent causing embolic damage. In open-heart patients, air, calcium, fat, or thrombus may be the source of embolization. Air emboli may occur at any time the left heart is opened, for example, in repair of atrial septal defects, ventricular septal defects, or aortic and mitral valvulotomies or replacements, or they may originate in the ECC system. Embolization can be suspected if the patient fails to awaken promptly and shows evidence of hemiparesis or has convulsions. In the event of a cerebral embolic episode, patients may require anticonvulsant therapy, reduction of body temperature, and tracheostomy. Patients with a deep level of unconsciousness have a poor prognosis. Fortunately, this complication is infrequent in experienced hands.

A more frequent problem (at least in the past), has been a diffuse neurological deficit characterized by a slow return of consciousness and partial motor paralysis. Such patients may require ventilatory assistance and help in eliminating tracheobronchial secretions. Slow recovery occurs in two to four days. The cause is probably related to poor cerebral capillary perfusion, but may be partially due to fibrin emboli. This diffuse neurologic deficit is more common after long (two-hour) total body perfusion.

Not all neurologic changes following open-heart operations are well understood. It has been suggested that some changes may be of a psychological nature. Neurologic deficits depend upon the extent of organic brain damage and the etiologic factors in individual cases.

11. *Liver malfunction.* Some patients become icteric after surgery, probably as the result of the effects of chronic congestive heart failure causing decreased liver function. When this is combined with the stress of ECC, further malfunction results. Recovery ordinarily follows in a few days, but occasional cases progress to death. Postoperative hepatitis has been unusual in our experience.

**Postoperative Care of Infants and Children.** The heart muscle in infants and children is of good tone, well supplied with blood, and thus withstands major surgery better than the damaged hearts of adults. In proportion to size, the amount of blood ejected by the heart per minute (the minute volume) in an infant is about twice that of the adult. The pulse rate is faster, being about 180 per minute at birth and about 120 per minute at one year of age.

The thorax at birth and for about two years thereafter is circular in shape; in the adult it is oval. Therefore, in the infant, the chest cannot be increased in diameter on inspiration, whereas in the adult it can. Hence, the infant has mainly abdominal (diaphragmatic) breathing, and is thus more liable to chest complications. Respiratory obstruction (and consequently anoxia) occurs more readily in the child than in the adult, because of certain anatomical differences in the respiratory passages. The oxygen demands of the infant are greater than the adult's. Also, the respiratory surface area of the lung for oxygen exchange is relatively small in the infant. These factors lead to a much faster respiratory rate in the infant in order that enough air may enter the lungs to supply the increased oxygen demand. Infants cannot withstand anoxia for as long a period as adults, because their residual air volume is relatively small. The weak and not so well-developed intercostal and diaphragmatic muscles of the small child and infant become fatigued much sooner and cannot so easily overcome respiratory difficulty. In the child, respiration is not as regular as in an adult; long pauses often occur at the end of inspiration instead of at the end of expiration.

The anatomical and physiological differences between children and adults will affect the postoperative observations and care of infants and children. The major emphasis of this chapter has been placed on the care of the adult patient. Further information about these anatomical and physiological differences and techniques of care for children can be obtained from standard medical and nursing textbooks of pediatrics.

## THE NURSING ROLE

**Initial Postoperative Period.** Initial nursing care consists of the following:

1. Vital signs are determined.
2. The patient is called by name and is told that his surgery is completed and that he is in the intensive care facility.
3. Skin color and temperature are noted to assess the degree of peripheral vasoconstriction.
4. Adequacy of peripheral pulses is ascertained.
5. Level of consciousness is determined.
6. The head of the bed is elevated to semi-Fowler's position to promote chest drainage and allow full lung expansion. Deep-breathing and coughing exercises are initiated.
7. Adults and older children are placed in open-top tents (infants are placed in isolettes and toddlers are placed in croupettes at this time).
8. The chest suction device is checked for adequate function and the level of drainage marked on the container.
9. The urinometer is attached to the drainage apparatus.
10. The central venous pressure catheter is attached to the manometer and pressure recorded from the reference point marked in the mid-axillary line. If an intra-arterial

catheter has been placed, the line is flushed with heparin-saline and connected to a recorder.

11. Apparatus for respiratory assistance (if needed) is attached.

12. The electrocardiographic monitoring electrodes (if needed) should be secured in place to allow good signals on the oscilloscope.

13. Laboratory, electrocardiographic, and x-ray technicians are summoned to conduct appropriate studies, etc.

**Subsequent Postoperative Care.** The postoperative care of the patient who has undergone cardiac surgery depends in large measure on the resolution of one or more of the complications discussed in this chapter in the section on "Principles of Treatment."

After the stability of the patient's condition has been ascertained, maintenance and supportive postoperative care is given. A chest x-ray is taken daily until the chest tube is removed. Hematologic and blood chemistry determinations mentioned in the preoperative preparation of the patient are made daily for three days in uncomplicated cases. An hourly cumulative intake-and-output sheet is kept. Maintenance and supportive care is as follows:

1. Use of IPPB, deep-breathing and coughing exercises.
2. Restriction of fluids.
3. Control of body temperature.
4. Antibiotic administration.
5. Prevention of pain and anxiety.
6. Range-of-motion exercises.
7. Back care to promote circulation and relieve muscle fatigue.
8. Mouth care, with small amounts of ice chips given if the patient complains of excessive thirst.
9. Environment kept conducive to comfort, sleep, and rest, with patient activities scheduled so as to minimize disturbances.

**Range-of-motion exercises.** The intended use of passive or active range-of-motion exercises should be discussed with the patient and demonstrated, if feasible, before operation. Range of motion is defined as the ability of a part of the body to move or be moved to a distance or range from its usual position. The extent of the range is determined by the anatomical structure of the part. In performing active assistive range-of-motion exercises, the nurse or therapist moves the patient's limbs through the range or assists the patient, where needed, in moving designated portions of his body through the required range of motion. In performing active range-of-motion exercises, the patient moves the portions of his body through the selected range of motion unassisted.

The following are recommended procedures for the patient to follow:

1. Start with arms straight out to side at shoulder level. Raise arms straight to ceiling, pulling and stretching the shoulder, neck, and arm muscles. Return to position even with the shoulder. Then stretch back as far as possible and swing forward to clasp hands. Then position arms down to side.

*Note:* In the case of a preoperative patient, this exercise should be performed in a standing position or sitting on the side of the bed. In the case of a postoperative patient, the exercise may be done in bed with the nurse assisting as necessary.

2. Raise shoulders up, circle them forward, down, and then pull back. The circular motion is used to loosen the chest, shoulder and upper back muscles. This exercise can be performed either in a sitting or standing position.

3. Clasp hands behind head and push elbows into the mattress. This exercise is to be performed lying flat in bed without a pillow, if possible.

**Breathing exercises.** These exercises should be begun preoperatively and continued postoperatively.

The following are recommended procedures for the patient to follow:

1. Place hands on ribs so that he can feel his chest move as he breathes.
2. Relax all abdominal muscles.
3. Suck in as much air as possible while expanding the chest.
4. Purse mouth, tighten abdominal muscles, and expel air. Cough.

## Bibliography

ABRAM, HARRY S.: Psychological Problems of Patients after Open-Heart Surgery. *Hospital Topics* XXXXIV:111–113, January 1966.

ENGEL, LEOPOLD: *The Operation.* McGraw-Hill Book Co., New York, 1958.

GANS, HENRY and KRIVIT, WILLIAM: Problems in Hemostasis During Open-Heart Surgery. *Arch. Surg.,* 90:731, 1965.

KEVY, SHERWIN, et al.: Hemorrhagic Defect in Open-Heart Surgery. Scientific exhibit presented at the clinical congress of the American College of Surgeons, Atlantic City, N.J., October 18–22, 1965.

KORNFELD, DONALD S., ZIMBERG, SHELDON, and MALM, JAMES R.: Psychiatric Complications of Open-Heart Surgery. *The New England Journal of Medicine,* 273:6:287–292, August 5, 1965.

LAWTON, GEORGE: *Straight to the Heart.* International Universities Press, New York, 1956.

McARDLE, KAREN H.: The Patient and the Bennett. In *The Nursing Clinics of North America,* pp. 143–152. W. B. Saunders Co., Philadelphia, March 1966.

MELTZER, LAWRENCE E., PINNEO, ROSE and KITCHELL, J. RODERICK: *Intensive Coronary Care, A Manual for Nurses.* The Charles Press, Philadelphia, 1965.

MODELL, et al.: *Handbook of Cardiology for Nurses,* fifth edition. Springer Publishing Co., New York, 1966.

NELSON, R. M., et al.: Effective Use of Prophylactic Antibiotics in Open-Heart Surgery. *Arch. Surg.,* 90:731, 1965.

PEDDIE, GEORGE H. and BRUSH, FRANCES E., (ed.): *Cardiovascular Surgery, A Manual for Nurses.* G. P. Putnam's Sons, New York, 1961.

REED, WILLIAM: Antibiotics and Cardiac Surgery. *The Journal of Thoracic and Cardiovascular Surgery,* 50:888–892, 1965.

Second National Conference on Cardiovascular Diseases, Cardiovascular Surgery. *The Heart and Circulation* I:597–631. Washington, D.C., 1964.

SHARP, A. A. and EGGLETON, M. J.: Haematology and the Extracorporeal Circulation. *Journal of Clinical Pathology,* 16:551–557, 1963.

Symposium on Nursing Problems of Persons with Cardiovascular Disorders, in *The Nursing Clinics of North America* I. W. B. Saunders Co., Philadelphia, March, 1966.

TAUSSIG, HELEN B.: *Congenital Malformations of the Heart,* vol. 1.

General Considerations. Harvard University Press, Cambridge, 1960.

TAUSSIG, HELEN B.: *Congenital Malformations of the Heart,* vol. II. Specific Malformations. Harvard University Press, Cambridge, 1960.

WULFSOHN, N. L.: *Aids to Pre and Postoperative Nursing,* second edition. Bailliere, Tindall and Cox, London, 1963.

*Films:*

1. "Disorders of the Heartbeat" (American Heart Association)
2. "Normal Heart Sounds and Innocent Murmurs" (United States Public Health Service)
3. "The Nurse's Role in Cardiopulmonary Resuscitation" (American Heart Association)
4. "Congestive Heart Failure in Infancy" (American Heart Association)
5. "Prescription for Life" (American Heart Association)
6. "Cardiac Arrhythmias" (Abbott Laboratories)

# CHAPTER XIII

# Acute Renal Failure and
# Renal Dialysis

BARBARA FELLOWS, R.N., M.N.

CHRISTOPHER R. BLAGG, M.D.

BELDING H. SCRIBNER, M.D.

Dialysis in the treatment of acute renal failure was first used by Dr. W. Koff in Holland in the early 1940's. Since that time many changes have taken place in dialysis equipment as well as the therapeutic approach to the problem of acute renal failure. Dialysis has evolved from a high-risk, expensive form of treatment to one that is relatively safe and economically feasible in many institutions. In the past, dialysis was considered the *last* form of treatment for a patient suffering from acute renal failure because of the inherent dangers of the procedure. Presently, either peritoneal or hemodialysis is one of the *first* procedures considered for patients with acute renal failure. This chapter will attempt to describe acute renal failure and its treatment by dialysis as used at the University of Washington Hospital, Seattle.

## THE PROBLEM

Most authors agree that acute renal failure can be defined as a condition in which the daily urine volume is less than 400 cc. Azotemia, however, sometimes develops rapidly despite normal urinary output. Causes of acute renal failure include:

1. *Prerenal failure* (circulatory insufficiency): blood loss; fluid and electrolyte imbalances; plasma loss; endotoxin shock; decreased cardiac output.

2. *Intrarenal:* acute tubular necrosis (which may follow prerenal failure); acute cortical necrosis; acute glomerulonephritis. Miscellaneous: papillary necrosis; multiple myeloma; polyarteritis nodosa and systemic lupus erythematosis; chronic renal disease presenting as apparent acute renal failure.

3. *Postrenal* (obstruction): *lower tract*—stricture; *upper tract* —bilateral calculi, blood clots, uric acid crystals; after bilateral retrograde catheterization; retroperitoneal fibrosis; cervical carcinoma or other pelvic carcinomas.

4. *Vascular occlusion: Arterial*—thrombosis, emboli; *venous* —thrombosis.

When a patient has oliguria, the physician first needs to exclude a reversible obstructive or vascular lesion and to treat any prerenal failure. Therefore, postrenal failure, vascular occlusion, and prerenal failure will be discussed first.

**Postrenal failure.** One of the first considerations in the treatment of acute renal failure must be to rule out postrenal or obstructive renal problems. It should be remembered that total anuria is common in postrenal failure, whereas it is very unusual in most other forms of acute renal failure.

Diagnostic measures which must be performed in order to exclude postrenal failure and so prevent the inevitable development of secondary renal damage include abdominal x-ray, cystoscopy, and ureteral catheterization. Additional information can be obtained by the introduction of 5–10 ml of dye via the ureteral catheter in order to delineate calyceal pattern and to assist in determination of kidney size and cortical thickness. A past history of renal calculi, urologic, or pelvic surgery can be causes to consider this diagnosis.

Prior to diagnosis or relief of the obstructive problem, dialysis may be necessary to control azotemia. If, however, diuresis follows relief of the obstruction, correction of uremia is rapid and electrolyte problems are more easily handled, because of the permitted higher fluid intake.

Nursing care of the patient with obstructive renal failure is basically the same as that of other patients in renal failure. However, symptoms of pain may be added to the observations made and should be reported immediately, for this may help in the diagnosis.

**Vascular occlusion.** Arterial and renal vein thrombosis are rare conditions. Renal vein thrombosis may arise from neoplasm, external compression, or in adults, renal amyloidosis. Sudden oliguria, proteinuria and renal failure occur along with edema of the lower limbs if the inferior vena cava is obstructed.

Renal artery thrombosis occurs particularly in elderly patients with advanced atheromatous vascular disease. A past history of cerebral or coronary thrombosis, or peripheral arterial disease is common. The outstanding symptom is severe pain in the renal area and flank.

Treatment of both of these occlusive conditions is anticoagulant therapy, in conjunction with rest and symptomatic treatment. Bilateral emboli to the renal arteries are most uncommon, but can occur in patients with heart disease. Immediate surgery is then necessary.

**Prerenal failure.** Conditions which reduce renal blood flow lead to decreased glomerular filtration rate and, therefore, decreased excretion of solutes. Metabolic waste products accumulate in the blood, resulting in acute tubular necrosis if proper treatment is not instituted early. In prerenal failure, correction of the circulation insufficiency results in diuresis; this is an important differential point between prerenal oliguria and acute *tubular necrosis.*

Great care must be taken by the physician to replace fluids, electrolytes, blood or plasma. If oliguria persists, signs of fluid overload must be carefully watched for. Monitoring of central venous pressure is a useful addition to the guidance obtained from the patient's history, skin turgor, pulse, blood pressure, urine volume, weight, hematocrit, electrolytes, and plasma protein concentration.

Nursing care of the patient with prerenal failure demands accurate calculations of intake and output. Daily weights are an invaluable aid in the determination of the patient's fluid status; to be of any value they must be accurate. Observing the patient for signs of fluid overload, such as dyspnea, is important and such evidence should always be brought to the attention of the physician. Proper explanation to the patient of why he must "save all urine" and "drink only fluids given to him" can be very helpful in his care. Reassurance to the patient that the urine output will increase and that he will soon be feeling better must be given cautiously. What may initially appear to be prerenal failure may well be the forerunner of a more serious renal problem. If prerenal failure is recognized and treated promptly by fluid and blood replacement, this state can usually be corrected. However, if circulatory insufficiency is allowed to persist without volume replacement, the patient may develop tubular necrosis.

In recent years there has been emphasis on the early recognition of prerenal failure as well as the need for adequate fluid replacement in those conditions leading to such failure. One useful solution in the management of these patients is mannitol. Mannitol, a carbohydrate, acts as a volume expander and as an osmotic diuretic. In patients with oliguria in whom the differential diagnosis between prerenal and renal failure is in doubt, judicious intravenous administration of mannitol will result in a diuresis, among those patients with prerenal failure. Prior to mannitol infusion, the patient's bladder should be catheterized to permit accurate measure of urine output. If diuresis ensues in response to mannitol, further treatment should be aimed at replacing the fluid, or electrolyte deficit, rather than continuing mannitol therapy. If diuresis does not occur after an intravenous dose of mannitol, the bladder catheter should be removed and the patient treated for acute tubular necrosis.

### Intrarenal failure

*Causes.* The most common form of acute intrarenal failure is *acute tubular necrosis*. This condition may be caused by the direct action of poisons (nephrotoxins) or, as previously stated, by *prolonged* circulatory insufficiency. Poisons such as carbon tetrachloride, mercury, arsenic, or lead cause necrosis of the tubular cells and prevent the transport of substances from the blood into the lumen of the tubule. Nephrotoxins also cause intense renal vasoconstriction with focal patches of renal ischemia, irregularly distributed.

*Acute cortical necrosis* is a very rare sequela of severe circulatory insufficiency and usually occurs as a complication of pregnancy.

*Acute glomerulonephritis* has many causes including reaction to infection with beta hemolytic streptococcus. Common clinical features of this disease are edema, weight gain, and oliguria; hypertension, increased venous pressure; and hematuria, and proteinuria. Prognosis is generally good; however, the longer the period of oliguria, the poorer the prognosis, particularly in adults.

Necrotizing papillitis, multiple myeloma, polyarteritis nodosa, and systemic lupus erythematosis may all present as acute renal failure; when they do the prognosis is extremely poor. Diagnosis of these conditions is often suggested by the presence of extrarenal clinical features. Renal biopsy can be invaluable for confirming the diagnosis and for establishing the prognosis.

Chronic renal disease may also present as apparent acute renal failure; in the past it also had a poor prognosis. However, with the advent of successful long-term dialysis programs, and the increasing success of renal transplantation, the outlook for a patient with chronic renal disease is much brighter.

*General treatment of acute tubular necrosis.* As in other types of renal failure, treatment includes proper replacement and maintenance of fluids and electrolytes. During the oliguric phase of renal failure, urea, creatinine, potassium, phosphates and other substances accumulate in the blood and extracellular fluid as a result of the catabolism of tissues and foodstuffs. There is also an accumulation of hydrogen ions, producing a fall in plasma pH and bicarbonate.

Successful treatment of renal shutdown depends to a large extent on the skill with which complications are anticipated and prevented. The complications to be prevented include pulmonary edema, water excess, potassium intoxication, acidosis and the uremic syndrome.

The main danger to life is a rising concentration of plasma potassium which may cause cardiac arrest. Any patient with acute renal failure, who begins to develop hyperkalemia, should be transferred immediately to a dialysis center. Hyperkalemia can be prevented in all but the most severely catabolic patients, hence, any treatment which will minimize catabolism is of value. In addition, removal of dead or traumatized tissue and collections of extravasated blood are essential. Prevention of acidosis will help control hyperkalemia by keeping potassium in the cells. Orally or rectally-administered cation-exchange resins may help remove excess potassium.

The other major imbalance associated with acute tubular necrosis is disturbance in sodium and/or water. Preventing water excess is difficult but essential. Water excess is characterized by low serum sodium concentrations. A falling serum sodium level indicates that the treatment plan is ineffective with respect to water restriction. Water depletion occurs less often in renal failure but can be suspected from elevated sodium levels.

Saline excess or extracellular volume excess can occur in any patient with renal failure and cause congestive heart failure and/or severe hypertension. The physical findings of such excess are weight gain and, later, edema. Saline depletion also can develop. Symptoms of saline depletion are hypotension, weakness, nausea, and vomiting. Low venous pressure is a more sensitive guide to this disorder, as is postural hypotension. Elevations of the hematocrit and serum proteins are characteristic of depletion states.

Patients with acute tubular necrosis sometimes develop thirst even in the presence of a low serum sodium level. They should not be allowed to drink water. Sucking a few ice chips made from hypertonic dextrose will help allay this feeling of thirst while at the same time providing needed calories.

Sodium restriction is essential in helping to prevent systemic and pulmonary edema. On the other hand, sodium may be needed to treat hyperkalemia, severe hyponatremia, and severe acidosis. Therefore, in order to avoid increasing the total body sodium above normal, attempts should be made to follow the principle that the only indication for giving sodium will be a definite decrease in the total body sodium. This may be accomplished by:

1. Treating hyponatremia by restricting water rather than by giving sodium.

2. Not giving sodium to patients with acute renal failure for the sole purpose of treating acidosis. Acidosis should be anticipated in each case of acute renal failure and every effort made to prevent its development. When the patient needs sodium to

replace losses, or a deficit, all sodium should be given in the form of sodium lactate or bicarbonate.

Anemia always develops in acute renal failure; it is due to increased red cell destruction and depressed bone marrow function. Usually this anemia requires no treatment except when the hematocrit drops below 25. The therapy necessary at this time is to administer red blood cells. Anemia usually persists during the first part of the diuretic phase but will eventually be corrected spontaneously.

The most common complication of uremia is infection. Every effort should be made to reduce the obvious sources of infection, e.g., by removing such unnecessary apparatus as urinary catheters. Pneumonia is often a problem that can often be prevented by good nursing care. Antibiotics should never be administered prophylactically but should be given only when an infection is identified. Care must also be taken to properly adjust the dose of toxic antibiotics which are excreted primarily by the kidneys (e.g., kanamycin).

Every effort should be made to start the patient on oral feeding as soon as possible. This not only eliminates the intravenous infusion as a source of infection but also allows the patient to ambulate freely without being hampered by bottles and tubing. Early ambulation is important if the pulmonary complications of uremia are to be avoided. With dialysis, the patient can be started on a palatable diet which is low in sodium, potassium, and protein.

The diuretic phase of acute renal failure begins when the urine volume reaches one liter in 24 hours. The early part of this phase can be troublesome and clinical improvement may be delayed for many days. Hemodialysis is often necessary during the diuretic phase and when the indications are present, it should never be postponed. Indications for dialysis include hyperkalemia and a BUN rising about 100 mg%. The therapeutic plan in establishing fluid balance is to compensate for various defects in renal regulation which develop as diuresis proceeds. The kidney may waste water, sodium, or potassium in an unpredictable pattern and these must be appropriately replaced.

The early diuretic phase is managed in the same manner as the oliguric phase, except that water restriction is less of a problem. Despite seemingly adequate intake, sodium depletion due to renal salt wastage may develop. Urine chloride will roughly reflect urine sodium during this time. Hematocrit determinations and measurement of body weight are needed serially to warn of saline depletion. Acidosis remains a potential problem. Potassium depletion may also be a complication at this time unless adequate maintenance therapy is provided. During this phase, patients may have a diuresis as large as 6 liters per day. The cause of this profound diuresis appears to be a combination of three mechanisms: an osmotic diuresis due to the high blood urea; tubular functional inadequacy; and the release of an accumulation of surplus fluid and electrolytes.

The post-diuretic phase is characterized by a normal urine output and has no distinct time of occurrence. It may take several months before this state is reached. Renal blood flow and glomerular filtration rate increase, and the ability to concentrate the urine (in conjunction with other tubular functions) tends to return toward normal, but may not do so completely.

Nursing care of patients in renal failure will be discussed subsequently.


## DIALYSIS

In our hospital, at the present time, dialysis is performed for patients in acute renal failure in order to prevent, rather than treat, uremia. By using this approach to the treatment of acute renal failure many of the complications of uremia can be reduced or eliminated, and the outlook for patient survival increased tremendously. Over the past 5 years, more than 200 patients with acute renal failure have been managed according to this philosophy. There have been no deaths due to technical complications. The mortality rate among these patients has averaged below 30% each year and appears to be determined mainly by the prognosis of the other diseases which are present in each particular case.

The overall management of the patient with acute renal failure is a difficult and complex problem which requires continuing experiences in all aspects of care of the critically ill patient. Although intensive dialysis is essential for optimal care, this alone will not ensure success.

**Principle of dialysis.** The principle of dialysis is that of bringing blood into contact with a semipermeable membrane through which diffusion of toxins takes place. The solutes in the solution of greater concentration pass through the membrane into the solution of lesser concentration. (Diffusion is described additionally on p. 231.) Figure 1 shows schematically the diffusion of urea from the blood, through the dialyzing membrane, while molecules of bicarbonate pass from the dialysate fluid into the blood. Sub-

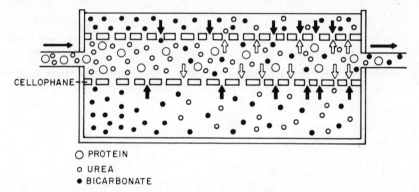

○ PROTEIN
○ UREA
● BICARBONATE

*Fig. 1. The principle of dialysis: diffusion of substances through a cellophane membrane.*

stances normally found in the blood such as sodium, calcium, and magnesium are placed in the dialysate fluid in such concentration that they will not be removed from the blood by dialysis. Substances which should be removed from the patient's blood, such as urea and creatinine, are absent from the dialysate fluid and therefore will be removed. In addition to removing substances, dialysis also permits the replacement of deficiencies. For example, a deficiency of bicarbonate can be corrected by placing this ion in the dialysate fluid. The semipermeable membrane used in hemodialysis is cellophane; in peritoneal dialysis the peritoneum serves as the membrane.

In our hospital, both hemodialysis and peritoneal dialysis are used in the treatment of acute and chronic renal failure. In acute renal failure the type of dialysis is often dependent on the patient's primary disease. Patients who have had recent abdominal surgery, severe respiratory distress, or who are extremely catabolic (all necessitating rapid removal of waste products), would be likely candidates for hemodialysis. Patients with *chronic* renal disease, who do not have a commitment for long-term dialysis, would probably be treated with peritoneal dialysis.

### A. *Hemodialysis*

#### 1. CANNULAS

When a patient is to be hemodialyzed, cannulas are inserted into an extremity of the patient. The exact placement of the cannula is dependent on available vessels. (Many patients with acute renal failure have multiple fractures of several extremities and are fed intravenously, thus reducing the number of available sites.)

The cannula is an appliance made of teflon and silastic and can be placed in the vessels of any extremity (Fig. 2). Teflon tips

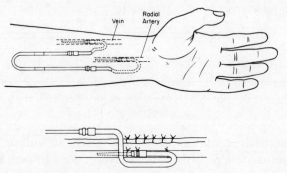

*Fig. 2. Schematic representation of cannulas in a patient's arm.*

(1½″ long) are inserted in a superficial artery and vein; these are attached to silastic tubing which is brought out through the patient's skin (Fig. 3). When dialysis is not being performed, the two cannula ends are connected by the use of a teflon joint. This creates an external shunt between the artery and vein as seen in Fig. 2. When the patient is to be dialyzed, the joint is opened and each end is connected to special fittings on the hemodialyzer (artificial kidney). When dialysis is stopped, the joint is reconnected for resumption of flow through the shunt. The indwelling cannulas eliminate the necessity for repeated cutdowns, and permit ready access to the patient's bloodstream when hemodialysis is indicated. In addition, the cannula may provide the only accessible vessel for intravenous infusions, and for blood collection.

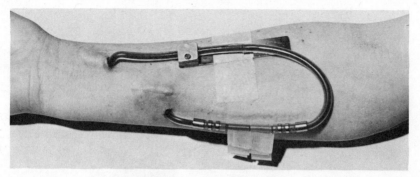

*Fig. 3. Cannulas in place in a patient's arm.*

The cannula should be cleaned twice a day with a hexachlorophene soap. The soap is used about the exit site of each cannula and left on the skin in order to decrease the chance of infection. The extremity is then cleansed with alcohol and redressed. Depending on the condition of the patient, the extremity may have to be immobilized to protect the system. The cannula is left in place until there is no further need for dialysis. At that time, the cannula is clamped for approximately 24 hours to allow clotting and it is then removed by the physician.

### 2. THE ARTIFICIAL KIDNEY

The artificial kidney currently in use in Seattle, is the modified two-layer Kiil (Fig. 4). Many other types of dialyzers can be used such as the twin coil, the "chronic" coil, and the Skeggs-Leonard dialyzers. Basically all dialyzers depend on the same principles: (a) the use of the patient's blood, (b) a cellophane membrane which is semipermeable, through which diffusion takes place between blood and dialysate fluid, and (c) a dialysate supply which runs over the cellophane membrane removing waste products from the patient's blood.

The modified two-layer Kiil consists of three polypropylene boards with grooves along which the dialysate fluid flows. When the dialyzer is assembled, there are two pieces of cellophane membrane in each layer between which the blood flows one way, and the dialysate fluid (outside of the cellophane membrane) flows in the opposite direction (Fig. 5).

The advantages of this type of dialyzer are many: (1) it can

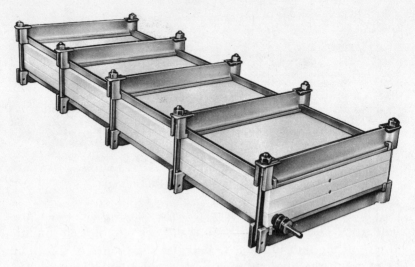

*Fig. 4. Modified two-layer Kiil dialyzer.*

be easily cleaned and assembled and the blood compartment readily sterilized; (2) it does not need to be filled or primed with blood before the patient goes on dialysis, as the system only holds between 300–400 cc of blood; (3) the patient is able to propel his blood through the dialyzer with his own arterial pressure, although, when necessary, a blood pump can be used to assist the flow; and (4) using this dialyzer, the techniques of hemodialysis have been simplified to the extent that it is a nurse-technician procedure.

The disadvantage of this type of dialyzer is the longer time re-

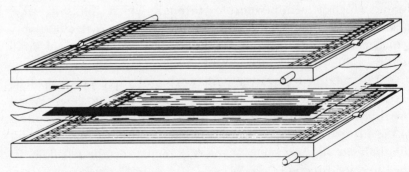

*Fig. 5. Schematic representation of the Kiil dialyzer showing blood between cellophane and the grooves through which the dialysate fluid flows.*

quired for dialysis, because of the smaller surface area. Blood flow rates through the Kiil dialyzer range from 100 to 250 cc/min, and are mainly dependent on the size of the cannulas used. Other dialyzers can achieve blood flow rates up to 500 cc/min. Dialysis, using a Kiil dialyzer, takes almost twice as long as some other types.

### 3. DIALYSATE SUPPLY SYSTEM

The dialysate supply system used for acute dialysis is a 385 liter refrigerated Sweden Freezer tank. The dialysate is pumped from the tank through rubber tubing into the dialyzer at a usual rate of 2 liters per minute. When the dialysate leaves the dialyzer, it is returned to the tank where it is recirculated. The dialysate fluid is kept at a temperature of 20° C. in order to decrease bacterial growth. Since the tank contains 385 liters of dialysate fluid, it is only necessary to change the fluid every 20–24 hours. At the end of dialysis, the waste products from the patient will remain in the dialysate in the tank. The advantage of this type of system is that it is mobile and can be moved to any place in the hospital. The dialysate fluid can be mixed according to the particular patient's needs.

### 4. PROCEDURE OF HEMODIALYSIS

After the physician has ordered the composition of the dialysate bath and a technician has made up the solution and assembled the equipment, the patient is moved to the intensive care unit for dialysis. The physician initiates the dialysis and it then becomes the nurse's responsibility to monitor procedure.

During dialysis of patients with acute renal failure, *regional* heparinization (in contrast to total heparinization) is required. The technique of regional heparinization consists of infusing heparin into the blood as it *leaves* the patient (to prevent the blood in the dialyzer from clotting) and at the same time adding protamine to the blood as it returns to the patient to neutralize the effects of the heparin. This method minimizes the risk of bleeding. The dosage of heparin to protamine varies between a 1:1 and a 1:2 ratio. The physician determines this ratio when he initiates the dialysis. The usual starting dose of each of these agents is 3000 units per hour (or 30 mg/hr). The dosage is adjusted according to the clotting times of the artificial kidney and of the patient as obtained during dialysis. The "kidney" clotting time should be over 40 minutes, and the "patient" clotting time should be as normal as possible. (Normal "patient" clotting times should be assessed before the patient is put on dialysis because of variations from patient to patient.) When patient bleeding problems no longer exist, *total* heparinization can be used. This technique consists of infusing heparin into the blood as it leaves the patient to go into the dialyzer. When using total heparinization, only "kidney" clotting times need to be determined since the concern is that the dialyzer does not clot. The "patient" clotting time will, of course, be prolonged.

### 5. MONITORING THE DIALYSIS

As noted, the nurse assumes the responsibility for continuous monitoring of the patient undergoing dialysis. The monitoring includes a series of written observations made every $\frac{1}{2}$ hour (Fig. 6).

Specifically, the nurse records the following information: a) the blood flow rate through the dialyzer; b) the dialysate flow rate; c) the temperature of the dialysate bath and the heating element (which warms the dialysate returning from the cooled storage tank); d) the rate of heparin and protamine delivery into the system; e) the blood pressure and other vital signs; f) negative pressure measurement.

In addition, the patient's clotting time and the kidney clotting time are recorded (Fig. 7).

### 6. MECHANICAL PROBLEMS DURING DIALYSIS

The nurse must be aware of disturbances related to equipment function. The following problems should be recorded promptly to the physician.

a. *Decrease in the patient's blood pressure*

A decrease in blood pressure might be the result of a blood leak in the dialysis circuit or excessive removal of fluid. If a blood leak exists, immediate action must be taken by the nurse to repair the circuit. If the leak is in the dialyzer, the nurse must stop the flow of blood from the patient to the dialyzer by clamping the line. Decreased blood pressure, due to excessive removal of fluid from the patient, may result from inappropriate dialysate concentrations.

## ACUTE HEMODIALYSIS LOG

On dialysis: Date _____ Hr _____ Name _____

Off dialysis: Date _____ Hr _____

*Predialysis   Postdialysis*

| Blood | | Total | | Potassium |
|---|---|---|---|---|
| _____ Pressure _____ | | Sodium _____ mEq/L | | Chloride _____ mEq/L |
| _____ Weight _____ | | Dextrose _____ Gm-mg% | | Calcium |
| Type of dialyzer _____ | | Sodium Bicar- | | Chloride _____ mEq/L |
| Tank size _____ | | bonate _____ mEq/L | | Magnesium |
| Priming blood _____ | | Sodium | | Chloride _____ mEq/L |
| Heparinization: | | Acetate _____ mEq/L | | Added |
| Total _____ | | Regional _____ | | Chemicals _____ |
| | | | | Time added _____ |

### MONITORING

| Time | Blood Flow | Dial Flow | Temperature Bath | Heater | Heparin Syringe (cc) | Protamine Syringe (cc) | Vital Signs | Neg. Press | Remarks |
|---|---|---|---|---|---|---|---|---|---|
| | | | | | | | | | |
| | | | | | | | | | |
| | | | | | | | | | |
| | | | | | | | | | |
| | | | | | | | | | |
| | | | | | | | | | |
| | | | | | | | | | |
| | | | | | | | | | |
| | | | | | | | | | |
| | | | | | | | | | |
| | | | | | | | | | |
| | | | | | | | | | |

*Fig. 6.*

## CLOTTING TIME

Name _____

Date _____

| PATIENT | | | KIDNEY | | | PUMP SETTING | |
|---|---|---|---|---|---|---|---|
| Time Drawn | Time Clotted | Clotting Time | Time Drawn | Time Clotted | Clotting Time | Heparin | Protamine |
| | | | | | | | |
| | | | | | | | |
| | | | | | | | |
| | | | | | | | |
| | | | | | | | |
| | | | | | | | |
| | | | | | | | |
| | | | | | | | |
| | | | | | | | |
| | | | | | | | |
| | | | | | | | |
| | | | | | | | |
| | | | | | | | |
| | | | | | | | |
| | | | | | | | |
| | | | | | | | |
| | | | | | | | |
| | | | | | | | |

*Fig. 7.*

b. *Abnormal clotting times*

These disturbances may be related to improper delivery of either heparin or protamine during regional heparinization leading to an incorrect ratio for the patient. Regional heparinization is a difficult procedure at best, and it is possible that not only may the ratio be incorrect for the patient, but abnormal clotting factors will also be present to exaggerate the problem. In this situation, the physician must change the ratio of heparin to protamine to correct the abnormality.

c. *Clotting in the artificial kidney or the cannula*

If a clot develops within the artificial kidney, another dialyzer must be obtained and put into use. The blood volume lost in the dialyzer must be replaced. Clots developing in a cannula can be removed by the physician. This is accomplished by instilling warmed heparinized saline (1:100 solution) into both the arterial and venous cannulas to dislodge the clots.

d. *Reduced blood flow through the dialyzer*

If the flow rate through the dialyzer becomes decreased, the patient's blood pressure should be checked and the circuit examined for disconnections or kinks. The physician should be notified promptly thereafter. A low systemic blood pressure (due to excess ultra filtration) is often the cause of reduced blood flow. The problem may also develop because of poor placement of the cannula or inadequate blood vessels. In these latter situations a blood pump can be attached to the system to improve the flow.

e. *Collapsed blood lines when using a blood pump*

This problem may indicate decreased systemic blood pressure, kinking of the blood lines (between the patient and the machine), or vessel spasm. The nurse should reduce the rate of the blood pump and then observe the circuit for problems (particularly the dialysate fluid for blood leaks). Frequent measurement of the patient's blood pressure is always important.

## PERITONEAL DIALYSIS

The technique of peritoneal dialysis employed on our service, for patients with acute renal failure, involves the insertion of a peritoneal catheter (through a customary paracentesis puncture) and the exchange of dialysis fluid by means of an automatic cycling machine.

**Peritoneal dialysis with an automatic cycling machine (Fig. 8).**

1. *Peritoneal catheter.* With the patient in a supine position, a "Trocath" peritoneal catheter (the type preferred in this institution) is inserted by the physician. The skin is prepared with iodine solution and aseptic techniques are employed. Following local anesthesia with 1% lidocaine, a minute (5 mm) skin incision is made below the umbilicus in the midline of the abdomen. Alternative sites for catheter insertion are the left or right abdomen near the iliac crests. The trocar is inserted through the skin inci-

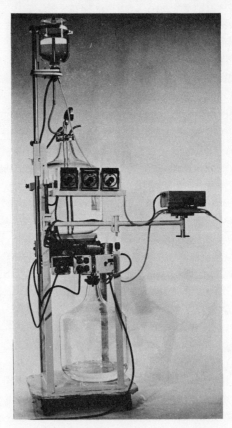

*Fig. 8. Automatic cycling machine used for peritoneal dialysis.*

sion and the peritoneum is then perforated without undue force. If the trocar meets resistance, a tract must be established for easy passage with the scalpel. The physician must use care in inserting the catheter to avoid the potential risk of perforating the bowel or of cutting a mesenteric artery by a sudden thrust of the trocar as it enters the peritoneal cavity. This threat can be avoided by puncturing the peritoneum with restrained force. The patient is then placed in a 45° sitting position which allows comfort and permits proper drainage of fluid. The patient may be turned without harm during the procedure.

After the dialysis has been completed, the catheter is removed and the skin incision swabbed with iodine. The wound is sealed by drawing the skin edges together with several gauze pads and sterile tape in order to prevent leakage.

2. *The automatic cycling machine* consists of a pumping system to deliver and remove the dialysing fluid, together with calibrated inflow and outflow bottles. In addition there are timers which automatically control the duration of the periods of inflow, diffusion, and outflow (Fig. 9).

When the dialysis is initiated, the physician sets the timing devices. The inflow time (i.e., the time to deliver the fluid into the peritoneal cavity) is usually about 5 minutes; the diffusion time (i.e., the period of actual dialysis) is 30 minutes; and outflow time (i.e., the return of fluid to the collection bottle) is approximately 15 minutes.

The sterile dialysis fluid is stored in a large bottle (a carboy holding 20 to 40 liters) which is heated by a hot plate to 38° C. This fluid is pumped into an elevated reservoir where the volume of fluid to be delivered to the patient is preset (the usual volume is two liters).

At time zero, a valve opens allowing this desired volume to flow into the abdomen. After 5 minutes, the valve closes and diffusion takes place for 30 minutes. The outflow valve then opens automatically and the fluid in the peritoneal cavity is allowed to flow into the outflow bottle. This latter flow which takes about 15 minutes is accomplished by gravity, assisted by a small vacuum pump. The entire cycle usually takes about 45 minutes, providing for an optimal dialysis flow rate of about 3 liters per

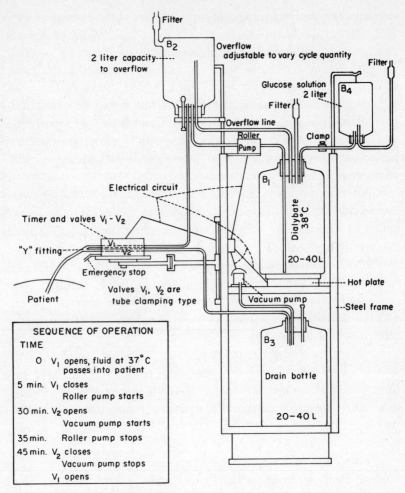

Filter

B₂
2 liter capacity to overflow

Overflow
adjustable to vary cycle quantity

Glucose solution
2 liter

Filter

B₄

Filter

Overflow line

Roller
Pump

Clamp

B₁

Dialybate
38°C

Electrical circuit

20–40L

Timer and valves V₁ - V₂

"Y" fitting

V₁
V₂

Emergency stop

Hot plate

Patient

Valves V₁, V₂ are
tube clamping type

Vacuum pump

Steel frame

SEQUENCE OF OPERATION

TIME

  0   V₁ opens, fluid at 37°C
        passes into patient

5 min.  V₁ closes
          Roller pump starts

30 min. V₂ opens
          Vacuum pump starts

35 min.   Roller pump stops

45 min. V₂ closes
          Vacuum pump stops
          V₁ opens

B₃

Drain bottle

20–40 L

*Fig. 9. Schematic diagram of automatic cycling machine.*

hour. If necessary, the outflow or any of the other cycles can be repeated as desired by the nurse.

**3. Monitoring peritoneal dialysis.** Unless the patient's condition warrants constant attention, the nurse need not remain at
the bedside during the complete procedure of peritoneal dialysis.
The nurse must verify, however, that the volume of fluid removed from the peritoneal cavity is equal to, or more than, the
amount put into the patient. The nurse caring for the patient
should check the system, at least after every full cycle. At these
times, the following information should be recorded (Fig. 10):

## PERITONEAL DIALYSIS LOG

Off dialysis: Date _____ Hr _____    Name _____

On dialysis: Date _____ Hr _____

Total hours _____

*Predialysis*          *Postdialysis*
_____              _____
*Blood Pressure*
_____ Supine _____
_____ Sitting _____
_____ Standing _____
_____ Weight _____

*Total infusion Volume*
_____
Onset _____ Liters
Inflow _____ Liters
Outflow _____ Liters
Blood Transfusion _____
Total Blood Drawn _____ ml

*Bath Composition*

Sodium Chloride _____ mEq/L

Sodium Acetate _____ mEq/L

Potassium Chloride _____ mEq/L

Calcium Chloride _____ mEq/L

Magnesium Chloride _____ mEq/L

Heparin _____ units/L

Dextrose _____ gm/mg%

Other Additions _____

_____

_____

| TIME | INFLOW | OUTFLOW | DIALYSATE TEMP. | REMARKS |
|------|--------|---------|-----------------|---------|
|      |        |         |                 |         |
|      |        |         |                 |         |
|      |        |         |                 |         |
|      |        |         |                 |         |
|      |        |         |                 |         |
|      |        |         |                 |         |
|      |        |         |                 |         |
|      |        |         |                 |         |
|      |        |         |                 |         |
|      |        |         |                 |         |
|      |        |         |                 |         |
|      |        |         |                 |         |
|      |        |         |                 |         |

*Fig. 10.*

a) inflow volume; b) outflow volume; c) dialysate temperature (to be kept between 36° and 40° C); d) leakage around the catheter?

**4. *Problems during peritoneal dialysis***

a. *Pain.* Patients frequently experience pain during the outflow cycle. This can usually be controlled by restarting the inflow along with the use of papaverine. In this situation the automatic cycling machine enables personnel to vary the volume of fluid administered, as well as the length of time for diffusion and outflow.

b. *Diaphragmatic pressure.* If the inflow volume of dialysate is excessive, or if all of the fluid is not removed from the peritoneal cavity with each outflow, excess pressure can develop against the diaphragm. This may decrease the normal excursion of the diaphragm and produce pulmonary complications. It is essential for the nurse to ascertain that a proper balance exists between inflow and outflow in order to prevent this threat. Extreme care should be taken to remove all fluid from the peritoneal cavity at each outflow period.

c. *Hypovolemia.* Occasionally, the fluid removed from the patient is greatly in excess of that administered. Continuation of this imbalance leads to a depletion of the body's fluids, which may be manifested by a fall in blood pressure, marked weight loss, and an obvious excess of fluid in the outflow bottle. This problem is corrected by parenteral fluid replacement.

The automatic cycling technique of peritoneal dialysis has several distinct advantages over the simple manual gravity system employed in many hospitals. The latter technique, which involves the connection and disconnection of multiple individual liter bottles, in order to deliver and return the dialysate, can be considered an open system with an inherent risk of infection. By using the closed sterile system of automatic cycling, the chance of infection is greatly reduced.

The automatic cycler also reduces nursing time to a minimum and decreases cost of fluid (made at the hospital in large 40 liter carboys at a fraction of the cost of 40 individual liter bottles).

This simplified method of peritoneal dialysis by an automatic cycling machine has enabled us to carry out this procedure easily in all areas of the hospital. Currently we have three chronic patients who are on a home peritoneal dialysis program using this same cycling machine, one for over 4½ years.

## THE NURSING ROLE

To see a patient arrive with multiple fractures, in a semi-comatose state, with hyperkalemia, oliguria and pulmonary edema due to acute renal failure, and then, several days later to observe him up in a wheelchair, alert and starting to regain his renal function, is a very exciting and rewarding experience. It is not difficult to imagine the limited survival time of this patient, or what complications may have developed without dialysis and good nursing care during the early stages of the illness.

Care of patients with acute renal failure treated with dialysis, compared to care without dialysis, differs only in degree. Both groups may present difficult nursing problems related to uremic complications; however, in the dialyzed patient the problems may be of a lesser degree and usually are easier to control.

Though nursing care of patients with acute renal failure is fundamentally the same as that given to any other critically ill patient, some areas of special importance are:

**Prevention of pulmonary complications.** Patients with uremia are highly susceptible to infections, particularly pneumonia; in fact, these complications frequently decide the ultimate outcome of the illness.

The high risk of pneumonia in patients with uremia is related to the presence of thick, tenacious pulmonary secretions along with depression of the cough reflex and sensorium. The nurse has an important responsibility in attempting to prevent this serious complication. The customary practices of early ambulation and turning the patient frequently are fundamental in this regard. Tracheal aspiration, tracheostomy, and positive pressure respirators are used commonly as prophylactic measures to prevent atelectasis. Mouth care is vitally important to prevent bacterial growth. Antiseptic mouth washes, as well as lubricants for sore mucous membranes, should be used frequently.

**Fluid balance.** Preservation of fluid balance is a basic aim in the treatment program. Precise intake and output recording, as well as accurate weighing of the patient, are essential guides in establishing fluid balance. These procedures are as necessary to the care of the patient in renal failure as is proper respiratory care. Weighing should not be relegated to auxiliary personnel alone, but should be carefully supervised by the nurse in charge of the patient.

**Diet.** Intravenous feedings are used until the patient can take food by mouth. During this period, thirst is a common complaint. This distressing symptom can sometimes be relieved by the use of glucose ice chips which are made by freezing 20%–50% glucose solution in an ice tray.

When oral intake is started, the diet is usually restricted to 20–40 G protein, 500 mg sodium and a low potassium content. Fluids are restricted to approximately 500 cc per day. The diet should be as high as possible in carbohydrate and fat in order to reduce the rate of endogenous protein breakdown. Hard candy, kept at the bedside, is useful in supplying added calories.

**Dialysis.** Prior to dialysis, the patient must be informed about the procedure. Because of mental confusion often associated with uremia, there is an unfortunate tendency to assume that the patient is unable to hear conversations, or that he is unaware of his surroundings. These assumptions should never be made and thoughtful communication with the patient must not be disregarded. Similarly, the patient's family should be informed of the dialysis and apprised of subsequent developments.

The nursing role in monitoring the dialysis has been described previously. It must be emphasized that the nurse's major responsibility during dialysis is to the patient and that management of the equipment is of lesser significance. Specifically, when a patient is put on dialysis, it does not mean that care of the machinery begins and good patient care ends. Physical care given the patient must not be interrupted because of dialysis. Dialysis does not bring an end to turning, coughing, deep breathing, mouth care, and the other elements of good nursing care. The oft-spoken comment, "I couldn't turn the patient because he was on dialysis" is absolutely false and every effort must be made to correct this damaging impression.

**The diuretic and recovery phases.** Although the oliguric phase has passed, efforts directed at preventing infection and pulmonary complications must not be abandoned, nor should accurate recording of intake and output, weight, and proper attention to diet, be neglected. In fact change in body weight is an important criterion in guiding therapy during the diuretic phase. If a patient loses weight rapidly and the urine volume is very high, a salt depletion state can develop. In this situation, the sodium intake usually has to be increased to levels considerably above normal, and the nurse can be instrumental in this regard by encouraging the patient to eat salty foods.

The recovery phase is often slow. Ambulation is desirable and should be encouraged. Reactive emotional depression may occur during the recovery period and the nurse can be of great assistance in helping the patient to combat this state.

## Dialysis training program

The orientation program employed at the University Hospital is conducted by the Renal Nursing Supervisor, with the assistance of her staff, during one 8-hour day. Its primary emphasis is on hemodialysis and the techniques used to insure patient care and safety. The expectations of the program are that the nurse will not only have a basic understanding of dialysis and its problems but also will be able to utilize the knowledge of the physician in charge of dialysis when necessary. It is emphasized during the orientation that the nurse's major responsibility is to the patient and that the management of the machinery is only an adjunct to his care. Technicians will be available to deal with any serious mechanical complication. The procedure of peritoneal dialysis is not emphasized in our hospital during the orientation program because of its simplicity. Approximately 30 minutes can be spent with a nurse explaining the automatic cycling machine and the complications which might arise.

For many nurses, one day of orientation is not enough. Our orientation program is flexible in order to provide added time, and a renal nurse can also be provided, as necessary, to assist the new nurse during her first period of caring for a dialysis patient.

Our intensive care units are set up to enable the nurse to assist in the dialysis procedure with a minimum of trouble. Equipment for cannulation is always kept in the unit ready for instant use. Materials such as clotting tubes, log sheets, and dialysate order sheets (Fig. 11) are stocked in the unit. Cards kept in the files provide ready reminders for the nurse on equipment needed to begin dialysis, how to measure clotting times, the equipment needed for a cannulation, how to monitor dialysis, and other procedures.

Communication among all members of the treatment team is vitally important and must be stressed. This communication must include for the nurse and technician such aspects as:

1. General plan of care for the patient.
2. Time and place of cannulation or insertion of peritoneal catheter.
3. Time and place of dialysis.
4. What does the physician want to accomplish during dialysis (e.g., how much fluid removal, lowering blood pressure, etc.)?
   a) Length of dialysis.
   b) Regional heparinization—what are the desired clotting times for the patient?
   c) Ultrafiltration—desired or not, and how much.
5. Whom to call in case of difficulties with the dialysis, cannula or catheter.

If these aspects of the procedure are made clear to all personnel involved with the dialysis procedure, reduction in wasted time and effort will be accomplished, better patient care will ensue, and fewer problems will be encountered.

The orientation program is shown below.

### ORIENTATION TO HEMODIALYSIS

This orientation is designed to familiarize the new staff nurse with the techniques and procedures of hemodialysis so that she is able to give satisfactory nursing care to patients undergoing hemodialysis. The emphasis in the orientation is on the technical aspects of dialysis, in order to make the nurse

## DIALYSATE ORDER FORM

Date of Dialysis _____ Time _____ Patient Name _____

### DIALYSATE COMPOSITION

_____ mEq/L Total Sodium (Na)     _____ _____

_____ mg% Dextrose     _____ _____
or

_____ gm%     _____ _____

_____ mEg/L Sodium Bicarbonate ($NaHCO_3$)    _____ _____

_____ mEq/L Sodium Acetate (NaAc)    _____ _____

_____ mEq/L Potassium Chloride (KCl)    _____ _____

_____ mEq/L Calcium Chloride ($CaCl_2$)    _____ _____

_____ mEq/L Magnesium Chloride ($MgCl_2$)    _____ _____

_____ mEq/L Sodium Chloride (NaCl)    _____ _____

_____ ml Lactic Acid    _____ml _____ml

_____ mg% Urea (BUN $\times$ 2 = Urea)    _____ _____

_____     Chemicals    _____ _____

_____     Regional Heparinization    _____   Negative Dialysate Pressure

_____     Constant Infusion Heparin    _____ _____

_____     Other

_____ M.D.
Signature

### FOR LABORATORY USE

| CHECK LIST ITEMS | Sent | Returned | DIALYSATE TEST | |
|---|---|---|---|---|
| Tubing Pliers | \_\_\_\_ | _____ | Total Base | _____ |
| Cannula Clamps | \_\_\_\_ | _____ | Chloride | _____ |
| Hemostats | \_\_\_\_ | _____ | Bicarbonate | _____ |
| Manometer, Hg | \_\_\_\_ | _____ | Potassium (TPB) | _____ |
| Manometer, Aneroid | \_\_\_\_ | _____ | | |
| Connectors (2) | \_\_\_\_ | _____ | | |
| Extra Drip Bulb | \_\_\_\_ | _____ | _____ | |
| Extension Cord | \_\_\_\_ | _____ | Technician | |
| | | | Dialysate Temp. in °C _____ | |

*Fig. 11.*

sufficiently comfortable with the equipment so that she can give the maximum amount of attention during dialysis to the patient and his needs. The primary objective of the technical orientation is to enable the nurse to preserve the safety of the patient at all times.

## PROGRAM

*Morning*
1. Discussion of acute and chronic dialysis programs, their philosophies and objectives.
2. Discussion and demonstration of cannulas and their care.
   a. Daily cannula care
   b. Cannula problems
   c. Return demonstration of cannula care
3. Acute renal failure.
   a. Etiology
   b. Most significant nursing care problems:
      1) Pulmonary complications
      2) Infections
      3) Fluid-electrolyte balance: restricted intake, measuring output, daily weight, B.P.
4. Principles of dialysis.
   a. The Kiil dialyzer
      1) General explanation of mechanics and dialysate
      2) Visit to Artificial Kidney Lab for observation
5. Observation of patients starting and ending dialysis.

*Afternoon*
6. The nurse's role in dialysis for acute renal failure.
   a. Intensive Care Unit
      1) Location of equipment
         a) For cannulation. Discussion of preparation
         b) For start and end of dialysis
      2) Ordering and obtaining other necessary equipment
      3) Kardex dialysis information. Reference manual
   b. Monitoring the equipment during dialysis
      1) Observation
      2) Discussion
      3) Return demonstration
   c. Recognizing problems during dialysis

1) Emergency measures: leaks; cannulas apart; heparin line off
2) Notifying the doctor: when to call, whom to call, how to reach him
   d. Regional and total heparinization
   1) How to do clotting times
   2) Bleeding problems, their prevention and treatment
7. Evaluation of orientation.

## Bibliography

BERNSTEIN, LIONEL M.: *Renal Function and Renal Failure.* The Williams Wilkins Co., Baltimore, 1965.

BLAGG, C. R.: The Management of Acute Reversible Intrinsic Renal Failure. *Postgrad. Med. J.,* 43:290–301, 1967.

BOEN, S. T.: *Peritoneal Dialysis in Clinical Medicine.* Charles C. Thomas, Springfield, Ill., 1964.

BOEN, S. T., CURTIS, F. K., TENCKHOFF, H. and SCRIBNER, B. H.: Chronic Hemodialysis and Peritoneal Dialysis. *Proc. European Dialysis and Transplant Assoc.,* 1:221, 1964.

BOEN, S. T., MULINARI, A. S., DILLARD, D. H. and SCRIBNER, B. H.: Periodic Peritoneal Dialysis in the Management of Chronic Uremia. *Trans. Amer. Soc. Artif. Int. Organs, 8:*256, 1962.

BROOKS, STEWART M.: *Body Water and Ions.* Springer Publishing Co., New York, 1961.

COLE, J. J., QUINTON, W. E., WILLIAMS, C., MURRAY, J. S. and SHERRIS, J. C.: The Pumpless Low Temperature Hemodialysis System. *Trans. Amer. Soc. Artif. Int. Organs, 8:*209, 1962.

DE WARDENER, H. E.: *The Kidney.* Little, Brown and Co., Boston, Mass., 1967.

FELLOWS, BARBARA JO.: The role of the nurse in a chronic dialysis unit. *Nursing Clinics of North America,* 1:577–586, No. 4, W. B. Saunders Co., Philadelphia, 1966.

MURRAY, J. S., HEGSTROM, R. M., PENDRAS, J. P., BURNELL, J. M. and SCRIBNER, B. H.: Continuous Flow Hemodialysis and Bypass Cannulas in the Management of Acute Renal Failure. *Trans. Amer. Soc. Artif. Int. Organs, 7:*94, 1961.

SCRIBNER, B. H.: *Fluid and Electrolyte Syllabus,* 124 pp.

SCRIBNER, BELDING H. and BLAGG, C. R.: Maintenance Dialysis. In Rapaport-Dausset, *Human Transplantation,* pp. 80–99. Grune & Stratton, 1968.

SCRIBNER, B. H., CANER, J. E. Z., BURI, R. and QUINTON, W.: The technique of continuous hemodialysis. *Trans. Amer. Soc. Artif. Int. Organs,* 6:88, 1960.

TRUSK, CAROL: Nursing Care of Hemodialyzed Patients with Acute Renal Failure. *Amer. J. Nursing,* 65:80, February 1965.

# Chapter XIV

# Hyperbaric Oxygenation

DORIS MOLBO, R.N., M.A.

JACK VAN ELK, M.D.

## THERAPEUTIC CONCEPT OF
## HYPERBARIC OXYGENATION THERAPY

The concept of hyperbaric oxygen therapy entered the field of experimental medicine after Boerema showed that a pig could live without blood (i.e., without hemoglobin) while it was breathing 100 per cent oxygen under a pressure of 3 atmospheres. Boerema also successfully used oxygen under pressure as a treatment for patients with gas gangrene, suggesting that this treatment may be effective in treating infections caused by anaerobic microorganisms.

The air we normally breathe contains about 21 per cent oxygen; at sea level the pressure of oxygen in the inhaled gas mixture that we call "air" is about 150 mm Hg. Because of mixture with the exhaled air in the mouth, nasal passages, larynx, and bronchi, the pressure of oxygen in the gas mixture in the pulmonary alveoli is usually just over 100 mm Hg. With efficient gas exchange in the alveoli, the pressure of oxygen in arterial blood leaving the lungs, usually termed the partial pressure of oxygen ($pO_2$), is also about 100 mm Hg.

Almost all oxygen in the blood is carried by the hemoglobin. Normally, the hemoglobin of arterial blood is nearly completely saturated with oxygen, and it is not able to carry more oxygen. Thus, the amount of oxygen, complexed with the hemoglobin of arterial blood in a patient with a normal heart and lungs, cannot be increased.

It is possible, however, to increase the amount of oxygen dissolved in the blood *plasma*. Normally, the oxygen dissolved in the blood plasma is very small, about 0.3 volume per cent. By increasing the oxygen content of the inhaled gas mixture from 21 per cent to 100 per cent, the pressure of oxygen in arterial blood ($pO_2$) can be raised from 100 mm to over 400 mm Hg. By raising the pressure of the environment to levels greater than sea level pressure, for instance to 2 or 3 atmospheres of pressure, the pressure of oxygen can be increased to over 2,000 mm Hg. At such greatly increased pressures, the oxygen carried in the blood plasma increases to about 6 volumes per cent.

In these considerations, it is important to keep in mind that the organs, tissues, and enzyme systems of the human body are "geared" to the oxygen content of air at sea level pressure (or 1 *atmosphere*). Raising the partial pressure of oxygen in arterial blood may result in toxic effects. At sea level pressure, 100 per cent oxygen is not tolerated by the human body for longer than about 24 hours. At a pressure of 3 atmospheres, 100 per cent oxygen usually is not tolerated for more than about 2 hours; some persons show toxic effects within a shorter period of time.

In human beings, the first signs of toxicity are usually manifested by central nervous system symptoms in the form of convulsions. Close observation may show earlier signs and symptoms including nausea, pallor, aloofness, and restlessness. These early signs of toxicity are completely reversible, and do not result in permanent damage. However, if oxygen administration at increased pressure is continued after the onset of such symptoms, permanent injury may occur. In this sense, hyperbaric oxygen can be regarded as a "drug." Too much oxygen at too great a pressure may be harmful, just as too high a dosage of digitalis or insulin is harmful.

The use of higher-than-sea-level pressure involves placement of the patient in a compartment called a pressure vessel or pressure chamber. Within such a protective chamber, higher than normal pressures are usually well tolerated, just as a diver suitably protected tolerates the increased pressure under water very well. When the pressure is decreased, or the diver surfaces too quickly, the possibility exists that gases, principally nitrogen, dissolved in the blood and in the tissues may be released as bubbles into the circulating blood. This condition is called "the bends" or decompression illness.

If one adheres strictly to the standard decompression tables developed by the United States Navy to show the relationship of time lapse to safe changes in atmospheric or water pressure, the risk of decompression illness is almost nonexistent. Because of strict adherence to these operating procedures, the patient who breathes oxygen in a pressurized therapeutic environment does not run the risk of decompression illness or "oxygen bends." The risk of decompression illness is further averted because the patient breathes oxygen instead of air during the decompression phase. (At Lutheran General Hospital we have not seen a single case of decompression illness due to improperly administered hyperbaric oxygen therapy.)

**Therapeutic indications**

It will probably take several more years before sufficient data will be available to reach conclusions with respect to the merits of hyperbaric oxygen therapy in specific disease states.

The value of hyperbaric oxygen for treatment of patients with gas gangrene is still not settled. Its use in treating patients with tetanus, also caused by an anaerobic organism, has been very disappointing.

Extensive studies are being carried out to assess the value of hyperbaric oxygen therapy for patients with arterial occlusive disease, such as coronary and cerebral artery occlusion, and for patients with occlusion of the arteries of the legs. Additionally, high-pressure oxygen therapy is being used on a trial basis for patients with frostbite and for other conditions in which the blood supply to a particular body area is diminished.

Heart surgery has been carried out while the patient was breathing oxygen under a pressure of 3 atmospheres. This procedure seems to be of particular value for those patients with congenital disorders causing cyanosis.

In several medical centers, radiation therapy or the administration of radiomimetic drugs (e.g., nitrogen mustard) in conjunction with hyperbaric oxygen has been used in the treatment of cancer. The therapeutic value of such combined treatment remains to be evaluated.

## Implementation of Therapy

Hyperbaric oxygen therapy is prescribed on an individual basis for each patient. The amount and duration of hyperbaric oxygen treatment is judged according to the disease entity, its location and severity, the total condition of the patient, his age, and his response to the hyperbaric environment. The evaluation of the patient during and after therapy is therefore critical, since it determines future therapy.

The entire time span within the hyperbaric environment varies from about one hour to 24 or 36 hours. In our hyperbaric unit at the present time, the usual duration of patient therapy is about 3 to $3\frac{1}{2}$ hours at an increased pressure of 28–30 pounds per square inch (psi). At lower pressures, however, the time period can be extended appreciably.

The time in the chamber may be divided into three phases: 1) the *compression* phase, during which the pressure is gradually increased from sea level pressure to 3 atmospheres absolute; 2) the therapeutic, or *"holding"* phase, during which the optimum therapeutic pressure is maintained for a specified period of time; and 3) the *decompression* phase, during which pressure is slowly decreased to 1 atmosphere and the patient and personnel are once again returned to normal environmental pressure.

The total duration of the *decompression* phase depends on the period of time under pressure and on the magnitude of the pressure. The United States Navy Diving Tables for decompression time are used as a guide of minimum safe limits. This means that the chamber is decompressed to a specific pressure within a specified time span and that there is a period of holding at the reduced pressure before further decompression proceeds. Because we are exposing an ill patient to pressure changes, the rate of compression and decompression must be slower and more gradual than that applied to healthy divers under similar pressures.

A pressure chamber large enough for the patient and required personnel is generally considered best for hyperbaric therapy. A single exception to this rule is that when hyperbaric oxygen is combined with radiation therapy, a pressure chamber large enough for only the patient is necessarily used. The patient receiving this combined form of therapy is in the hyperbaric environment a relatively short period of time.

## Uniqueness of Therapy

Hyperbaric oxygenation therapy superimposes unusual conditions of stress on both patient and personnel. Uniquely, personnel who enter the chamber with the patient share many of the conditions of the therapy with the patient, such as the increased pressure environment, breathing oxygen by mask, and the feeling of being isolated from the outside world.

**Increased pressure environment.** Patient and personnel experience the physical changes due to increasing environmental pressure inherent in the compression phase. One of these disturbances is a sense of ear fullness and at times eardrum pain, due to slow equalization of the chamber pressure through the eustachian tube to the middle ear. During the period of *holding,* such ear sensations are usually absent. There is usually no diminution of auditory ability. Another physical change experienced early in the compression phase is an increase in environmental temperature. During the "holding" period, the chamber temperature is maintained at an optimum 72° F. The beginning of the decompression period again produces ear fullness and a decrease in the environmental temperature.

Throughout all phases, a noise may be heard which is similar in decibel volume to the well-known noise from certain air conditioning equipment. No other physical changes are experienced at the therapeutic pressure level.

**Breathing oxygen by mask.** Patients within the hyperbaric chamber breathe 100 per cent oxygen by mask from the beginning of the *compression* phase, throughout the *holding* phase, and until the completion of the *decompression* phase. In our unit, personnel within the chamber breathe 100 per cent oxygen by mask for 15 minutes during a typical *holding* phase and during the entire decompression phase. Personnel therefore co-experience the feel and smell of an oxygen mask, the drying effect of oxygen on nasal and oral secretions, the eye irritations created by an ill-fitting mask, and the barriers of communication that a mask imposes.

**Feeling of isolation.** Although certain forms of isolation are recognized and accepted by the healing professions as adjunctive to therapy, the isolation seldom involves the personnel caring for the patient with the same intensity experienced within a hyperbaric environment.

Visual and auditory contact *can* be made with the world outside the chamber through numerous glass port windows and by the use of an intercommunication system. Personnel *can* enter and leave the pressurized chamber via air-locks (while observing decompression time). Various materials, including drugs and instruments, can be passed in and out of the chamber through a small "pass-through" lock. Despite these modes of contact and communication, the patient and personnel within the chamber *are* isolated. They cannot leave the chamber area for a prescribed time period and are dependent on the group outside, because they cannot have contact with those outside the chamber unless the latter make themselves visible and/or communicate.

Routine messages are given frequently to the chamber occupants concerning oxygen usage, pressure, and temperature. However, personnel and patients within the chamber note that they especially appreciate any spontaneous auditory interruptions into their environment. Even the acutely ill patient responds to this contact, which often serves to focus or reorient a wavering sensorium. Messages to the patient from his doctor, friends, or family, as well as direct communication by a relative or news from the engineer, such as, "It's snowing outside," may be well-received messages. However, this always implies that those outside the chamber are sensitively aware of the inside emotional climate at the time and that they adapt their communication content, inflection, and manner of speaking to fit the occasion. (The recognition of music as bane or balm in a therapeutic setting is apparent.)

The hyperbaric environment imposes unusual responsibilities on those physically isolated from the therapeutic scene to remain in close contact by accurate interpretation of both verbal and nonverbal cues. An empathic core group is capable of minimizing isolation factors for all involved in the therapeutic hyperbaric environment.

## Similarities to any Intensive Care Unit

Identification of existing or possible problems within the unit, planning for their elimination or alleviation, and continuing training to cope effectively with emergency situations, are ever present considerations. Within the hyperbaric unit this means experience with ECG, monitoring, and defibrillating equipment. All equipment involving electrical switches is eliminated from the hyperbaric environment. The actual machinery is placed outside the chamber; sensing electrodes and the electrodes for defibrillating shock are permitted inside; special wiring takes the signal from the inside to the outside or vice versa. This means that the members of the group responsible for the equipment outside must function as one with the emergency-stressed group (or individual) inside the chamber. It means instantaneous action when faced with cardiac arrest, the irrationally violent patient, or other catastrophes. Thus, coordination of activities of those within the chamber with those outside the chamber is vital.

The physical intensity and isolation of the hyperbaric environment focuses attention upon many problem areas. They concern problems of sensory deprivation, social interaction, communication, subjective evaluation, and interdependent relationships. We believe these problems are also common to *all intensive care and clinical units,* though often unidentified or obscured by mobility of personnel, multiplicity of responsibility, or other factors. They are described here as identified within the hyperbaric environmental situation.

**Sensory deprivation.** Behavioral scientists have linked some confusional and disoriented states in hospitalized patients with the isolating or monotonous immobilization imposed upon them. Leiderman has identified the cataract patient, the deaf patient, the orthopedic patient, the very young patient, the elderly surgical patient, and the paralyzed respirator patient as being especially vulnerable to such situations.

The hyperbaric environment also requires an awareness of

the factors of sensory deprivation and modalities for combating them. Initially in the planning-construction stages of a hyperbaric unit, attention must be paid to factors of light and brightness, color and color values, and special qualities of height, breadth, and balance. This applies not only to the interior of the chamber, but also the chamber exterior and the room in which it is contained. Noise volume, door and window placement, communicating systems, air circulation, and temperature regulation are other important factors to be considered in planning.

Personnel caring for the patient within a hyperbaric environment are cognizant of structuring time spans within the therapy periods; of encouraging verbal communication even though discouraged by a mask; of maintaining visual contact with a minimal incidence of turning from the patient, leaving the patient's range of vision, or walking out of the periphery of the patient's unit; of reenacting familiar social situations such as the "office break," whether it involves water, fruit juice, or coffee and a sweet roll; of frequently stimulating and reorienting the acutely ill or toxic patient; of providing human tactile stimuli, especially to those patients who cannot move and whose fingers or hands no longer convey tactile messages or who are restrained by intravascular needles or cannulae. Isolating factors and monotonous or reduced stimuli are modified by sensitive and skilled interactions of personnel with patient and of personnel with one another.

**Communication.** Verbal communication is often *not* the most frequently used communicative expression of the ill. In times of emotion and stress there is usually poverty of verbal language; nonverbal communication of the gesture, facial expression, body movement, and tactile contact become the message-bearing mediums. In the hyperbaric environment the oxygen mask further discourages verbal communication; it destroys voice inflection and therefore content emphasis. Thus, interpretation of patient communication is primarily dependent on recognizing the presence of his handicap and a particular patient's unique nonverbal cues. These may be vague, may expand his verbal statements, or may seem to be incongruent to their content. Understanding the patient is dependent on a realization that "the patient who is plagued by pain and disabilities must speak in what he believes to be the 'language' of his auditor," as he tries to make that person understand him. Ultimately, success of patient communication is dependent upon the existent interpersonal relationship that enhances the patient's ability to express himself accurately, verbally, or nonverbally, and that permit him to do this openly, without fear of censure.

**Subjective observations.** Continuing clinical evaluation and judgments prevail whenever responsibility of therapy exists. They become more difficult when that responsibility is shared. Despite laboratory determinations and monitored data, many evaluations of the patient are subjective. The color of an extremity, or its temperature, demand relative and absolute judgments during different phases of the therapy or day-to-day subjective discriminations. The communication of pain and its interpretation and evaluation are always subjective. Especially important in the hyperbaric environment, subjective evaluations of the patient's tolerance for continued oxygen often must be made for the patient who is toxic, fatigued, febrile, anxious, or fearful, or who is a diabetic. Symptoms of any of these conditions must be continually evaluated and differentiated from those which would indicate imminent oxygen toxicity. Since restlessness, nausea, or emesis may be symptoms for all these states, the difficulty, and yet the necessity, for correct judgment is apparent. Everyone's perceptual ability narrows and becomes distorted during times of emergency and stress. When trust exists between the patient and those caring for him, and when those caring for him feel trust toward him and the core group, then distortions of observation and judgment are minimized.

**Interdependent relationships.** The aforementioned factors are influenced by the quality of the *intra*-actions of the core group and their *inter*-actions with the patient. In the final analysis, the actions of the group are influenced by the therapy itself. The uncertainty of medical research, its unknown effects, and its rigid controls can deeply affect the ways in which the group views the patient's future and provides his present therapy. The enthusiasm or faith in a form of therapy has been described as "the placebo effect." The manner and expectations of those extending care to the patient have unmeasured effects on the therapeutic potentials of the therapy itself.

The patient in any therapeutic setting is dependent on others for safe care. The patient in the hyperbaric environment must trust *many* others. He is also dependent on many others for their understanding concern. He may be an acutely ill patient who accepts the therapy as a last emergency measure; he may be in extreme pain; he may fearfully face death; he may angrily denounce the possibility of mutilation because of his disease, or he may actively mourn his disability. The medical and nursing professions, being deeply involved in all life-saving measures, sometimes forget that for the intensive care patient the life-adjusting measures for the future may be equally critical and overwhelming. When life is assured to the gas gangrene patient, but the reality of that life means the lack of an important right hand, his restored life may seem worthless to him. Within the life-saving environment, and at the very time when the personnel are still focused on life *saving,* he may question or refute the value of his life. Fear, pain, and despondency influence any therapy; they are especially critical factors in the kinds of patients receiving hyperbaric oxygen therapy because of the nature of their disease process and because such patients are subjected to a new kind of treatment procedure.

Thus, the creation and maintenance of both a safe and sensitive environment for each patient is necessary. Empathic interactions between patient and personnel can enhance open communication and accurate subjective observation. Intra-actions of the group itself enhance their individual and combined abilities to care for the patient and to influence the environment of therapy. They permit adaptability and flexibility in a changeable environment and increase the possibilities for new approaches and creative ideas.

"If people, young or old, can build groups with standards that reward and strengthen honest self-expression and self-acceptance, creativity, mutual helpfulness, and the capacity to cope with conflicts (within the self or with others), then the members of such groups will assimilate these values as conditions of membership." (*Benne*)

In an era when many physical modalities of resuscitation and therapy exist, it is tempting to credit all therapeutic benefits to them. Yet the unknown and unmeasured variable in all therapy exists in the interactions of the personnel, the patient, and his family within the therapy environment, and in their interdependence.

## THE NURSING ROLE

The hyperbaric nurse cannot realize her full therapeutic function in the care of each individual patient without fully accepting the knowledge that she is neither dependent on others nor independent of others; she is maturely *inter*dependent in her functions and relationships with the patient and with others. Too few nurses and doctors work together in a manner that potentiates the effectiveness of each profession's function. Yet the existence of such a relationship among all personnel in a hyperbaric oxygen therapy unit is imperative if optimal therapy is to be extended to the patient and a stable clinical research setting is to be assured. The success and future of hyperbaric oxygen therapy may well be measured in relation to the sensitivities, abilities, and creativity of an interrelated group of individuals. In our unit this core group comprises a doctor, nurses, a technician familiar with the physiology of increased environmental pressure, engineers, a biochemist, and a secretary. Its united focus is the patient.

### Bibliography

BENNE, KENNETH D.: The Uses of Fraternity. *Daedalus,* 90, 2:239–240, 1961.

KAPLAN, STANLEY: Laboratory Procedures as Emotional Stress, *J.A.-M.A.* 161:677–681, 1956.

KASPER, AUGUST: The Psyche Doctor, the Soma Doctor and the Psychosomatic Patient. *Bulletin of the Menninger Clinic,* 16, 3:77–83, 1952.

KAUFMAN, M. RALPH and ABRAHAM FRANZBLAU: The Emotional Impact of Ward Rounds. *N.Y. State J. Med.,* 57, 19:3193–3205, 1957.

LEIDERMAN, HERBERT, MENDELSON, JACK H., WEXLER, DONALD and SOLOMON, PHILIP: Sensory Deprivation, Clinical Aspects. *A.M.A. Arch. Int. Med.,* 101, 2:389–396, 1958.

Schottstaedt, Wm. W., Pinsky, Ruth H., Mackler, David, and Wolf, Stewart: Sociologic, Psychologic and Metabolic Observations on Patients of a Metabolic Ward. *Am. J. Med.,* 25, 2:248–257, 1958.

Shapiro, A. K.: A Contribution to the History of the Placebo Effect. *Behavioral Science,* 5, 2:109–135, 1960.

# CHAPTER XV

# Organ Homotransplantation

KATHLEEN S. FELIX, R.N.
BETSY MARSHALL, R.N., B.S.
ALBERT RUBIN, M.D.

The replacement of diseased organs by homotransplantation is likely to be one of the major steps in medical progress during the next decade. Although successful transplantation has already been achieved with the liver, kidneys, and heart, the field of organ transplantation is still in its infancy. At the present time renal transplantation is performed in several medical centers with sufficient frequency to merit a brief discussion here of the principles and problems involved in this one area of organ transplantation.

## THE PROBLEM

Patients with chronic renal disease whose kidney function is not adequate to maintain life are candidates for renal transplantation. The ultimate decision regarding transplantation depends on the extent and degree of damage to *other* organ systems, and the ability to obtain an adequate donor kidney.

## ASSESSMENT OF THE PROBLEM

**Patient selection.** Exact assessment of renal function is essential. It is vital to distinguish temporary reduction in renal function that is superimposed on chronic disease from irreversible destruction of the kidneys. For example, a secondary infection of the urinary tract, or a concomitant infection elsewhere in the body, may embarrass already diminished renal function to the point of *apparent* complete failure. Such infection can sometimes be suspected from x-ray studies and sputum, urine, and blood cultures. Microscopic examination of the urine can also help elucidate the problem. Ordinary light and phase-contrast microscopy are supplemented with fluorescent techniques using acridine orange to distinguish the types of cells and casts present. If infection is demonstrated, vigorous antibiotic therapy may improve renal function and obviate the need for transplantation. Frequently, the underlying renal disease (especially in congenital malformation), precludes eradication of infection.

Patients with advanced renal disease most often have evidence of multiple system involvement, and *each* system must be studied carefully prior to the decision for transplantation. The major manifestations which accompany renal disease are found in the cardiovascular, hematopoietic, and central nervous systems. Hypertension and congestive heart failure are frequent sequelae of kidney disease, and the degree of impaired cardiovascular function must be known specifically.

**Donor selection.** At the present time, the kidney to be transplanted is obtained either from live donors (usually relatives), or from cadavers. It is not within the scope of this discussion to debate the moral and philosophical problems concerned with living donors. In the event that a living donor is to be selected, it is essential that the physicians and nurses be in close harmony with responsible members of the patient's family in deciding on the donor. The details and consequences of the procedure must be discussed and fully understood. Nurses are an invaluable aid in this regard. If the hospital has a program for obtaining cadaver kidneys, the nurse's role is central in such procurement. Information must be gathered daily regarding potential deaths and clearance obtained for use of kidneys immediately after death, because the time between death and transplantation is of utmost importance. Only an integrated physician-nurse team can insure success of a cadaver-kidney program.

## PRINCIPLES OF TREATMENT

### Preoperative preparation

Before transplantation can be contemplated, the patient must be brought to an optimal state for surgery:

a. Particular emphasis must be given to the control of hypertension and heart failure. Antihypertensive therapy is employed carefully, and extreme fluctuation of blood pressure must be avoided. Since disturbed renal function leads to water and salt retention, careful management of this problem must be undertaken before surgery. Digitalization is accomplished with the realization of the high risk of toxicity in patients with impaired renal function and electrolyte imbalances.

b. Severe anemia, secondary to hematopoietic depression from azotemia, is anticipated in most patients. This anemia must be corrected (partially, at least) prior to the surgical procedure. Hematocrits of more than 25, and preferably about 30, should be obtained.

c. Acidosis should be controlled with the use of sodium bicarbonate.

d. Adequate hydration must be maintained without the creation of edema. It is important to determine the maximum amount of urine the patient is capable of excreting without gaining weight. If the patient continues to gain weight in spite of fluid restriction, or if symptomatic uremia develops rapidly, peritoneal dialysis or hemodialysis must be performed in preparation for transplantation. If transplantation is feasible within a short period of time, peritoneal dialysis is usually attempted, but if long-term maintenance is anticipated, hemodialysis is preferable because of the reduced incidence of complications.

e. To minimize the risk of infection, phisohex baths and shampoos are given daily for two days before surgery.

### Postoperative care

a. Because of the body's inherent defense against the introduction of foreign tissue and the associated threat of rejection of the transplanted organ, immuno-suppressive therapy is essential. Treatment with agents which suppress the antigen-antibody response created by foreign tissue is usually instituted prior to the implant or immediately thereafter. Steroids, Imuran, and cobalt irradiation are the most common techniques employed for this purpose. These suppressive methods distinctly lower the body's resistance to infection, and strict isolation techniques are vital to the success of the post-transplantation period.

b. Renal function must be assessed on a continuous basis in the immediate postoperative period. Such assessment includes:

1. Total urine volume (via cystostomy, lymphatic and ureterostomy drainage).

2. Measurement of urinary protein, specific gravity, and pH.

3. Daily urine culture.

4. Repeated urea and creatinine clearances.

5. Daily stretcher (or bed) weights.

6. Determination of BUN and electrolytes (serum and urinary), at frequent intervals of the first 24–48 hours and then once daily.

c. The patient must be observed and followed carefully for signs of beginning rejection of the transplanted kidney. The development of fever, decreased urinary output, increased urinary protein, or laboratory evidence of diminishing renal function all are reflections of possible rejection, and immuno-suppressive therapy must be adjusted in the event that rejection is occurring.

**Convalescent care**

a. After successful transplantation, a period of convalescence ensues, during which time renal function studies are continued and optimum drug therapy is determined. During this phase the patient is instructed to follow a daily routine which is continued after discharge. The program includes daily measurement of weight, temperature, urine volume, and protein. Simple record-keeping of this information and other pertinent data, including medication, is undertaken by the patient.

b. The patient is cautioned to avoid obvious sources of infection, for example, large crowds, individuals with upper respiratory infections, and the like. The practice of scrupulous cleanliness is stressed. Careful perineal care is especially important in females.

**Care after discharge**

The patient is followed by the same physician-nurse team at each visit. A routine physical examination is performed with emphasis on kidney size and tenderness. Renal function tests and hematologic studies are obtained. The urine sediment is stained with acridine orange and examined by fluorescent microscopy.

## THE NURSING ROLE

The nurse member of the physician-nurse team is involved in the total care of the patient from the time of initial hospitalization through the stages of evaluation, acceptance of the operation and postoperative care, convalescence, and post-discharge follow-up. During this long period the nurse develops a close relationship with the patient and his family, which has bearing on the outcome of this major attempt at prolonging life.

**a. Evaluation.** Nurses should be specifically trained in the correct technique for collecting urine for cultures and in the details of microscopic examination of the urine. Urine for culture is collected in customary sterile containers from a midstream specimen obtained after an antiseptic wash. Examination of urinary sediment under fluorescent microscopy is performed by nurses in our unit.

**b. Acceptance of the operation.** Obviously, the patient and his family face a major decision when the transplantation is proposed by the physician. The nursing role, in clarifying details of the operation and its sequelae, is crucial at this point. Similarly, if a live donor is involved, careful, unhurried discussion must be planned between the family and the physician-nurse team.

**c. Preoperative.**

1. As stated, it is important in the preoperative period to determine the maximum amount of urine the patient can void without gaining weight from the fluid intake. This balance requires utmost diligence on the part of the nurse in maintaining accurate intake and output records and in determining precise daily weights.

2. Many patients require either peritoneal dialysis or hemodialysis in preparation for surgery. The details of dialysis are considered in Chapter XIII, "Acute Renal Failure and Renal Dialysis." (In our unit, nurses perform and supervise these dialyses.)

**d. Postoperative care.**

1. *Isolation technique.* Strict reverse isolation techniques must be maintained during the postoperative period (i.e., the protection of the patient from infection by personnel, equipment, or environment). The transplantation suite must include all supplies and equipment that may be necessary in normal or emergency care.

All surface areas of the suite are scrubbed with S.B.T.-12 within 24 hours prior to surgery and then every 8 hours while the suite is occupied.

Equipment is either autoclaved or cleaned with S.B.T.-12 before it is placed in the anteroom of the suite.

Personnel entering the anteroom *must* don sterile boots, cap, mask, and gown, and perform a surgical scrub.

The duration of isolation is determined by the absence of clinical infection, the stabilization of the white count, and the removal of drainage tubes.

2. *Patient care.*

a. The volume of fluid replacement is determined every 30 minutes according to the output during that same period. The output measurement includes drainage from the gastrointestinal tract (Levine tube), the operative site (lymphatic drainage in dressings), and urinary volume (cystostomy, ureterostomy).

b. The urine is carefully measured and tested for amount of protein as well as specific gravity and pH. Urinary electrolytes are usually determined every 8 hours.

c. Urine cultures are obtained each day.

d. The body weight is obtained daily and recorded, preferably with a bed scale.

These data are carefully recorded (see Fig. 1).

**Bibliography**

SCHREINER, G. E. and MAHER, J. F.: Uremia. Thomas Co., 1961.

RAPPAPORT, F. T. and DAUSSET, J.: Human Transplantation. Grune and Stratton, Inc. 1968.

STARZL, T. E.: Experience in Renal Transplantation. Saunders Co., 1963.

## Fig. 1.

POST RENAL TRANSPLANTATION RECORD

Recipient_____ Age_____ Blood Type_____

Donor_____ Age_____ Blood Type_____

| | | | | | | | | | |
|---|---|---|---|---|---|---|---|---|---|
| | Date | | | | | | | | |
| | Days Post-op | | | | | | | | |
| | Temperature | | | | | | | | |
| | Blood Pressure | | | | | | | | |
| | Weight | | | | | | | | |
| | Clinical | | | | | | | | |
| | | | | | | | | | |
| | Intake | | | | | | | | |
| | Output (Urine) | | | | | | | | |
| | Output (Total) | | | | | | | | |
| **D** | Imuran | | | | | | | | |
| **R** | Steroids | | | | | | | | |
| **U** | | | | | | | | | |
| **G** | Anti-Hypertensives | | | | | | | | |
| **S** | Antibiotics | | | | | | | | |
| | Other | | | | | | | | |
| | BUN | | | | | | | | |
| **B** | Hematocrit | | | | | | | | |
| **L** | WBC | | | | | | | | |
| **O** | Differential | | | | | | | | |
| **O** | Platelets | | | | | | | | |
| **D** | Creatinine Clearance | | | | | | | | |
| | Urea Clearance | | | | | | | | |
| | Electrolytes | | | | | | | | |
| | | | | | | | | | |
| | | | | | | | | | |
| | | | | | | | | | |
| | Serum Saved | | | | | | | | |
| | 24 hr. Protein | | | | | | | | |
| **U** | gms/24 hrs. | | | | | | | | |
| **R** | Sediment | | | | | | | | |
| **I** | Protein | | | | | | | | |
| **N** | Cultures | | | | | | | | |
| **E** | Electrolytes | | | | | | | | |

*443*

# Appendix

EQUIPMENT AND SUPPLIES FOR AN INTENSIVE CARE UNIT

*Editor's note:* In preparing this book, each of the contributors was asked to include a list of the equipment and supplies that they deemed essential in the practice of their specialties within a modern intensive care unit. In reviewing these lists it was apparent that while there were occasional differences regarding certain ancillary items, the basic needs were very similar in each instance and that no purpose would be served by repeating the lists within each chapter. For this reason, the following consensus was prepared for use here.

**Equipment:**

*Equipment required for the unit but* NOT *for each patient individually*

1. Automatic respirators including at least one pressure cycled (e.g., Bird, Bennett, etc.) and one volume controlled (e.g., Emerson, Air Shields, etc.) device
2. Breathing bags suitable for use with face masks or endotracheal tubes (e.g., Ambu bag)
3. Cardiac monitors with slave oscilloscopes at the bedsides
4. Electrocardiographic machine
5. DC defibrillator which can be used for synchronized precordial shock or emergency defibrillation
6. Pacemaker equipment, battery operated
7. Automatic rotating tourniquet machine
8. Portable x-ray machine or portable image intensifier in the unit or readily available from nearby site
9. Bed scale or weighing litter
10. Hypothermia machine
11. Mist generators (ultrasonic and conventional forced-air types)

12. Laryngoscope with detachable blades
13. Lamp, operating type (e.g., Castle)
14. Large wall clock with sweep second hand
15. Open-top tent with nebulizer attachment
16. Intra-arterial pressure system
17. Litters with side rails
18. Portable intravenous standards
19. Telephone alarm system
20. Centrifuge for hematocrit determinations
21. Pressure infuser
22. Telethermometer
23. Gram scale for weighing dressings

*Equipment required for* EACH *patient*

1. Bed, either motor driven or stretch type, with siderails
2. Overhead intravenous fixture ("skyhook")
3. Lights and lamps, overhead and examination types
4. Over-bed table
5. Bedside cabinet
6. Call bell
7. Urinometer and attachment
8. Commode, portable
9. Cardiac arrest board
10. Multiple electrical outlets, separately fused, including a 220 V line for x-ray, etc.

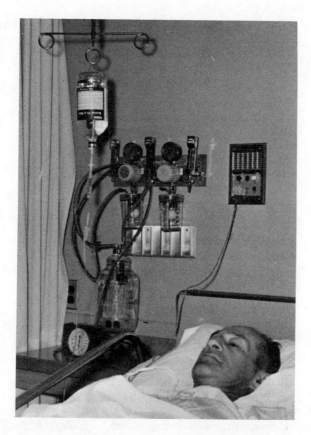

THE OVERHEAD, BUILT-IN BEDSIDE CONSOLE

*Fig. 1*

1. Suction with variable control for nasotracheal and gastrointestinal suction
2. Suction with variable control for thoracotomy drainage
3. Oxygen outlet with regulator and humidifier
4. A shelf for:
    Oxygen and suction catheters
    Dressings and tape
    Padded tongue blades
    Hemostats
    Hoffman clamp
    Electrodes for cardiac monitoring
    Airways
    Tourniquets
5. Sphygmomanometer, either built in or on wall shelf

**Arrangement of Equipment**

The individual patient unit and necessary equipment can be arranged according to the particular medical or surgical problem to be treated. For example, if a patient in shock is to be admitted to the intensive care facility, a patient unit might be prepared in a manner schematically depicted in Fig. 2.

1. Hypothermia unit
2. Bird respirator
3. Recessed suction and oxygen
4. Overhead intravenous hanger
5. Central venous pressure manometer
6. Cardiac monitor unit and defibrillator
7. Heart-rate meter (if not incorporated into cardiac monitor)
8. Over-bed cardiac table with small supplies
9. Urimeter
10. Folding shelf with current data records
11. Chart box
12. Telethermometer
13. Stethoscope
14. Gram-scales

**Supplies**

Because intensive care is predicated on efficiency, most authors recommend that equipment and supplies be packaged in individual trays, or containers, which are clearly marked and stored together for immediate use.

**Prepared trays**

Trays containing all necessary supplies and equipment are recommended for the following studies or procedures:

1. Central venous pressure
2. Intra-arterial pressure
3. Bronchoscopy
4. Tracheostomy
5. Venous cutdowns
6. Peritoneal dialysis
7. Minor surgery
8. Venesection and blood administration
9. Cardiac monitoring (e.g., electrodes, paste)

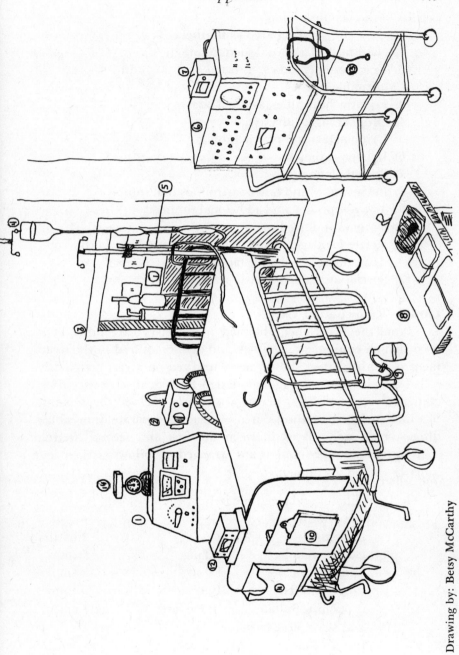

Drawing by: Betsy McCarthy

*Fig. 2*

   10. Transvenous pacing

**Prepared containers**

 1. Nasotracheal and oral suction catheters
 2. Tracheostomy tubes, assorted sizes including those with inflatable cuffs
 3. Endotracheal tubes, assorted sizes
 4. Oropharyngeal airways
 5. Urinometers and plastic tubing
 6. Urinary catheters
 7. Polyethylene tubing
 8. Levine tubes and other gastrointestinal tubing
 9. 3-way stopcocks, and additional tubing
 10. Syringes and needles
 11. Sterile bandages, small and large gauze flats, kerlix rolls, Ace bandages, adhesive tape, gloves
 12. Special instruments sets

## Cardiac Resuscitation Cart

From the experience obtained in coronary care units, it is clear that all equipment, supplies, and drugs required in the treatment of cardiac arrest should be centralized on a cart (popularly called a crash cart). A suggested design for a cardiac resuscitation cart involves a mobile structure with three shelves, the topmost of which can serve as a work area. A series of separate drawers for drug storage are situated between the first and second shelves. The equipment and supplies are arranged as follows:

*Top Shelf:*

 1. Defibrillator and electrode jelly
 2. Tray containing:

| | | |
|---|---|---|
| Lidocaine | 2% | 2 bottles |
| Isoproterenol | 0.2 mg | 3 amps |
| Epinephrine | 1.0 cc | 2 amps |
| Propanolol Hcl | 1 mg/cc | 3 amps |
| Protamine Sulfate | 50 mg/5cc | 1 vial |

5 cc, 10 cc, 50 cc syringes
Intracardiac needle (#22 gauge)
$H_2O$ for injection
NaCl for injection

*In Drawers:*

| | | |
|---|---|---|
| Adrenaline Cl | 1:100 | 10 amps |
| Pronestyl | 10 cc | 3 amps |
| Dilantin | 100 mg | 1 vial |
| Solu Cortef | 100 mg | 2 |
| Solu Medrol | 40 mg | 2 |
| Solu Medrol | 125 mg | 1 |
| Decadron | 4 mg | 2 |
| Calcium Cl | 10 ml | 4 amps |
| Calcium Gluconate | 10 ml | 2 amps |
| Isuprel | 1.0 mg | 4 amps |
| Isuprel | 0.2 mg | 5 |
| Isuprel Glossetts | 10 mg | 10 |
| Aminophyllin | 500 mg | 2 amps |
| Aramine | 100 mg | 3 |
| Wyamine | 30 mg | 2 |
| Ouabain | 0.5 mg | 4 amps |
| Levophed | 4 cc | 4 amps |
| Cedilanid | 0.8 mg | 2 amps |
| Digoxin | 0.5 mg | 6 amps |
| Na HCO$_3$ | 50 cc | 10 amps |

*Second Shelf:*

1. Central venous pressure set
2. Sterile gloves and sterile drapes
3. Pacemaker
4. Pacemaker catheters (transvenous and transthoracic)
5. Endotracheal tray (tubes, adapters, airways, and laryngo-scope)

*Third Shelf:*

1. Venesection tray
2. 500 ml 5% D/W—1 bottle
3. 500 ml 5% NaHCO$_3$—1 bottle
4. Solution administration set—1
5. #17 Med Intracath radiopaque—3
6. Arm board
7. Tourniquets

# Index

# 466 Index

Respirators, pressure-cycled or pressure limited (cont.)
Sterilization, 44-46
Types of, 27-28
Weaning from respirator support, 35
Respirators, volume-controlled, 23, 30-32, 33-35, 43-46, 81
Adequate ventilation, 43-44
Benefits of positive pressure breathing, 31-32
Complications, 30-32
Description and use, 30-31
Nursing care, 43
Patient management, 33-35
Sterilization, 44-46
Types, 30
Weaning from respiratory support, 35
Respiratory acidosis
in respiratory failure, 24-25
Respiratory depression, 24-25, 129
in hypothyroidism, 220
Respiratory failure
See Pulmonary function tests
See Blood gas studies
Causes of, 5-6
Clinical course, 5
Definition, 1
Respiratory function, normal, 2
Control of, 4-5
Respiratory insufficiency
Clinical manifestations, 7
Cerebral effects, 353
in chest surgery, 352-353, 357
in head injury, 327-328
Treatment of conscious patient, 13-17
Treatment of unconscious patient, 17-37
Respiratory Insufficiency and Failure, 1
Alveolar ventilation, 348
Assessment of the problem, 6-12
Clinical disorders of respiratory function, 3-5
Drug therapy, 35-36
in chest surgery, 347-349
in children and infants, 383
Normal respiratory function, 2

Nursing role, 38-48
post heart surgery, 382-383
Prevention of infection, 46
Principles of treatment, 12-37
Problem, 1-6
Pulmonary function tests, 7-12
Summary of patient management, 36-37
Respiratory stimulants, 36
Respiratory therapy, mechanical, 23, 26-35, 127-128, 162-163
See also Respirators, pressure cycled
See also Respirators, volume controlled
Adequacy of ventilation, 33, 44-45
Benefits of, 31-32
Complications of, 32-34
Drug therapy, 34-36
Patient management, 33-35
Weaning from respirator, 35
Resuscitation, mouth-to-mouth, 17, 23
Rheumatic heart disease, 144-145
Rotating tourniquets
See Tourniquets, rotating
Ringer's lactate solution, 161

Sedatives, 4-5, 143, 183-184, 189
Seizures
See Convulsions, control of
See Head injuries
See Motor activity,
Sensory deprivation, 102
Septic emboli, 145
Septic shock
See Bacteremic shock
Serum glutamic oxalacetic transaminase (SGOT), 54-55, 140, 182
Serum glutamic pyruvic transaminase, 54-55, 182
Shock, 153
See Anaphylactic shock
See Bacteremic shock
See Cardiogenic shock
See Hypovolemic shock
Assessment of the problem, 154-159
Drug therapy, 164-166
Equipment needed for care, 167
Fluid replacement, 160-162, 169-170